Musculoskeletal Disease Associated with Diabetes Mellitus

Masaaki Inaba
Editor

Musculoskeletal Disease Associated with Diabetes Mellitus

Springer

Editor
Masaaki Inaba
Graduate School of Medicine
Osaka City University
Osaka
Japan

ISBN 978-4-431-55719-7 ISBN 978-4-431-55720-3 (eBook)
DOI 10.1007/978-4-431-55720-3

Library of Congress Control Number: 2015958784

Springer Tokyo Heidelberg New York Dordrecht London

Printed on acid-free paper

Springer Japan KK is part of Springer Science+Business Media (www.springer.com)

Preface

Although the title of this book is *Musculoskeletal Disease Associated with Diabetes Mellitus*, it describes not only bone and muscle disease but also its association with various metabolic abnormalities in diabetes. In the past decade, we have made substantial progress in accumulating evidence on the important role of bone and muscle as an endocrine organ in the development of abnormal glucose metabolism and in the progression of atherosclerotic changes in diabetes mellitus. Although diabetic osteopathy is characterized by various forms of bone abnormalities, increased fracture rate due to osteoporosis is the most important of those because it has been shown to increase mortality. It had been believed that diabetic patients, particularly those with type 2 diabetes, maintained bone mineral density normal for their age; however, recent epidemiological data indicate a higher bone fracture rate related to bone mineral density in diabetic patients, both type 1 and type 2, to which impaired bone quality and preferential occurrence of cortical porosis might contribute. Furthermore, the importance of sarcopenia is increasingly recognized from the standpoint of impaired longevity or mortality in diabetic patients, because muscle has now been established not only as a target organ of insulin to regulate various aspects of metabolism including glucose towards a normal level but also as an endocrine organ that regulates systemic metabolism in a diabetic state, in addition to the maintenance of activities of daily living.

To continue to improve our understanding of this newly developing area, this book therefore summarizes the current state of the art in this field. Each contributing author was asked to review the available data on each topic and the strategies to protect abnormalities of bone and muscle metabolism of a diabetic state in a comprehensive way. Owing to this design of the book, there might be some overlap of descriptions as well as some redundancy from one chapter to another.

We are most appreciative of the efforts of my colleague Dr. Masanori Emoto for his magnificent effort to improve the quality of the section on muscle, and we thank Ms. Yoko Arai and Ms. Chihiro Haraguchi at Springer Japan for their editorial assistance. This book is clearly the result of an enormous effort by authors who responded positively to the call by an editor to produce their chapters in spite of their other, urgent work. I am truly grateful for their commitment.

Osaka, Japan Masaaki Inaba, M.D.

Contents

Part I
Bone Diseases

Chapter 1
Bone Disease Associated with Diabetes Mellitus: Particularly Focusing on Its Contribution to the Development of Atherosclerosis

Masaaki Inaba

Abstract Bone abnormality associated with diabetes mellitus (DM) is characterized by its low bone turnover status (Krakauer et al. Diabetes 44(7):775–782, 1995). Suppression of bone turnover occurs in DM by several mechanisms, such as (i) the impaired secretion of parathyroid hormone (Inaba et al. Am J Kidney Dis 39 (6):1261–1269, 2002; Inaba et al. Am J Kidney Dis 38(4 Suppl 1):S139–S142, 2001) and (ii) osteocyte/osteoblast deficit, which are caused by the sustained high glucose condition (Inaba et al. Osteoporos Int 7 (suppl 3): S209–S212, 1997) or insulin/insulin-like growth factor-1 deficiency (Wettenhall et al. Diabetes 18:280–284, 1969). Therefore, DM is recently recognized as the disease which causes often adynamic bone disease (ABD), which cause higher fracture rate in spite of no apparent reduction in bone mass (Vestergaard Osteoporos Int 18: 427–44, 2007). The decrease in the number and activity of osteeoblasts/osteocytes impaired the secretion of fibroblast growth factor (FGF)-23 from the cells (Yoda et al. J Clin Endocrinol Metab 97(11):E2036–E2043, 2012), resulting in the development of hyperphosphatemia due to phosphate overloading. Furthermore, ABD is a major risk factor for vascular calcification by diminishing the capacity of bone to adsorb surplus calcium and phosphate in circulation (London et al. J Am Soc Nephrol 15(7):1943–1951, 2004).

Therefore, it is recognized that the suppression of bone turnover with the deficit of osteocyte/osteoblast might enhance atherosclerotic change by disturbing phosphate/calcium metabolism in DM patients.

Keywords Diabetes • Bone • Atherosclerosis • Adynamic bone disease (ABD) • FGF-23

M. Inaba, M.D., Ph.D. (✉)
Department of Metabolism, Endocrinology and Molecular Medicine, Osaka City University Graduate School of Medicine, 1-4-3, Asahi-machi, Abeno-ku, Osaka 545-8585, Japan
e-mail: inaba-m@med.osaka

M. Inaba (ed.), *Musculoskeletal Disease Associated with Diabetes Mellitus*,
DOI 10.1007/978-4-431-55720-3_1

1.1 Characteristics of Osteopathy in Diabetes Mellitus (DM)

Bone disease associated with DM develops as the combined forms of various disorders of calcium (Ca) metabolisms, such as impairment of Ca absorption, osteoblast/osteocyte deficit, and increased urinary Ca excretion [9]. As glycemic control becomes poorer, Ca loss into urine as a result of hyperglycemia and/or glycosuria could be greater, resulting in the development of secondary hyperparathyroidism [9]. Although bone resorption is enhanced by this mechanism, it should be emphasized that bone formation by osteoblast/osteocyte is not sufficient to compensate for the increased bone resorption [10]. Therefore, impaired bone formation due to osteoblast/osteocyte, for which insulin/insulin-like growth factor (IGF)-1 deficiency and sustained exposure to high glucose are mainly responsible, is now established as the main factor for the development diabetic osteopathy [11, 12]. Furthermore, together with the suppressive effect of sustained high glucose condition on parathyroid function, bone turnover might be suppressed so severely to easily develop ABD.

1.1.1 Enhanced Bone Resorption in the Early Stage of Poorly Controlled DM Patients: Its Significance on the Progression of Atherosclerosis

Bone resorption is associated with the release of phosphate, in addition to calcium, from bone because of the dissolution of hydroxyapatite. Supportive of this notion that serum phosphate is partly originated from the release of bone is our recent reports [13] that cinacalcet administration significantly suppressed serum phosphate level in hemodialysis patients and our finding that administration of denosumab suppressed serum phosphate by approximately 10 % (unpublished results). Of great interest, our data demonstrated that groups of hemodialysis patients who exhibited higher serum active PTH(1-84) fraction [14] and bone alkaline phosphatase [15], and significant bone loss [16] showed significantly higher all-cause mortality than those without bone loss. Administration of cinacalcet to 5/6-nephrectomized hyperparathyroid rats protected against the development of vascular calcification at aortic arch [17]. In humans, aortic calcification is often observed in CKD patients, particularly in those with increased bone resorption resulting from renal hyperparathyroidism. Furthermore, Together with our data indicating that, even in non-CKD postmenopausal osteoporotic women, administration of risedronate attenuated age-related increase of pulse wave velocity (PWV), a clinically relevant marker for arterial wall stiffening [18], the data indicating the significant protective effect of bisphosphonate against the development of acute myocardial infarction in osteoporotic patients [19], the increased release of phosphate from bone is capable of directly damaging vascular endothelial cells and inducing vascular smooth muscle cells to dedifferentiate into osteoblasts to cause vascular calcification [20]. Our previous study [20] showed that increase of phosphate levels from 1.4 to 2.0 mM caused calcification of vascular muscle cells in vitro after 14 days of culture, and that phosphate entry inside the cell is the trigger to induce dedifferentiation of vascular muscle cells to osteoblasts to develop calcification. Furthermore, increased phosphate load into circulation is known to deteriorate renal function to decrease glomerular filtration rate and increase proteinuria/albuminuria [21]. This mechanism might be involved in the harmful effect of phosphate to accelerate vascular injury in DM patients.

Therefore, al least in the early stage of DM patients under poorly controlled conditions, it is suggested that poor glycemic control increases urinary loss of calcium, stimulate bone resorption by inducing secondary hyperparathyroidism and that the resultant increased phosphate release from bone causes vascular damage, directly and indirectly by kidney damage, in DM patients.

1.2 Mechanism of Osteoblast/Osteocyte Deficit in DM Ostepotahy

1.2.1 Effect of High Glucose on the Proliferation of Osteoblast/Osteocyte and Their Responsiveness to PTH/Vitamin D

Sustained 7-day exposure to high glucose significantly inhibited growth of human osteoblast-like MG-63 cells in a dose-dependent manner, in contrast with the insignificant suppression of high mannitol, osmolality control [10]. The mechanism for the suppression of osteoblasts by high glucose is explained by the direct suppressive effect of high glucose on cell proliferetaion through an intracellular accumulation of soribitol [10] and its indirect effect to attenuate IGF-1 stimulation of cell growth. In agreement with these data, the number of osteoblasts/osteocyte is reported to decrease significantly, resulting in the development of ABD in DM patients. Osteoblasts, in response to PTH and 1,25-dihydroxyvitamin D, an active form of vitamin D, increase intracellular cytosolic Ca^{++} and osteocalcin production/ secretion in vitro. Sustained 7-day exposure to high glucose significantly impaired the responsiveness of human osteoblast-like MG-63 cells to these hormones in a dose-dependent manner, in contrast with the insignificant suppression of high mannitol, osmolality control [22, 23]. These data may suggest that high glucose condition and/or insulin/IGF-1 deficiency impaired the proliferation and the cell responsiveness of osteoblast/osteocyte to cause ABD in DM patients.

1.2.2 *Effect of Increased Calcium Load to Cause Vascular Calcification in DM Patients with DM*

In vitro system, calcium level in culture medium, independent of phosphate level, stimulates calcification of vascular smooth muscle cells in a dose-dependent manner, suggesting the direct effect of calcium on vascular calcification. The enhancement of aortic calcification by increased calcium load is also evidenced in vivo in hemodialysis patients, although the aortic calcification score was significantly affected by bone turnover status [8]. Since administration of calcium-containing phosphate binder to CKD patients is known to induce vascular calcification significantly more than non-calcium containing phosphate binder [24]. Although the direct effect of calcium load to enhance vascular calcification is hypothesized on the basis of in vitro study, the main mechanism by which calcium load to stimulate vascular calcification in human subjects is explained by its indirect effect to suppress bone turnover by suppressing parathyroid function [8, 25]. As bone turnover status becomes slower, the rate of bone calcification could be progressed too high to adsorb more calcium/phosphate from circulation. This phenomenon could easily elevate serum calcium/phosphate to cause ectopic calcification including vascular wall. We recently reported that replacement of calcium carbonate (CaC), a calcium-containing phosphate binder, with lanthanum carbonate (LaC), a non-calcium containing phosphate binder, increased serum PTH and bone turnover markers in hemodialysis patients with suppressed serum PTH$\leqq$150 pg/mL [26], along with the re-appearance of double tetracycline labeling on bone biopsy specimens obtained from such hemodialysis patients [27]. Therefore, it is suggested that LaC normalized CaC-induced suppression of parathyroid function and bone turnover by decreasing calcium overloading.

The positive associations between calcium load and PWV or aortic calcification were stronger in ABD patients than in those with normal bone turnover, indicating that the presence of ABD conferred significantly greater influence of calcium load on the development of aortic calcification and arterial wall stiffening [8, 25]. Conversely, the presence of an active bone was associated with lower aortic stiffness and better aortic capacitive function. Taken these data collectively, it is suggested that ABD might be a significant risk for the development of vascular calcification. Since ABD has no significant bone formative activity with the degree of bone mineralization too high to be mineralized further. Excess calcium and phosphate in the blood are hypothesized to be preferentially adsorbed into bones. However, patients with low bone turnover rate such as ABD show markedly reduced capacity of bone to adsorb calcium and phosphate into bones and are prone to ectopic calcification such as vascular calcification. Therefore, it is suggested that DM patients, in whom ABD might occur preferentially, have higher risk for atherosclerotic changes including vascular calcification. These data may suggest that DM patients should be monitored for the low bone turnover status using bone alkaline phosphatase (BAP) or tartrate-resistant acid phosphatase (TRACP)-5b, which are bone markers whose levels do not apparently increase upon the deterioration of kidney function [28]. However, bone markers, which derive from collagen metabolism, apparently increase in uremic serum independent of bone turnover [28].

1.3 Vascular Calcification as a Definite Risk for Cardiovascular Mortality

Vascular calcification is more prevalent in DM patients. Among DM patients, DM patients on hemodialysis exhibited significantly higher prevalence than DM non-CKD patients or non-DM hemodialysis patients, either at medial calcification or aortic calcification [29, 30]. In terms of the association between aortic calcification and mortality, Kaplan-Meier analysis we performed showed that either all-cause mortality or cardiovascular mortality was significantly greater in patients with aortic calcification compared to those without ($P < 0.0001$, log-rank test) [31]. Multivariate Cox proportional hazards analysis found that the presence of aortic calcification was significantly associated with increased all-cause mortality (hazard ratio, 2.07; 95 % confidence interval, 1.21–3.56; $P < 0.01$) and increased cardiovascular mortality (hazard ratio, 2.39; 95 % confidence interval, 1.01–5.66; $P < 0.05$) after adjustment for age, hemodialysis duration, presence of diabetes, serum albumin level, and C-reactive protein level [31]. Furthermore, the association of medial calcification at small artery with all-cause mortality was also reported. Therefore, either in DM or non-DM patients, vascular calcification is established as a definite risk for all-cause mortality and cardiovascular mortality.

1.4 Conclusion

It is concluded that DM is a disease which is prone to phosphate overloading to increase serum phosphate, which significantly increase all-cause and cardiovascular mortality by inducing vascular calcification, and thus recommended that maintenance of bone turnover state within normal range is most important to accommodate phosphate loading to prevent atherosclerosis in DM patients.

Conflict of Interest Masaaki Inaba declares that he has no conflict of interest.

References

1. Krakauer JC, McKenna MJ, Buderer NF, Rao DS, Whitehouse FW, Parfitt AM (1995) Bone loss and bone turnover in diabetes. Diabetes 44(7):775–782
2. Inaba M, Nagasue K, Okuno S, Ueda M, Kumeda Y, Imanishi Y, Shoji T, Ishimura E, Ohta T, Nakatani T, Kim M, Nishizawa Y (2002) Impaired secretion of parathyroid hormone, but not

refractoriness of osteoblast, is a major mechanism of low bone turnover in hemodialyzed patients with diabetes mellitus. Am J Kidney Dis 39(6):1261–1269
3. Inaba M, Okuno S, Nagasue K, Otoshi T, Kurioka Y, Maekawa K, Kumeda Y, Imanishi Y, Ishimura E, Ohta T, Morii H, Kim M, Nishizawa Y (2001) Impaired secretion of parathyroid hormone is coherent to diabetic hemodialyzed patients. Am J Kidney Dis 38(4 Suppl 1):S139–S142
4. Inaba M, Nishizawa Y, Shioi A, Morii H (1997) Importance of sustained high glucose condition in the development of diabetic osteopenia: possible involvement of the polyol pathway. Osteoporos Int 7(suppl 3):S209–S212
5. Wettenhall REH, Schwqarz PL, Bornstein J (1969) Actions of insulin and growth hormone on collagen and chondroitin sulfate synthesis in bone organ cultures. Diabetes 18:280–284
6. Vestergaard P (2007) Discrepancies in bone mineral density and fracture risk in patients with type 1 and type 2 diabetes – a meta-analysis. Osteoporos Int 18:427–444
7. Yoda K, Imanishi Y, Yoda M, Mishima T, Ichii M, Yamada S, Mori K, Emoto M, Inaba M (2012) Impaired response of FGF-23 to oral phosphate in patients with type 2 diabetes: a possible mechanism of atherosclerosis. J Clin Endocrinol Metab 97(11):E2036–E2043
8. London GM, Marty C, Marchais SJ, Guerin AP, Metivier F, de Vernejoul MC (2004) Arterial calcifications and bone histomorphometry in end-stage renal disease. J Am Soc Nephrol 15 (7):1943–1951
9. Leman J Jr, Lennon EJ, Piering WR, Prien EL Jr, Ricinati ES (1970) Evidence that glucose ingestion inhibits net renal tubular reabsorption of calcium and magnesium in man. J Lab Clin Med 75:578–585
10. Terada M, Inaba M, Yano Y, Hasuma T, Nishizawa Y, Morii H, Otani S (1998) Growth-inhibitory effect of a high glucose concentration on osteoblast-like cells. Bone 22:17–23
11. Rico H, Hernandez ER, Cabranes JA, Gomez-Castresana F (1989) Suggestion of a deficient osteoblastic function in diabetes mellitus: the possible cause of osteopenia in diabetics. Calcif Tissue Int 45:71–73
12. Yamada S, Inaba M, Okada S, Imanishi Y, Mori K, Emoto M, Ishimura E, Nishizawa Y (2010) Association of glycated albumin, but not glycated hemoglobin, with calcaneus quantitative ultrasound in male hemodialysis patients with type 2 diabetes mellitus. Metabolism 59 (3):390–394
13. Kurajoh M, Inaba M, Okuno S, Nagayama H, Yamada S, Imanishi Y, Ishimura E, Shoji S, Yamakawa T, Nishizawa Y (2011) Reduction of whole PTH/intact PTH ratio as a predictor of bone metabolism in cinacalcet treatment of hemodialysis patients with secondary hyperparathyroidism. Osteoporos Int 22(3):923–930
14. Inaba M, Okuno S, Imanishi Y, Ishimura E, Yamakawa T, Shoji S (2013) Increased active PTH(1-84) fraction as a predictor of poor mortality in male hemodialysis patients. Osteoporos Int 24(11):2863–2870, Kobayashi I, Life Sci
15. Kobayashi I, Shidara K, Okuno S, Yamada S, Imanishi Y, Mori K, Ishimura E, Shoji S, Yamakawa T, Inaba M (2012) Higher serum bone alkaline phosphatase as a predictor of mortality in male hemodialysis patients. Life Sci 90(5–6):212–218
16. Kohno K, Inaba M, Okuno S, Maeno Y, Maekawa K, Yamakawa T, Ishimura E, Nishizawa Y (2009) Association of reduction in bone mineral density with mortality in male hemodialysis patients. Calcif Tissue Int 84(3):180–185
17. Kawata T, Nagano N, Obi M, Miyata S, Koyama C, Kobayashi N, Wakita S, Wada M (2008) Cinacalcet suppresses calcification of the aorta and heart in uremic rats. Kidney Int 74 (10):1270–1277
18. Okamoto K, Inaba M, Furumitsu Y, Ban A, Mori N, Yukioka K, Imanishi Y, Nishizawa Y (2010) Beneficial effect of risedronate on arterial thickening and stiffening with a reciprocal relationship to its effect on bone mass in female osteoporosis patients: a longitudinal study. Life Sci 87(23–26):686–691, Bis &AMI
19. Kang JH, Keller JJ, Lin HC (2013) Bisphosphonates reduced the risk of acute myocardial infarction: a 2-year follow-up study. Osteoporos Int 24(1):271–277

20. Jono S, McKee MD, Murry CE, Shioi A, Nishizawa Y, Mori K, Morii H, Giachelli CM (2000) Phosphate regulation of vascular smooth muscle cell calcification. Circ Res 87(7):E10–E17
21. Zoccali C, Ruggenenti P, Perna A, Leonardis D, Tripepi R, Tripepi G, Mallamaci F, Remuzzi G, REIN Study Group (2011) Phosphate may promote CKD progression and attenuate renoprotective effect of ACE inhibition. J Am Soc Nephrol 22(10):1923–1930
22. Inaba M, Terada M, Koyama H, Yoshida O, Ishimura E, Kawagishi T, Okuno Y, Nishizawa Y, Otani S, Morii H (1995) Influence of high glucose on 1,25-dihydroxyvitamin D3-induced effect on human osteoblast-like MG-63 cells. J Bone Miner Res 10(7):1050–1056
23. Yoshida O, Inaba M, Terada M, Shioi A, Nishizawa Y, Otani S, Morii H (1995) Impaired response of human osteosarcoma (MG-63) cells to human parathyroid hormone induced by sustained exposure to high glucose. Miner Electrolyte Metab 21(1–3):201–204
24. Toussaint ND, Lau KK, Polkinghorne KR, Kerr PG (2011) Attenuation of aortic calcification with lanthanum carbonate versus calcium-based phosphate binders in haemodialysis: a pilot randomized controlled trial. Nephrol (Carlton) 16(3):290–298
25. London GM, Marchais SJ, Guérin AP, Boutouyrie P, Métivier F, de Vernejoul MC (2008) Association of bone activity, calcium load, aortic stiffness, and calcifications in ESRD. J Am Soc Nephrol 19(9):1827–1835
26. Inaba M, Okuno S, Nagayama H, Yamada S, Ishimura E, Imanishi Y, Shoji S (2015) Restoration of parathyroid function after change of phosphate binder form calcium carbonate to lanthanum carbonate in hemodialysis patients with suppressed serum parathyroid hormone. J Ren Nutr 25(2):242–246
27. Yajima A, Inaba M, Tominaga Y, Tanaka M, Otsubo S, Nitta K, Ito A, Satoh S (2013) Impact of lanthanum carbonate on cortical bone in dialysis patients with adynamic bone disease. Ther Apher Dial 17(Suppl 1):41–48
28. Yamada S, Inaba M, Kurajoh M, Shidara K, Imanishi Y, Ishimura E, Nishizawa Y (2008) Utility of serum tartrate-resistant acid phosphatase (TRACP5b) as a bone resorption marker in patients with chronic kidney disease: independence from renal dysfunction. Clin Endocrinol (Oxf) 69(2):189–196
29. Ishimura E, Okuno S, Kitatani K, Kim M, Shoji T, Nakatani T, Inaba M, Nishizawa Y (2002) Different risk factors for peripheral vascular calcification between diabetic and non-diabetic haemodialysis patients – importance of glycaemic control. Diabetologia 45(10):1446–1448
30. Taniwaki H, Ishimura E, Tabata T, Tsujimoto Y, Shioi A, Shoji T, Inaba M, Inoue T, Nishizawa Y (2005) Aortic calcification in haemodialysis patients with diabetes mellitus. Nephrol Dial Transplant 20:2472–2478
31. Okuno S, Ishimura E, Kitatani K, Fujino Y, Kohno K, Maeno Y, Maekawa K, Yamakawa T, Imanishi Y, Inaba M, Nishizawa Y (2007) Presence of abdominal aortic calcification is significantly associated with all-cause and cardiovascular mortality in maintenance hemodialysis patients. Am J Kidney Dis 49(3):417–425

Chapter 2
RETRACTED CHAPTER: Various Kinds of Bone Disease in Diabetes: Rheumatic Conditions

Hitoshi Goto

Abstract Diabetes mellitus (DM) is a chronic systemic disease with a wide range of complications in the musculoskeletal system. Diabetic patients suffer from diverse rheumatic conditions, which are common and, while not life threatening, are an important cause of morbidity, pain, and disability that affect their quality of life. Joints affected by diabetes include peripheral joints and the axial skeleton. This article reviews the rheumatic conditions that are associated with DM and the pathophysiologic relationships that might link these conditions (Table 2.1). A number of fibrosing conditions of the hands and shoulder are recognized, including limited joint mobility, Dupuytren's contracture, flexor tenosynovitis, carpal tunnel syndrome, and adhesive capsulitis. Charcot osteoarthropathy is an important cause of deformity and amputation associated with peripheral neuropathy. Diabetes patients are more prone to diffuse idiopathic skeletal hyperostosis, osteoarthritis, diabetic muscle infarction, crystal-induced arthritis, osteoporosis, sarcopenia, and complex regional pain syndrome (CRPS) type 1. Management of these conditions requires early recognition and close liaison between diabetes and rheumatology specialists.

Keywords Rheumatic conditions • Diabetes mellitus • Joint • Hand • Shoulder • Muscle • Bone

2.1 Limited Joint Mobility (Diabetic Cheiroarthropathy)

Limited joint mobility (LJM), or diabetic cheiroarthropathy, is characterized by thick, tight, waxy skin, mainly on the dorsal aspect of the hands, with flexion contracture of the metacarpophalangeal and interphalangeal joints (Fig. 2.1). It is a common complication of type 1 and type 2 diabetes mellitus (DM). The prevalence of LJM ranges between 30 and 58 % among patients with type 1 DM and between 45 and 76 % among those with type 2 DM, as compared between 4 and 20 % among individuals without DM [1–5]. LJM is usually painless; however, in

H. Goto, M.D. (✉)
Graduate School of Medicine, Osaka City University, 1-4-3, Asahi-machi, Abeno-ku, Osaka 545-8585, Japan
e-mail: goto@msic.med.osaka-cu.ac.jp

M. Inaba (ed.), *Musculoskeletal Disease Associated with Diabetes Mellitus*,
DOI 10.1007/978-4-431-55720-3_2

Table 2.1 Rheumatic complications of DM

Conditions unique to DM
Diabetic muscle infarction
Conditions occurring more frequently in DM
Limited joint mobility
Dupuytren's contracture
Stenosing flexor tenosynovitis (trigger finger)
Adhesive capsulitis of shoulder
Carpal tunnel syndrome
Neuropathic arthropathy
Conditions sharing risk factors of DM and metabolic syndrome
Diffuse idiopathic skeletal hyperostosis
Osteoarthritis
Gout
Pseudogout
Calcific periarthritis of shoulder
Osteoporosis
Sarcopenia

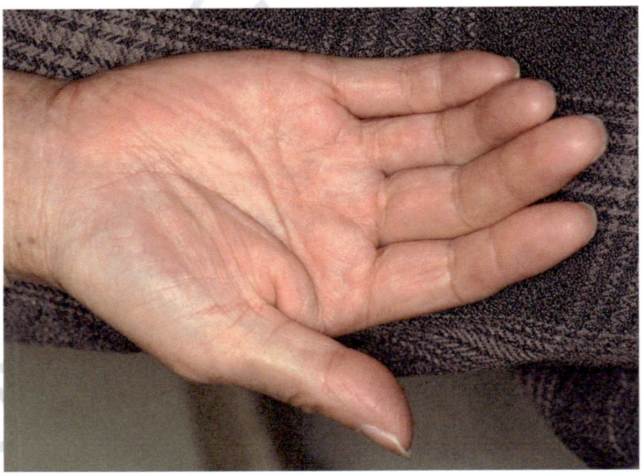

Fig. 2.1 Limited joint mobility. Flexion contracture of the metacarpophalangeal and proximal interphalangeal joints in fingers

the early stage, slight pain and paresthesia may develop. LJM is diagnosed based on the presence of the characteristic clinical signs on physical examination. The prayer sign is defined as an inability to oppose the palmar surfaces of the hands and fingers with the wrists dorsiflexed. The tabletop sign is defined as the entire surface of the palm and fingers cannot make contact with a flat surface when patients lay their palms on a tabletop with the fingers spread apart. The long duration of DM and poor glycemic control possibly predispose patients to developing LJM and influencing its progression as LJM is associated with the presence of retinopathy and nephropathy [6]. The pathophysiology is thought about as follows. Increased glycosylation and degradation of collagen in the skin and periarticular tissues, diabetic microangiopathy, and diabetic neuropathy have been implicated as contributing factors [7]. The treatment of LJM is mainly physical therapy to increase the range of motion. Improved glycemic control may not reverse the conditions but may help to prevent future progression.

2.2 Dupuytren's Contracture

Dupuytren's contracture is characterized by palmar or digital thickening, tethering, pretendinous bands, and flexion contractures of the fingers (Fig. 2.2). In patients with diabetes, both genders are equally affected, and the ring and middle finger are more commonly involved, while in nondiabetic patients, men are more likely affected, and the small finger is more involved. The prevalence of Dupuytren's contracture in diabetic patients ranges between 16 and 42 % [8, 9] compared with 13 % in the general population [10]. The prevalence is higher in patients who are older and with a longer duration of DM. Patients with Dupuytren's contracture should be evaluated for DM, as 13–39 % of them are found to have DM [11]. The pathophysiology of Dupuytren's contracture is likely to be multifactorial. Genetic predisposition explains the higher prevalence in some population over others. Trauma, long-term hyperglycemia, microangiopathy, and ischemia are also important factors. Microvascular disease and ischemia will result in increased production of oxygen free radicals. Ischemia also stimulates platelets and macrophages to produce different cytokines such as interleukin 1, tumor necrosis factor, and growth factors, such as platelet-derived growth factor, epidermal growth factor, connective tissue growth factor, vascular endothelial growth factor, and basic fibroblast growth factor, resulting in local collagen overproduction and fibrosis [12].

Treatment consists of optimizing glycemic control and physiotherapy. Recently, injections of collagenase clostridium histolyticum have been developed for the treatment of Dupuytren's contracture. Hurst et al. in 2009 [13] did a prospective,

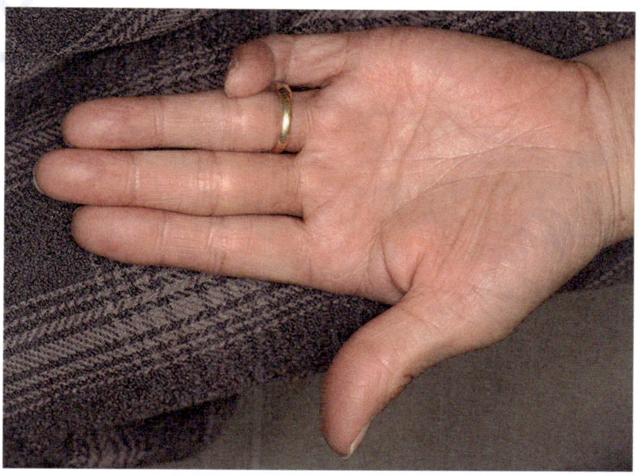

Fig. 2.2 Dupuytren's contracture in the small finger characterized by palmar thickening, tethering, pretendinous bands, and flexion contractures

randomized, and placebo-controlled trial of 308 patients with Dupuytren's contracture, 6.5 % of whom had DM; up to three collagenase injections significantly reduced fixed flexion contractures and improved the joint range of motion. There were no recurrences after follow-up of up to 90 days. Only three serious adverse events were reported in this study, including two tendon ruptures and one case of complex regional pain syndrome. Surgery is required if the hand function is severely compromised.

2.3 Stenosing Flexor Tenosynovitis (Trigger Finger)

Flexor tenosynovitis is caused by fibrous tissue proliferation in the tendon sheath (Fig. 2.3) leading to limitation and restriction of the movement of the tendon, also known as trigger finger. The prevalence of flexor tenosynovitis is estimated at 11 % in diabetic patients, compared with less than 1 % in nondiabetic individuals [14]. Patients with DM are more likely to have multiple digit involvement. It most commonly involves the ring, middle fingers, and thumb. The occurrence of flexor tenosynovitis correlates significantly with the duration of DM, but not with glycemic control [15]. Treatment of flexor tenosynovitis includes modification of activities, splinting, NSAIDs, corticosteroid injection into the tendon sheath, and surgical release [16].

2.4 Carpal Tunnel Syndrome

Carpal tunnel syndrome (CTS) is an entrapment neuropathy caused by compression of the median nerve within the carpal tunnel. It is estimated to occur in 3.8 % of the general population [17]. The prevalence of CTS in diabetic patients is higher and

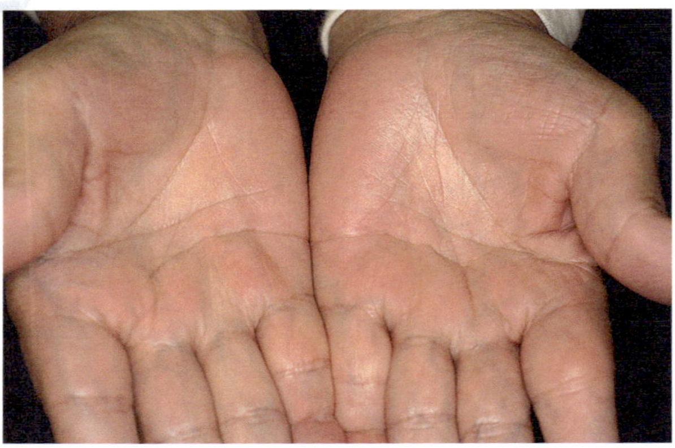

Fig. 2.3 Stenosing flexor tenosynovitis in the right small finger and the left ring finger characterized by fibrous tissue proliferation in the palmar tendon sheaths

estimated to occur in 14 % of patients without diabetic polyneuropathies and up to 30 % in those with diabetic polyneuropathies [18]. CTS prevalence increases as the DM duration extends. Increased prevalence of CTS in diabetes suggests the presence of intrinsic nerve pathology in addition to mechanical compression. The intrinsic nerve factors include loss of normal regenerative ability in the peripheral nerve because of microangiopathy, macrophage dysfunction, abnormalities in the retrograde cell body reaction, Schwann cell dysfunction, or decreased expression of neurotrophic factors and their receptors [19]. CTS manifests as pain, tingling, and paresthesia of the thumb, index, middle fingers, and the radial aspect of the ring finger. The symptoms may be improved by shaking or flicking the wrists known as "flick sign." A reduction of the pinch strength caused by the atrophy of the thumb ball and function of the affected hand may occur (Fig. 2.4). Symptoms tend to worsen at night. Bilateral CTS is common, but the symptoms may not occur simultaneously in both hands. It is usually diagnosed by history and clinical examinations, by percussion of the median nerve at the wrist (Tinel's test), by asking the patient to do wrist dorsiflexion (Phalen's test), or by employing the hand elevation test which is conducted by asking the patient to raise the affected hand and holding it in that position for 1 min. The test is considered positive if the patient experiences tingling and numbness in the median nerve distribution area [20, 21]. The diagnosis of CTS is confirmed by a nerve conduction study. Imaging studies, including magnetic resonance imaging (MRI) and ultrasonography (US), can be useful for this purpose. US is a simple, easy-to-perform, and noninvasive procedure. It has been implicated in the diagnosis of CTS as it can demonstrate the thickening of the median nerve, the flattening of the nerve within the tunnel, and the bowing of the flexor retinaculum, which are all features that indicate the presence of CTS. Several studies have concluded that the cross-sectional area is the most predictive measurement, but there is debate regarding the level within the tunnel

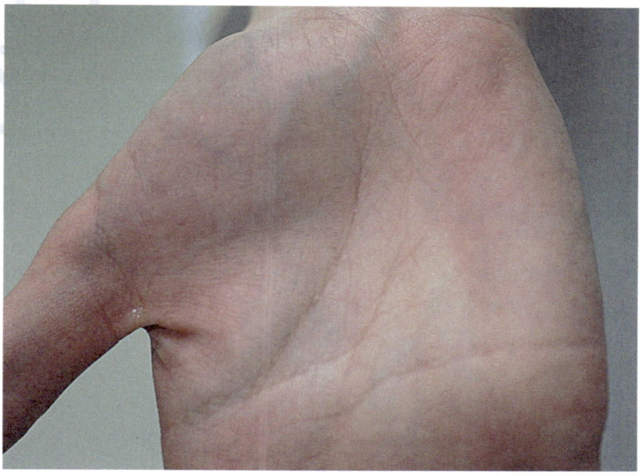

Fig. 2.4 The atrophy of the thumb ball due to median nerve palsy caused by carpal tunnel syndrome

that this measurement should be taken and what constitutes abnormal values. The sensitivity of US is 64.7 % [22]. An MRI will demonstrate swelling of the median nerve and increased signal intensity on T2-weighted images, indicating accumulation of the axonal transportation, myelin sheath degeneration, or edema, which are the signs to look out for when diagnosing CTS. An MRI shows the severity of the nerve compression and has a sensitivity of 96 %. However, its specificity is extremely low at 33–38 % [22]. The treatment options for CTS include splinting and local injection of corticosteroids or NSAIDs. Although corticosteroid treatment is effective in reducing inflammation and edema, it limits the tenocyte function by reducing collagen and proteoglycan synthesis, thus reducing the mechanical strength of the tendon and ultimately leading to further degeneration [23]. When conservative treatment fails, surgery is indicated. Surgery is performed more frequently among patients with DM and is estimated to be 4–14 times higher than the general population [24].

2.5 Adhesive Capsulitis of the Shoulder (Frozen Shoulder)

Adhesive capsulitis, or frozen shoulder, or shoulder periarthritis is characterized by progressive painful restriction of the shoulder movements, especially the external rotation and abduction. The prevalence in diabetic patients ranges 10–29 % [5, 16], as compared with 3–5 % of the age-matched controls [25]. The presence of shoulder adhesive capsulitis increases the incidence of DM and may be a presenting symptom. Connie et al. in 2008 studied the prevalence of a diabetic condition (DM and prediabetes) and adhesive capsulitis of the shoulder which revealed that a patient presenting with adhesive capsulitis had a 71.5 % chance of having a diabetic condition (38.6 % chance of being diabetic and a 32.95 % chance of being prediabetic) [26]. The natural history of the condition is characterized by three phases: pain, adhesion or stiffness, and recovery phases. Among diabetics, it occurs at a younger age, is less painful, lasts longer, and responds less well to treatment [27]. Bilateral involvement is more frequent in patients with diabetes than in nondiabetic subjects (33–42 % vs. 5–20 %) [28]. It occurs more in older patients with longer disease duration. Shoulder adhesive capsulitis is found to be associated with other diabetic complications such as limited joint mobility, autonomic neuropathy with either type of DM, and with myocardial infarction in patients with type 1 DM [5]. The exact mechanism is unknown, but it is thought that excessive glucose concentration in diabetic patients can lead to a faster rate of collagen glycosylation and cross-linking in the shoulder capsule, restricting shoulder range of motion [29]. Management of shoulder adhesive capsulitis in the painful early phase consists of adequate analgesia, intra-articular corticosteroid injections, and an appropriately graded exercise program. During the adhesive phase, physical therapy and operative treatments (arthroscopic capsular release or open surgical release) are used.

2.6 Diffuse Idiopathic Skeletal Hyperostosis

Diffuse idiopathic skeletal hyperostosis (DISH) is a condition that is characterized by diffuse calcification and ossification of the ligaments and enthesis (Figs. 2.5 and 2.6). The prevalence of DISH in type 2 DM was reported at 13–40 %, while in general population, 2.2–3.5 %. The prevalence of metabolic syndrome is higher among patients with DISH [16]. It most commonly affects the spine, particularly the thoracic spine. Patients with DISH are rarely symptomatic. However, it can cause spinal rigidity and impingement of nearby structures and nerves, resulting in hoarseness, stridor, sleep apnea, and dysphagia. It also can occur in extraspinal sites with prominent bony reactions at ligamentous and tendinous insertions, particularly in the pelvis, greater trochanters, patellae, and calcaneus. The diagnosis of DISH is based on radiologic features that are usually based on Resnick and Niwayama's 1976 criteria: (1) flowing ligamentous calcifications involving at least four contiguous vertebral bodies, (2) preservation of intervertebral disk space, and (3) absence of changes of degenerative spondylosis or spondyloarthropathy. The exact mechanism of DISH is not known. However, insulin, growth hormone, and growth factor (IGF-1) are proposed as factors that promote bone growth in DISH. Also, atherosclerosis, which is common in metabolic syndrome, will lead to damage in the endothelium and aggregation of platelets that result in increased levels of IGF-1 and then more osteoblast proliferation and bone formation. The treatment of DISH is symptom based and generally limited to analgesia as needed. Rarely, surgical

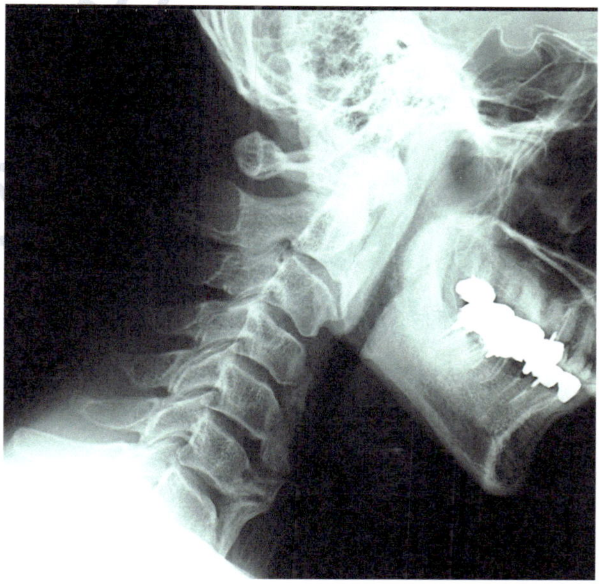

Fig. 2.5 The anterior longitudinal ligamentous calcifications of cervical vertebrae in diffuse idiopathic skeletal hyperostosis

removal of impinging bone bridges is undertaken when critical functions, such as swallowing, are compromised.

2.7 Osteoarthritis

Osteoarthritis (OA) is a very common form of arthritis in adults. Several risk factors are described for OA, including obesity, which is part of metabolic syndrome and not uncommon in DM. Dahaghin et al. [30] described an association between diabetes and hand osteoarthritis that was noted in people aged 55–62 years and was absent in other age groups. Peripheral neuropathy may increase the risk of advanced, aggressive forms of osteoarthritis. Recently, an association between knee osteoarthritis and diminished lower extremity vibratory perception was identified [31]. However, there is no clear evidence that supports DM or metabolic syndrome as risk factors for developing early or severe hip or knee OA [32].

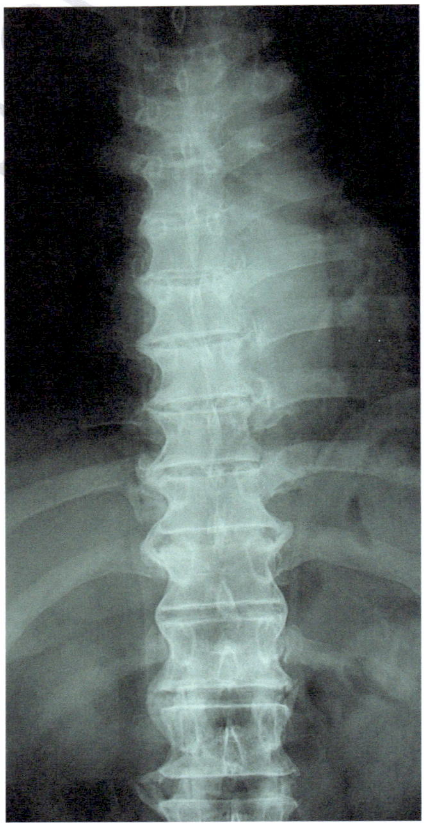

Fig. 2.6 The ligamentous calcifications of thoracolumbar vertebrae in diffuse idiopathic skeletal hyperostosis characterized by no lesion in heart side of thoracic vertebrae

2.8 Neuropathic Osteoarthropathy (Charcot Osteoarthropathy)

Neuropathic osteoarthropathy, also known as Charcot osteoarthropathy, is a progressive destructive process affecting the bone and joint structure associated with various diseases in which neuropathy occurs. However, DM is by far the most common etiology. It mainly affects the foot and ankle in diabetic patients. It is a devastating, limb-threatening condition resulting in dramatic deformities and recurrent ulceration that may ultimately lead to amputation. The pathogenesis of neuropathic osteoarthropathy remains debatable. It may result from repeated trauma, often minor, in the setting of decreased sensation due to a sensory neuropathy which results in increased damage with microfractures. An alternative possibility is that the neuropathy triggers an increased blood flow or distal hyperemia that results in stimulation of osteoclasts with increased bone resorption, osteoporosis, fractures, and joint damage. Recently, inflammation has been identified as another factor in the development of neuropathic osteoarthropathy. The release of proinflammatory cytokines leads to increased expression of the polypeptide receptor activator of nuclear factor-κB ligand (RANKL). RANKL triggers the synthesis of the nuclear transcription factor nuclear factor-κβ, and this in turn stimulates the maturation of osteoclasts from osteoclast precursor cells. At the same time, NF-κβ stimulates the production of the glycopeptide osteoprotegerin from osteoblasts [33]. The proinflammatory cytokines, RANKL, NF-κβ, and osteoclasts will result in increased osteolysis. The neuropathic osteoarthropathy is characterized by acute and chronic phases. In the acute phase, the foot is warm, edematous, and erythematous, mimicking cellulitis. Pain may or may not be present, depending on the degree of neuropathy. The chronic phase is characterized by deformity of the foot with abnormal pressure on the plantar surface due to the collapse of the plantar arch and the development of a rocker bottom deformity. Calluses may form which are liable to ulcerations, especially in the midfoot. The plain radiographs may not be useful in an acute phase; however, they may demonstrate excessive destruction in the chronic phase (Fig. 2.7). An MRI may show bone marrow edema, bone bruising,

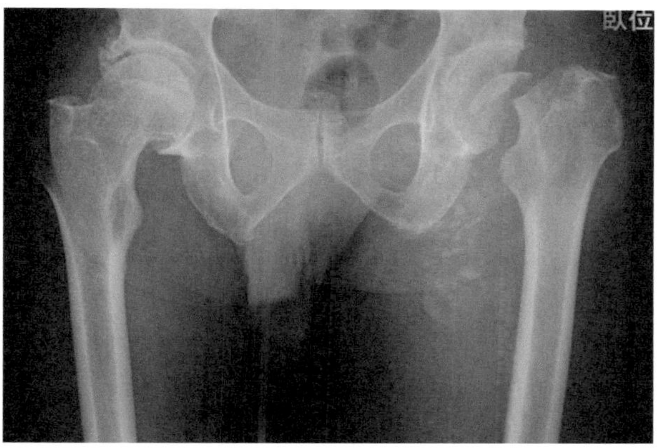

Fig. 2.7 The severe destructive lesion in the left hip joint due to Charcot osteoarthropathy

or microfractures. If osteomyelitis is a clinical possibility, radionuclide bone scanning, such as indium-111-leukocyte (111In-WBC) scanning and technetium-99m-methylene diphosphonate (99mTc-MDP) bone scanning, virtually excludes the osteomyelitis if both studies have negative results. Treatment involves weight-bearing limitations for at least 3 months for healing [34]. NSAIDs, calcitonin, and bisphosphonates may be used. Bisphosphonates inhibit the osteoclastic resorption, may have direct anti-inflammatory properties, and might slow or even stop the bony destruction. However, the data are weak to support their use as a routine treatment for acute neuropathic osteoarthropathy [35]. Surgical treatment may be required when this conservative treatment fails. Moreover, surgery in the presence of DM and diabetic complications carries higher risk for complications.

2.9 Osteoporosis

Patients with diabetes mellitus (DM) are at higher risk of bone fracture relative to their bone mineral density (BMD). A number of reports indicate a higher prevalence of vertebral fracture (VF) in those with type 2 DM (T2DM) than in those without, irrespective of the insignificant difference in BMD between patients with or without T2DM. Meta-analysis studies reported that T2DM patients exhibited a higher fracture rate, particularly in appendicular bones, despite their comparable BMD, suggesting the possible involvement of impaired bone quality, but not BMD, in the development of bone fragility. It is recognized that the higher fracture rate in T2DM patients is explained by increased cortical porosity, as shown by high-resolution peripheral quantitative computed tomography (HR-pQCT) or quantitative ultrasound (QUS) device [36].

It has been recently recognized that serum parathyroid hormone (PTH) plays an important role in the development of cortical porosity, which starts to increase in chronic kidney disease (CKD) patients as they progress to stage 3, for whom evidence shows a higher fracture rate at the femur neck. Since T2DM patients are complicated with stage 3 CKD more often than non-DM patients, it is important to examine whether DM by itself or in association with CKD might be a more important contributing factor to the development of cortical porosity [36].

2.10 Frailty, Sarcopenia

Frailty is a pre-disability condition that can be defined clinically. The major factors leading to frailty are sarcopenia and a decline in executive function. Stressors precipitate frail individuals into a state of disability. Diabetics develop the conditions necessary for frailty earlier than other aging individuals. Appropriate treatment of diabetes mellitus and frailty precursors can result in a slowing of the aging process [37].

2.11 Diabetic Muscle Infarction

Diabetic muscle infarction is a rare complication of DM. It is usually reported in association with long-standing, poorly controlled DM, particularly patients with type 1 DM, in the presence of microangiopathic complications such as retinopathy, nephropathy, or neuropathy. Patients with diabetic muscle infarction usually present with acute pain with swelling (and a palpable mass in 34–44 % of the patients) in an extremity that persists at rest and worsens with exercise and expands during a period of days to weeks without any prior history of trauma. The thigh muscles are commonly involved. However, the calf muscles, upper extremity, and abdominal wall muscles have also been reported. The diagnosis is established based on a clinical presentation and radiological finding. Laboratory studies generally demonstrate an elevated ESR and normal or mildly elevated WBC counts. Measurements of creatine kinase (CK) may be normal or elevated. Therefore, CK is not a reliable marker. The MRI is the diagnostic test of choice for diabetic muscle infarction. MRI findings demonstrate diffuse edema and swelling of multiple thigh or calf muscles, often in more than one compartment. Muscle biopsy should be reserved for patients with an atypical clinical presentation. The biopsy will demonstrate muscle necrosis and edema, phagocytosis of the necrotic muscle fibers, granulation tissue, and collagen deposition. Findings at advanced stages include replacement of the necrotic muscle fibers by the fibrous tissue, myofiber regeneration, and mononuclear cell infiltration [38]. The underlying pathophysiology remains incompletely understood. The most likely hypothesis is that muscle infarction is caused by vascular disease such as arteriosclerosis and diabetic microangiopathy. Hypercoagulability resulting from alteration of the coagulation–fibrinolytic system and endothelial dysfunction in DM has been proposed as a potential pathogenic mechanism [38]. The treatment involves bed rest, analgesics, and aggressive control of DM. Other medical therapies that have been suggested as being beneficial include antiplatelet agents such as low-dose aspirin, dipyridamole, NSAIDs, and nifedipine; however, there are no randomized control trials to support the use of these agents. Vigorous physical therapy should be avoided since it may lead to an exacerbation. Patients usually recover spontaneously over a period of weeks to months of bed rest, although the recurrence rate in the same or the contralateral extremity is approximately 40 % in all treatment groups [39].

2.12 Crystal-Induced Arthritis

2.12.1 Gout

Gout is a condition that is characterized by hyperuricemia, which is defined as urate levels >6.8 mg/dl (≥360 mmol/L), and monosodium urate crystal deposition in the joints. It has two stages: an acute stage characterized by recurrent attacks of arthritis and a chronic stage that manifests as chronic tophaceous gout. The relationships between hyperuricemia, gout, and metabolic syndrome have been evaluated in several studies. It has been demonstrated that the prevalence of the metabolic syndrome among patients with hyperuricemia or gout is higher than the others. Insulin resistance and type 2 DM have also been noted to be associated with gout. It was found that the incidence of insulin resistance in gout patients increased by as much as 35 % over individuals without gout [40]. Recently, it was shown that both gout and type 2 DM share most of the common genetic risk factors and that there exists a mutually interdependent effect with regard to higher incidences between these two diseases [41]. Indeed, hypertension, chronic kidney disease, and hyperlipidemia are not uncommon in patients with DM, which are known risk factors for gout. Hyperuricemia was found to be a risk factor for the development of DM. Vidula et al. [42] evaluated the impact of serum uric acid levels on the future risk of developing type 2 diabetes independent of other factors, and they reported that as the level of uric acid increases, the incidence of DM also increases. These associations persisted in both genders and were independent of other known risk factors including age, BMI, alcohol consumption, smoking, physical activity level, hypertension, and levels of glucose, cholesterol, creatinine, and triglycerides [38]. Hyperuricemia may lead to endothelial dysfunction and nitric oxide inhibition, which in turn contribute to insulin resistance and thus diabetes. An alternative possibility is that the higher insulin levels associated with prediabetes can reduce renal excretion of uric acid.

2.12.2 Calcium Pyrophosphate Dihydrate Crystal Deposition Disease (Pseudogout)

Calcium pyrophosphate dihydrate (CPPD) crystal deposition in the hyaline or fibrous cartilage may be asymptomatic and identified by plain radiography which detects the calcification characteristic of CPPD. It may manifest as acute or chronic inflammatory arthritis. DM is considered as a possible risk factor for CPPD deposition disease. This is based on a small collection of cases [43]. Nevertheless, the association of CPPD disease with DM has not been proven.

2.12.3 Basic Calcium Phosphate Crystal Deposition Disease

Basic calcium phosphate (BCP) crystal depositions can occur in the intra-articular and periarticular components known as calcific tendonitis or calcific periarthritis. It most commonly affects the shoulder in which BCP crystals deposit predominantly in periarticular areas resulting in tendonitis or bursitis. The incidence of calcific shoulder periarthritis is increased in DM. Shoulder calcifications were detected in 31.8 % of patients with DM, while only 10 % in controls without DM [44]. The diagnosis is made by a proof of the crystal in synovial fluid but it may not be easy, as BCP crystals are not detected even by polarized light microscopy. Therefore, the diagnosis depends upon excluding of the other causes. There is no specific treatment. Analgesics, NSAIDs, and joint aspirations with or without glucocorticoid injections are used. Calcific tendonitis may coexist with adhesive capsulitis in the shoulder.

2.12.4 Complex Regional Pain Syndrome Type 1 (Reflex Sympathetic Dystrophy)

Complex regional pain syndrome type 1 (CRPS 1), or reflex sympathetic dystrophy (RSD), is characterized by localized or diffuse pain in the upper or lower extremity usually associated with swelling, vasomotor disturbances, and trophic skin changes including loss of hair, skin color changes, skin temperature changes, and skin thickening. The condition may occur after minimal trauma or even spontaneously. DM may predispose one to CRPS 1. Walling [45] conducted a review on 387 patients with CRPS 1 and found that 28 patients have secondary CRPS 1 and DM was the commonest associated disease (in 11 out of 28). Treatments have been used with variable results, including analgesics, physiotherapy, intravenous bisphosphonates, calcitonin, oral corticosteroids, and sympathetic ganglion blocks.

2.13 Conclusions

DM is associated with various rheumatic conditions. Recognition of these conditions is important, as they affect the patient's quality of life. Several rheumatic conditions are more prevalent or caused by the long-term metabolic consequences of DM. Some of the rheumatic conditions associated with DM may be presented before the diagnosis of DM is established. Therefore, management of these conditions requires early recognition and close liaison between diabetes and rheumatology specialists.

References

1. Pal B, Anderson J, Dick WC, Griffiths ID (1986) Limitation of joint mobility and shoulder capsulitis in insulin- and non-insulin-dependent diabetes mellitus. Br J Rheumatol 25 (2):147–151
2. Rosenbloom AL, Silverstein JH, Lezotte DC, Richardson K, Mccallum M (1981) Limited joint mobility in childhood diabetes mellitus indicates increased risk for microvascular disease. N Engl J Med 305(4):191–194

3. Fitzcharles MA, Duby S, Waddell RW, Banks E, Karsh J (1984) Limitation of joint mobility (cheiroarthropathy) in adult noninsulin-dependent diabetic patients. Ann Rheum Dis 43 (2):251–254
4. Starkman HS, Gleason RE, Rand LI, Miller DE, Soeldner JS (1986) Limited joint mobility (LJM) of the hand in patients with diabetes mellitus: relation to chronic complications. Ann Rheum Dis 45(2):130–135
5. Arkkila PE, Kantola IM, Viikari JS, Ronnemaa T, Vahatalo MA (1996) Limited joint mobility is associated with the presence but does not predict the development of microvascular complications in type 1 diabetes. Diabet Med 13(9):828–833
6. Aljahlan M, Lee KC, Toth E (1999) Limited joint mobility in diabetes. Postgrad Med 105 (2):99–101, 105–106
7. Wyatt LH, Ferrance RJ (2006) The musculoskeletal effects of diabetes mellitus. J Can Chiropr Assoc 50(1):43–50
8. Ardic F, Soyupek F, Kahraman Y, Yorgancioglu R (2003) The musculoskeletal complications seen in type II diabetics: predominance of hand involvement. Clin Rheumatol 22(3):229–233
9. Cagliero E, Apruzzese W, Perlmutter GS, Nathan DM (2002) Musculoskeletal disorders of the hand and shoulder in patients with diabetes mellitus. Am J Med 112(6):487–490
10. Carson J, Clarke C (1993) Dupuytren's contracture in pensioners at the Royal Hospital Chelsea. J R Coll Physicians Lond 27(1):25–27
11. Lennox IA, Murali SR, Porter R (1993) A study of the repeatability of the diagnosis of Dupuytren's contracture and its prevalence in the Grampian region. J Hand Surg Br 18 (2):258–261
12. Childs SG (2005) Dupuytren's disease. Orthop Nurs 24(2):160–163, quiz 164–165
13. Hurst LC, Badalamente MA, Hentz VR et al (2009) Injectable collagenase clostridium histolyticum for Dupuytren's contracture. N Engl J Med 361(10):968–979
14. Leden I, Schersten B, Svensson B, Svensson M (1983) Locomotor system disorders in diabetes mellitus. Increased prevalence of palmar flexortenosynovitis. Scand J Rheumatol 12 (3):260–262
15. Yosipovitch G, Yosipovitch Z, Karp M, Mukamel M (1990) Trigger finger in young patients with insulin dependent diabetes. J Rheumatol 17(7):951–952
16. Lebiedz-Odrobina D, Kay J (2010) Rheumatic manifestations of diabetes mellitus. Rheum Dis Clin North Am 36(4):681–699
17. Atroshi I, Gummesson C, Johnsson R, Ornstein E, Ranstam J, Rosen I (1999) Prevalence of carpal tunnel syndrome in a general population. JAMA 282(2):153–158
18. Perkins BA, Olaleye D, Bril V (2002) Carpal tunnel syndrome in patients with diabetic polyneuropathy. Diabetes Care 25(3):565–569
19. Kennedy JM, Zochodne DW (2005) Impaired peripheral nerve regeneration in diabetes mellitus. J Peripher Nerv Syst 10(2):144–157
20. Amirfeyz R, Gozzard C, Leslie IJ (2005) Hand elevation test for assessment of carpal tunnel syndrome. J Hand Surg Br 30(4):361–364
21. Ahn DS (2001) Hand elevation: a new test for carpal tunnel syndrome. Ann Plast Surg 46 (2):120–124
22. Ibrahim I, Khan WS, Goddard N, Smitham P (2012) Carpal tunnel syndrome: a review of the recent literature. Open Orthop J 6:69–76
23. Scutt N, Rolf CG, Scutt A (2006) Glucocorticoids inhibit tenocyte proliferation and tendon progenitor cell recruitment. J Orthop Res 24(2):173–182
24. Makepeace A, Davis WA, Bruce DG, Davis TM (2008) Incidence and determinants of carpal tunnel decompression surgery in type 2 diabetes: the Fremantle Diabetes Study. Diabetes Care 31(3):498–500
25. Manske RC, Prohaska D (2008) Diagnosis and management of adhesive capsulitis. Curr Rev Musculoskelet Med 1(3–4):180–189
26. Tighe CB, Oakley WS Jr (2008) The prevalence of a diabetic condition and adhesive capsulitis of the shoulder. South Med J 101(6):591–595

27. Griggs SM, Ahn A, Green A (2000) Idiopathic adhesive capsulitis. A prospective functional outcome study of nonoperative treatment. J Bone Joint Surg Am 82-A(10):1398–1407
28. Crispin JC, Alcocer-Varela J (2003) Rheumatologic manifestations of diabetes mellitus. Am J Med 114(9):753–757
29. Hsu JE, Anakwenze OA, Warrender WJ, Abboud JA (2011) Current review of adhesive capsulitis. J Shoulder Elbow Surg 20(3):502–514
30. Dahaghin S, Bierma-Zeinstra SM, Koes BW, Hazes JM, Pols HA (2007) Do metabolic factors add to the effect of overweight on hand osteoarthritis? The Rotterdam Study. Ann Rheum Dis 66(7):916–920
31. Shakoor N, Agrawal A, Block JA (2008) Reduced lower extremity vibratory perception in osteoarthritis of the knee. Arthritis Rheum 59(1):117–121
32. Burner TW, Rosenthal AK (2009) Diabetes and rheumatic diseases. Curr Opin Rheumatol 21 (1):50–54
33. Rogers LC, Frykberg RG, Armstrong DG et al (2011) The Charcot foot in diabetes. Diabetes Care 34(9):2123–2129
34. Boddenberg U (2004) Healing time of foot and ankle fractures in patients with diabetes mellitus: literature review and report on own cases. Zentralbl Chir 129(6):453–459
35. Richard JL, Almasri M, Schuldiner S (2012) Treatment of acute Charcot foot with bisphosphonates: a systematic review of the literature. Diabetologia 55(5):1258–1264
36. Mishima T, Motoyama K, Imanishi Y et al (2015) Decreased cortical thickness, as estimated by a newly developed ultrasound device, as a risk for vertebral fracture in type 2 diabetes mellitus patients with eGFR of less than 60 mL/min/1.73 m. Osteoporos Int 26(1):229–236
37. Morley JE (2008) Diabetes, sarcopenia, and frailty. Clin Geriatr Med 24(3):455–469
38. Trujillo-Santos AJ (2003) Diabetic muscle infarction: an underdiagnosed complication of long-standing diabetes. Diabetes Care 26(1):211–215
39. Kapur S, Brunet JA, Mckendry RJ (2004) Diabetic muscle infarction: case report and review. J Rheumatol 31(1):190–194
40. Yoo HG, Lee SI, Chae HJ, Park SJ, Lee YC, Yoo WH (2011) Prevalence of insulin resistance and metabolic syndrome in patients with gouty arthritis. Rheumatol Int 31(4):485–491
41. Lai HM, Chen CJ, Su BY et al (2012) Gout and type 2 diabetes have a mutual inter-dependent effect on genetic risk factors and higher incidences. Rheumatology (Oxford) 51(4):715–720
42. Bhole V, Choi JW, Kim SW, De Vera M, Choi H (2010) Serum uric acid levels and the risk of type 2 diabetes: a prospective study. Am J Med 123(10):957–961
43. Louthrenoo W, Sukitawut W (1999) Calcium pyrophosphate dehydrate crystal deposition: a clinical and laboratory analysis of 91 Thai patients. J Med Assoc Thai 82(6):569–576
44. Mavrikakis ME, Drimis S, Kontoyannis DA, Rasidakis A, Moulopoulou ES, Kontoyannis S (1989) Calcific shoulder periarthritis (tendinitis) in adult onset diabetes mellitus: a controlled study. Ann Rheum Dis 48(3):211–214
45. Walling HW (2011) Clinical differentiation of primary from secondary hyperhidrosis. J Am Acad Dermatol 64(4):690–695

Chapter 3
Fracture Risk in Diabetes

Masahiro Yamamoto and Toshitsugu Sugimoto

Abstract Meta-analyses have revealed that the relative risk of hip fractures in patients with type 1 and type 2 diabetes mellitus is higher than that in nondiabetic subjects. The risk of fracture in diabetic patients increases along with a decrease in bone mineral density (BMD) similarly to those in nondiabetic patients. However, the observed risk of fracture is higher than the expected one by BMD in both type 1 and type 2 diabetic patients, indicating that precise estimation of bone fragility by BMD values in patients with diabetes is difficult. Bone strength consists of BMD and bone quality; for this reason, poor bone quality is the most suitable and explicable cause for elevated fracture risk in this population. Bone quality indicators closely related to bone fragility are required to be identified to establish a diagnostic method for osteoporosis in diabetic patients.

Keywords Bone quality • Low bone turnover • Vertebral fracture pentosidine • Advanced glycation end products (AGEs)

3.1 Introduction

With the development of insulin therapy for diabetic patients after the discovery of insulin in 1921, microvascular diseases, such as diabetic retinopathy, diabetic neuropathy, and diabetic nephropathy, were identified as the complications of diabetes mellitus. In the same period, in 1948, Albright reported that diabetic patients who had been exposed to poor blood glucose over a long period developed osteoporosis for the first time. However, the underlying mechanisms of these associations remained unknown.

M. Yamamoto (✉) • T. Sugimoto
Internal Medicine 1, Shimane University Faculty of Medicine, 89-1 Enya-cho, Izumo, Shimane 693-8501, Japan
e-mail: masa-ya@med.shimane-u.ac.jp

M. Inaba (ed.), *Musculoskeletal Disease Associated with Diabetes Mellitus*,
DOI 10.1007/978-4-431-55720-3_3

3.2 Bone Mineral Density in Diabetic Patients

Measurement of bone mineral density (BMD) is an established method for assessment of bone strength. The association between decreased BMD measured by dual-energy X-ray absorptiometry (DXA) and fracture rate was found in postmenopausal osteoporosis. In 1991, osteoporosis was defined as "a disease that is characterized by low bone mass, microarchitectural deterioration of bone tissue leading to enhanced bone fragility, and consequent increase in fracture risk" [1], and the diagnosis criterion of osteoporosis primarily based on bone density was established. In contrast, there was less information on BMD value of diabetic patients. Diabetes mellitus is classified into two major types: type 1 diabetes mellitus (T1DM), which is caused by a loss of ability to secrete insulin that possesses anabolic action of bone, and type 2 diabetes mellitus (T2DM), which develops in the presence of underlying insulin resistance. In T1DM, BMD measured in the femoral neck or the lumbar vertebrae has been reported to be significantly lower than the respective value in age and body mass index-matched nondiabetic subjects [2, 3]; these findings were consistently confirmed in other reports [4, 5]. A meta-analysis published in 2007 showed that BMD Z-scores (the age-adjusted BMD) of hip and spine in T1DM patients were lower than those in nondiabetic participants [6]. In contrast, the BMD values at these sites in T2DM patients were inconsistent; early reports with small number of patients showed that BMD values were lower than, equivalent to, or higher than those in the control groups [7–10]. However, successive reports from large-scale studies indicated that BMD values in these subjects were significantly higher than in nondiabetic populations [11, 12]. The meta-analysis including these studies revealed that the BMD Z-score in T2DM patients was higher than those in nondiabetic population, unlike in the case of that in T1DM patients [6].

3.2.1 The Risk of Fracture in Diabetic Patients

The relationship between the presence of diabetes and risk of fracture has been investigated by the clinical type of diabetes. In the patients with T1DM, the risk of hip fractures after adjustment for confounding factors has been reported to be significantly higher in female patients compared with that in nondiabetic subjects [13, 14]. Two meta-analyses confirmed the consistent relationship between the presence of diabetes and risk of fracture [6, 15]. In contrast, the findings obtained from the patients with T2DM confused us for a long time: some reports indicated that the risk of hip fractures is increased in T2DM. However, others showed the opposite results. Two meta-analyses concluded that the risk of hip fracture in T2DM is significantly higher than that of nondiabetic subjects, although their BMD was higher compared to the control group [6, 15]. Taken together, these findings suggest that diabetes mellitus is an underlying disease for secondary osteoporosis because the risk of fracture is increased in diabetic patients irrespective of their diabetic clinical type.

3.2.2 *Characteristics of the Risk of Fracture in Diabetes Mellitus*

Vestergaard et al. found out some interesting results in their report [6]. The predicted odds ratios for the relative risk of fracture in T1DM and T2DM patients, when estimated by the Z-score, were 1.42 and 0.77, respectively. However, the observed values were 6.94 and 1.38, respectively, indicating that the risk of hip fractures in the patients with diabetes was higher compared to the risk predicted by BMD, irrespective of the diabetic type. On the other hand, Schwartz et al. observed that the rate of hip fractures over a period of 10 years in T2DM patients aged 75 years was higher at any BMD of the femoral neck than that in nondiabetic population of the same age [16]. This finding suggested that it is difficult to assess bone fragility in diabetic patients by BMD that is the conventional and golden standard method for diagnosis of osteoporosis.

Occurrence of hip fracture needs excess external force such as falls. The risk of falls is increased in the diabetic patients with diabetic retinopathy, diabetic peripheral neuropathy, orthostatic hypotension, or hypoglycemia and in those on insulin therapy with an HbA1c of <6 % [17–21]. However, the risk of fracture in T2DM patients is higher than that in nondiabetic subjects, even when statistical adjustment for the history of falls was performed [22], suggesting that the increased risk of falls is not a major factor in the increased risk of fractures in diabetic patients. On the other hand, vertebral fractures may be a susceptible sign of the presence of bone fragility, because these fractures can be caused by mild external forces generated during the course of daily activities without any obvious injury such as falls. In T2DM patients, the relative risk of vertebral fractures is significantly higher than that in nondiabetic subjects (Fig. 3.1), despite BMD being markedly higher than that in nondiabetic patients, irrespective of sex [23] (Fig. 3.2), and significant association is not found between BMD and risk of vertebral fractures [23, 24] (Fig. 3.3). In addition, studies in T1DM patients have shown that, unlike the control group, there is no significant relationship between fracture severity and BMD Z-score [25]. Taken together, the observed risk of fracture is higher than the estimated one by BMD of these patients [6, 15, 16, 23], suggesting that pathophysiologic mechanisms not able to be assessed by BMD underlie in bone fragility of diabetic patients, irrespective of the clinical type of diabetes.

Osteoporosis is defined as "a skeletal disorder characterized by compromised bone strength predisposing a person to an increased risk of fracture," and bone strength consists of "BMD" and "bone quality" [26] (Fig. 3.4). Estimation of bone strength by BMD is difficult for diabetic subjects; therefore, poor bone quality is the

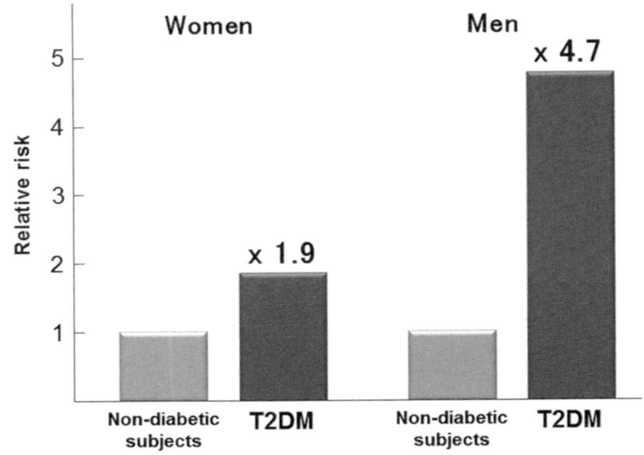

Fig. 3.1 Associations between the presence of T2DM and vertebral fractures. The relative risk of vertebral fractures in T2DM patients is significantly higher than that in nondiabetic subjects in both genders after adjustment for age, BMI, and L2–4 BMD (From Ref. [23])

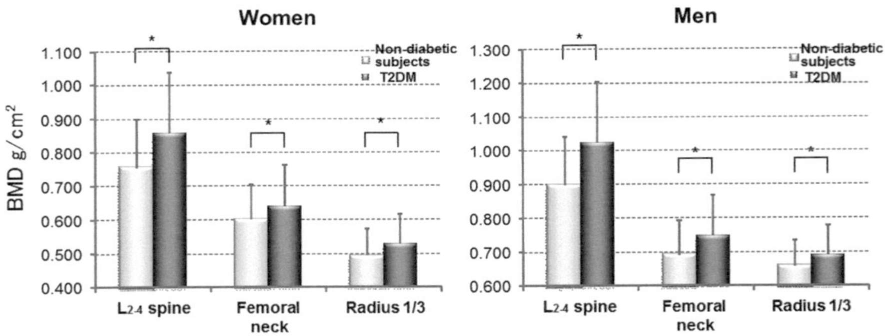

Fig. 3.2 Comparison of BMD between control subjects and patients with T2DM. BMD values at any site in T2DM patients are significantly higher than those of nondiabetic subjects in both genders. * $P < 0.05$ (From Ref. [23])

most suitable and explicable cause for elevated fracture risk in this population and may be a diabetes-specific mechanism for bone fragility.

3.3 Mechanism of Decreased Bone Quality in Diabetic Patients

Bone quality is divided into material properties and geometrical properties (Fig. 3.4): the former reflects the physical characteristics of the bone, and the latter indicates the morphological characteristics of the bone. Material properties include the “bone matrix” composed mainly of collagen; “bone turnover,” which shows the metabolic rate at which old bone tissue is absorbed and replaced by new bone

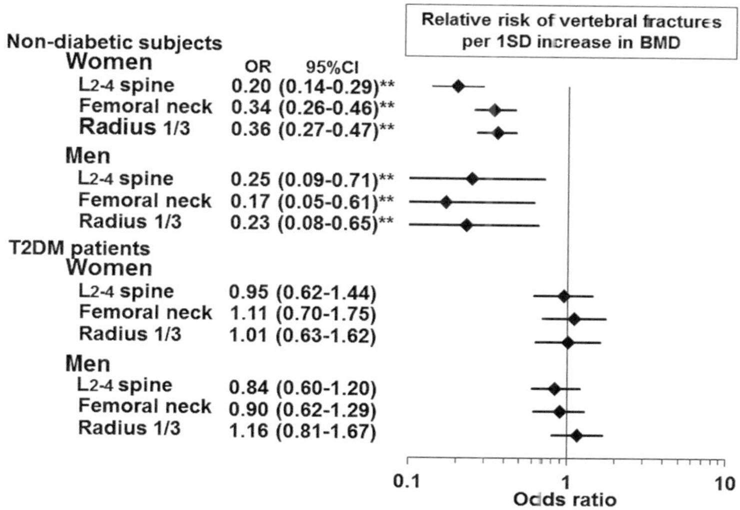

Fig. 3.3 Association between BMD and vertebral fractures in nondiabetic subjects and patients with T2DM. In contrast to nondiabetic subjects, the association between BMD and risk of vertebral fracture is not observed in T2DM patients. ** $P < 0.01$ (From Ref. [23])

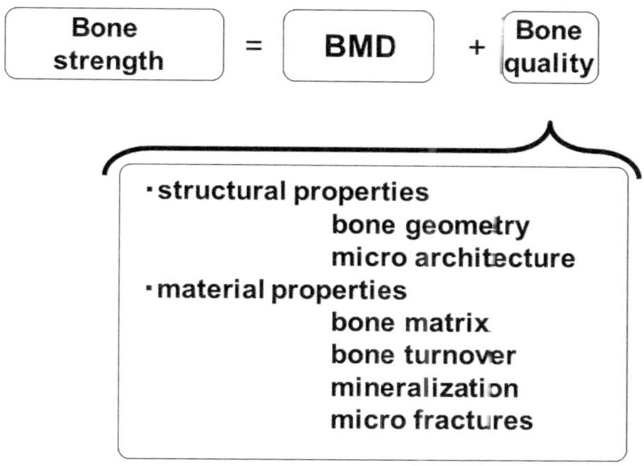

Fig. 3.4 Definition of bone strength. Bone strength consists of "BMD" and "bone quality," the latter includes structural properties and material properties (From Ref. [26])

tissue; "mineralization" of the bone tissue; and "microfractures," which are cracks confirmed using electron microscopy. The geometrical properties include "bone geometry" of the cortical bone on a macroscopic level and "microarchitecture" of the trabecular bone on a microscopic level [26]. Specific factors which are clinically associated with the risk of fracture independent of BMD are etiologic causes of deterioration of bone quality and may serve as a powerful clue for elucidating the pathology of bone fragility in diabetic patients.

3.3.1 Deterioration of the Bone Matrix and Bone Fragility

Type I collagen is the main constituent protein of the bone matrix; the formation of cross-links between neighboring collagen molecules by enzymatic reaction changes it into stabilized collagen fiber, which determines the mechanical strength of the bone tissue. Pentosidine, one of the advanced glycation end products (AGEs) which is known to be increased in diabetic patients, is composed of lysine and arginine cross-linked by a pentose. Saito et al. showed that pentosidine was increased in bone collagen content just before the onset of diabetes in spontaneously diabetic rats and that bone strength measured by three-point bending fixture test in the diabetic group was significantly decreased compared to that in the control group [27, 28]. Indeed, the negative correlation between bone strength and bone pentosidine content has been confirmed in nondiabetic patients with hip fracture [29, 30]. These findings suggest that hyperglycemic condition pathologically promotes the excessive glycosylation of bone collagen that is assumed to form cross-linking between collagen fibers by a non-enzymatic mechanism. This change in material properties of bone collagen may be a plausible cause for poor bone quality, that is, deteriorated bone strength that cannot be assessed by BMD.

Bone content of pentosidine is significantly and positively correlated with its serum concentration [31]. Clinical studies showed that increased serum and urinary pentosidine concentrations were related to an increased risk of vertebral as well as clinical fractures independent of BMD in T2DM patients [32, 33] (Fig. 3.5). These observations indirectly suggested that advanced glycation of bone collagen in patients with diabetes also deteriorates material property of bone tissue. A microindentation method recently reported directly measures material properties of bone based on the depth of the dimple impacted by the testing probe on the tibia [34]. This method revealed that bone material strength of T2DM women was significantly lower than that of age-matched nondiabetic postmenopausal women

	OR (95%CI)
Vertebral fractures	
serum pentosidine	2.50 (1.09-5.73)*
urinary pentosidine	5.93 (2.08-16.9)**
Clinical fractures	
urinary pentosidine	1.42 (1.10-1.83)**

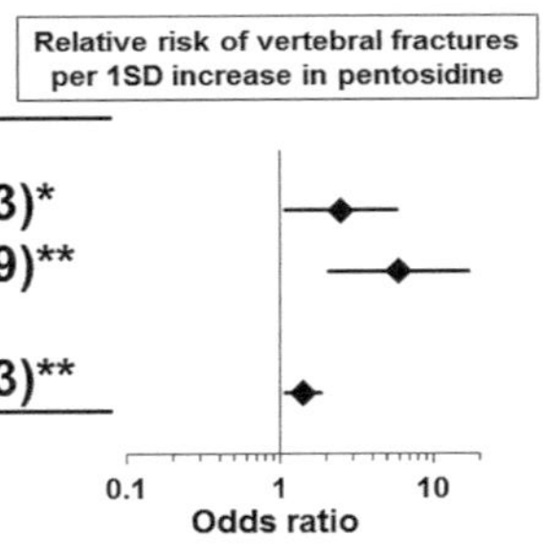

Fig. 3.5 The association between serum or urinary pentosidine levels and vertebral as well as clinical fractures in T2DM patients. Increased serum and urinary pentosidine concentrations were related to an increased risk of vertebral as well as clinical fractures independent of BMD after adjustment for multiple variables at least including age, BMI, HbA1c, renal function, and BMD. * $P < 0.05$, ** $P < 0.01$

[35], which directly revealed the presence of poor bone quality caused by deteriorated material property of the bone tissue in T2DM patients.

3.3.2 Bone Turnover and Bone Fragility

The collagen products as well as the factors for mineralization, which are secreted from osteoblast during its maturity, and the collagen degradation products derived from bone tissue resorption by osteoclasts are indices for bone turnover. Parathyroid hormone (PTH) and the bone formation as well as resorption markers in T2DM patients are significantly lower than those in nondiabetic subjects (Fig. 3.6), indicating that these patients possess suppressed bone turnover [36, 37]. The subgroup with relatively lower bone formation in addition to lower PTH levels has a higher risk of vertebral fracture independent of BMD compared to the subgroup with relatively higher these values. This finding suggests that low bone turnover accompanied with decreased bone formation causes deterioration of the bone quality. Decreased ratio of osteocalcin (OC) to bone alkaline phosphatase (BAP), which is secreted proteins, the former from mature osteoblasts or osteocytes and the latter from pre-osteoblasts, is associated with increased risk of vertebral fracture

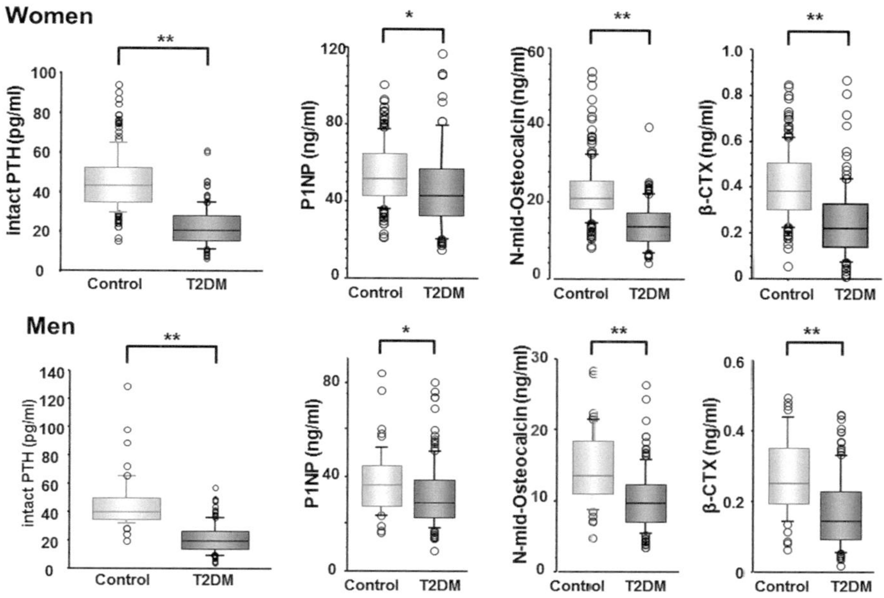

Fig. 3.6 Comparison of intact PTH and bone metabolic markers values between controls and T2DM patients. Parathyroid hormone (PTH) and the bone formation as well as resorption markers in T2DM patients are significantly lower than those in nondiabetic subjects. *, $P < 0.01$; **, $P < 0.001$ (From Ref. [36])

independent of BMD [38], suggesting that maturation disorders of osteoblast may be involved in the poor bone quality.

In addition, various factors for regulating bone turnover are reported to be involved in a risk of fracture independent of BMD. Insulin-like growth factor-1 (IGF-1), which is abundantly present in both circulating blood and bone matrix, is an important local factor for promoting the proliferation and differentiation of osteoblasts [39, 40]. IGF-1 activates the canonical Wnt/β-catenin pathway by increasing the concentration of intracellular β-catenin via promoting the degradation of glycogen synthase kinase-3 (GSK-3) after binding to the insulin receptor substrate (IRS-1) [41]. The serum IGF-1 level in female T2DM patients is lower than that in nondiabetic subjects [42], which is related to an increased risk of vertebral fractures independent of BMD [42, 43].

Sclerostin is a protein secreted by osteocytes that binds to the osteoblast LDL receptor-related proteins 5 and 6 (LRP5/6) and suppresses the canonical Wnt/β-catenin pathway by inhibiting receptor complex formation. Elevated sclerostin level is significantly associated with an increased risk of vertebral fractures, independent of BMD and bone turnover [42, 44].

The receptor for AGEs, which is presented on specific cell surface, recognizes AGEs as ligands [45] and is involved in the progression of diabetic complications such as diabetic nephropathy [46]. The studies on osteoblast derived from mice showed that hyperglycemia and AGEs suppress osteoblastic differentiation and mineralization accompanied with enhanced expression of RAGE [47–49] and that BMD was decreased in RAGE-deficient animals [50], suggesting that the AGEs-RAGE axis is involved in bone formation. Splicing variant of this receptor lacking a membrane-spanning portion is known as endogenous secretory RAGE (esRAGE), which acts as "decoy receptor" inhibiting RAGE on the cell membrane from binding to AGEs outside the cell [51] (Fig. 3.7). Irrespective of sex, the conditions of low esRAGE values and relatively low esRAGE values compared to AGEs are associated with an increased risk of vertebral fractures that are independent of BMD [52]. These findings suggest that AGEs are associated not only with glycation-induced physical changes to bone tissue but also with the pathogenesis of decreased bone quality through the biological effects mediated by RAGE.

These findings indicate that inhibitory factors for bone formation are associated with fracture risk independent of BMD. Under the low bone turnover coupled with low bone formation, hyperglycosylated bone collagen or microfractures may accumulate in the bone matrix. As a result of these metabolic disorders, bone fragility may increase due to deterioration of bone material properties.

3.3.3 Structural Properties of Bone and Bone Fragility

Bone strength of cylindrical bones such as the extremities and femoral neck rises as the external diameter and cortical bone thickness increase. The distal one-third of the radius in men with T2DM is narrower than that in nondiabetic patients [53]. In

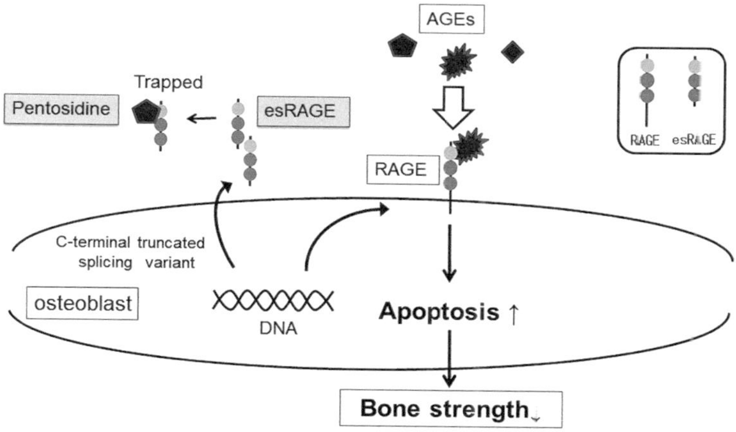

Fig. 3.7 The relationship between advanced glycation end-products (AGEs) and RAGE as well as esRAGE. Splicing variant of receptor for AGEs (RAGE) lacking a membrane-spanning portion is known as endogenous secretory RAGE (esRAGE), which acts as "decoy receptor" inhibiting RAGE on the cell membrane from binding to AGEs outside the cell. *AGEs* advanced glycation end-products, *RAGE* receptor for AGEs, *esRAGE* endogenous secretory RAGE

addition, diabetic patients with higher or equal HbA1c values of 7.5 % have narrower external diameters of the femoral neck and a higher hazard ratio for fractures [54]. Recent progress in diagnostic imaging technology, high-resolution peripheral quantitative computed tomography (HR-pQCT), has shown that T2DM patients with fractures have significantly advanced cortical porosity at the radius as well as the tibia compared to those without fracture [55, 56] and revealed that the bone strength of these patients calculated by bone geometry of the cortical bone is decreased. In addition, trabecular bone score (TBS), which reflects finesses of cancellous bone structure, is significantly lower in T2DM patients with major fractures than that without fracture [57], indicating that exacerbated microarchitecture also affects bone strength. Because diminished bone strength caused by bone morphology is not reflected by BMD, deterioration of structural bone quality is also considered as one of the crucial pathogeneses of increased bone fragility in diabetic patients.

3.4 Diabetic Therapy and Bone Fragility

Achieving favorable control of blood glucose may be effective in preventing fractures through keeping appropriate bone turnover, because improvement of blood glucose recovers decreased marker levels of bone formation [58, 59]. However, some antidiabetic agents have been reported to influence bone turnover negatively. Large-scale surveys indicated that insulin secretagogue and metformin were not associated with the risk of fracture, rather reduce it [60–63]. Several studies showed that patients with insulin therapy have a higher risk of fractures than those with other antidiabetic therapies [19, 60–65], which is considered as an adverse effect of insulin deficiency or poor blood glucose control. Glucose-dependent insulinotropic polypeptide (GIP) [66, 67] and glucagon-like peptide-1 (GLP-1) [68, 69], which are called incretins, have been reported to increase bone mass in genetically modified animals. However, unlike the result from the first meta-analysis among short-term administration of various dipeptidyl peptidase-4 (DPP-4) inhibitors [70], a recent clinical study of long-term outcomes after treatment with certain DPP-4 inhibitors has been reported to show an increased risk of fractures [71]. In addition, results of GLP-1 treatment on increase in BMD in animal studies are inconsistent with those in clinical studies [72]. To date, established conclusion that incretin treatment decreases the risk of fractures in diabetic patients has not been obtained. Treatment with dapagliflozin, one of the sodium-glucose co-transporter 2 (SGLT2) inhibitors, did not significantly decrease BMD compared to that with metformin as control drug during 2 years' administration [73]. In contrast, thiazolidine is known to suppress differentiation of undifferentiated mesenchymal cells into osteoblasts via activation of peroxisome proliferator-activated receptor gamma (PPARγ), and it results in decreasing bone formation. Meta-analyses have shown that the patients treated with thiazolidine have a significantly decreased BMD at lumbar vertebrae or femoral neck, compared with those treated with other hypoglycemic agents, irrespective of sex [74, 75], and that their fracture risk of hip, extremities, and all of osteoporotic fractures is significantly higher than those treated with non-thiazolidine agents [74, 76, 77].

3.4.1 Therapeutic Effect of Osteoporosis Drugs for Diabetic Patients

None of the clinical studies have clarified whether osteoporosis drugs can prevent fractures in diabetic patients. When considering the pathological state of osteoporosis in diabetic patients, bone fragility in patients with diabetes may be rescued by improvement of bone formation or material properties. In the subanalysis of the MORE study, which demonstrated the preventive effect of raloxifene on vertebral fracture in postmenopausal osteoporotic women, the risk of vertebral fracture in the subgroup with diabetes at the baseline is lower than that with the nondiabetic subgroup [78]. When a nondiabetic animal model which experimentally induced pentosidine was treated with raloxifene, bone strength recovers presumably through decreasing bone content of pentosidine [79]; therefore, raloxifene administration to diabetic patients is expected to improve the material properties of the bone matrix and prevent fractures. On the other hand, the risk of fracture in diabetic patients also increases along with decrease in BMD [16]; therefore, agents which are capable of increasing BMD may be useful in preventing fractures. Teriparatide, the only current agent promoting bone formation, decreased bone pentosidine content in addition to increasing BMD in nondiabetic animal model [80]. Teriparatide may be useful as a treatment for osteoporosis in diabetic patients, because of its pleiotropic effects, including recovery of impaired bone turnover in diabetic patients and improvement of bone matrix quality. On the other hand, bisphosphonates, which suppress bone absorption, increase BMD in T2DM patients whose bone turnover decreased, similarly to nondiabetic subjects [81], suggesting that these drugs may particularly possess advantage for preventing fracture in the diabetic patients with decreased BMD.

3.5 Conclusion

Statistical confirmation of increased risk of fracture in patients with diabetes reminds us that diabetes is one of the crucial underlying illnesses for secondary osteoporosis. This increased risk of fracture may be affected by bone extrinsic factor, such as the increased risk of falls associated with diabetic complications or treatment. However, decreased bone quality may be a major cause of bone fragility in diabetic patients, because of the increased risk of atraumatic fractures such as vertebral fractures and the presence of more excessively increased risk of fracture than expected by BMD. The bone fragility observed in diabetic patients is caused by unique pathogenesis in diabetes, suggesting that osteoporosis in diabetic patients may be one of the diabetic complications and that specific diagnostic criteria for this osteoporosis are required. Further researches are needed to develop easy tools for assessment of bone strength of diabetic patients such as bone quality markers closely related to bone fragility.

References

1. Anonymous (1991) Consensus development conference: prophylaxis and treatment of osteoporosis. Am J Med 90(1):107–110
2. Tuominen JT, Impivaara O, Puukka P, Ronnemaa T (1999) Bone mineral density in patients with type 1 and type 2 diabetes. Diabetes Care 22(7):1196–1200
3. Kemink SA, Hermus AR, Swinkels LM, Lutterman JA, Smals AG (2000) Osteopenia in insulin-dependent diabetes mellitus; prevalence and aspects of pathophysiology. J Endocrinol Invest 23(5):295–303
4. Campos Pastor MM, Lopez-Ibarra PJ, Escobar-Jimenez F, Serrano Pardo MD, Garcia-Cervigon AG (2000) Intensive insulin therapy and bone mineral density in type 1 diabetes mellitus: a prospective study. Osteoporos Int 11(5):455–459
5. Lopez-Ibarra PJ, Pastor MM, Escobar-Jimenez F, Pardo MD, Gonzalez AG, Luna JD et al (2001) Bone mineral density at time of clinical diagnosis of adult-onset type 1 diabetes mellitus. Endocr Pract 7(5):346–351
6. Vestergaard P (2007) Discrepancies in bone mineral density and fracture risk in patients with type 1 and type 2 diabetes – a meta-analysis. Osteoporos Int 18(4):427–444
7. Isaia G, Bodrato L, Carlevatto V, Mussetta M, Salamano G, Molinatti GM (1987) Osteoporosis in type II diabetes. Acta Diabetol Lat 24(4):305–310

8. Wakasugi M, Wakao R, Tawata M, Gan N, Koizumi K, Onaya T (1993) Bone mineral density measured by dual energy x-ray absorptiometry in patients with non-insulin-dependent diabetes mellitus. Bone 14(1):29–33
9. Barrett-Connor E, Holbrook TL (1992) Sex differences in osteoporosis in older adults with non-insulin-dependent diabetes mellitus. JAMA 268(23):3333–3337
10. Weinstock RS, Goland RS, Shane E, Clemens TL, Lindsay R, Bilezikian JP (1989) Bone mineral density in women with type II diabetes mellitus. J Bone Miner Res 4(1):97–101
11. van Daele PL, Stolk RP, Burger H, Algra D, Grobbee DE, Hofman A et al (1995) Bone density in non-insulin-dependent diabetes mellitus. The Rotterdam study. Ann Intern Med 122 (6):409–414
12. Schwartz AV, Sellmeyer DE, Ensrud KE, Cauley JA, Tabor HK, Schreiner PJ et al (2001) Older women with diabetes have an increased risk of fracture: a prospective study. J Clin Endocrinol Metab 86(1):32–38
13. Forsen L, Meyer HE, Midthjell K, Edna TH (1999) Diabetes mellitus and the incidence of hip fracture: results from the Nord-Trondelag health survey. Diabetologia 42(8):920–925
14. Nicodemus KK, Folsom AR (2001) Type 1 and type 2 diabetes and incident hip fractures in postmenopausal women. Diabetes Care 24(7):1192–1197
15. Janghorbani M, Van Dam RM, Willett WC, Hu FB (2007) Systematic review of type 1 and type 2 diabetes mellitus and risk of fracture. Am J Epidemiol 166(5):495–505
16. Schwartz AV, Vittinghoff E, Bauer DC, Hillier TA, Strotmeyer ES, Ensrud KE et al (2011) Association of BMD and FRAX score with risk of fracture in older adults with type 2 diabetes. JAMA 305(21):2184–2192. doi:10.1001/jama.2011.715, 305/21/2184 [pii]
17. Weber G, Beccaria L, de'Angelis M, Mora S, Galli L, Cazzuffi MA et al (1990) Bone mass in young patients with type I diabetes. Bone Miner 8(1):23–30
18. Nelson DA, Jacober SJ (2001) Why do older women with diabetes have an increased fracture risk? J Clin Endocrinol Metab 86(1):29–31
19. Ivers RQ, Cumming RG, Mitchell P, Peduto AJ (2001) Diabetes and risk of fracture: the blue mountains eye study. Diabetes Care 24(7):1198–1203
20. Patel S, Hyer S, Tweed K, Kerry S, Allan K, Rodin A et al (2008) Risk factors for fractures and falls in older women with type 2 diabetes mellitus. Calcif Tissue Int 82(2):87–91
21. Schwartz AV, Vittinghoff E, Sellmeyer DE, Feingold KR, de Rekeneire N, Strotmeyer ES et al (2008) Diabetes-related complications, glycemic control, and falls in older adults. Diabetes Care 31(3):391–396. doi:10.2337/dc07-1152, doi:dc07-1152 [pii]
22. Bonds DE, Larson JC, Schwartz AV, Strotmeyer ES, Robbins J, Rodriguez BL et al (2006) Risk of fracture in women with type 2 diabetes: the women's health initiative observational study. J Clin Endocrinol Metab 91(9):3404–3410
23. Yamamoto M, Yamaguchi T, Yamauchi M, Kaji H, Sugimoto T (2009) Diabetic patients have an increased risk of vertebral fractures independent of BMD or diabetic complications. J Bone Miner Res 24(4):702–709. doi:10.1359/jbmr.081207
24. Yamamoto M, Yamaguchi T, Yamauchi M, Kaji H, Sugimoto T (2007) Bone mineral density is not sensitive enough to assess the risk of vertebral fractures in type 2 diabetic women. Calcif Tissue Int 80(6):353–358
25. Zhukouskaya VV, Eller-Vainicher C, Vadzianava VV, Shepelkevich AP, Zhurava IV, Korolenko GG et al (2013) Prevalence of morphometric vertebral fractures in patients with type 1 diabetes. Diabetes Care. doi:10.2337/dc12-1355
26. Anonymous (2001) Osteoporosis prevention, diagnosis, and therapy. JAMA 285(6):785–795
27. Saito M, Fujii K, Mori Y, Marumo K (2006) Role of collagen enzymatic and glycation induced cross-links as a determinant of bone quality in spontaneously diabetic WBN/Kob rats. Osteoporos Int 17(10):1514–1523
28. Saito M, Marumo K (2013) Bone quality in diabetes. Front Endocrinol 4:72. doi:10.3389/fendo.2013.00072
29. Saito M, Fujii K, Soshi S, Tanaka T (2006) Reductions in degree of mineralization and enzymatic collagen cross-links and increases in glycation-induced pentosidine in the femoral neck cortex in cases of femoral neck fracture. Osteoporos Int 17(7):986–995

30. Saito M, Fujii K, Marumo K (2006) Degree of mineralization-related collagen crosslinking in the femoral neck cancellous bone in cases of hip fracture and controls. Calcif Tissue Int 79 (3):160–168. doi:10.1007/s00223-006-0035-1
31. Odetti P, Rossi S, Monacelli F, Poggi A, Cirnigliaro M, Federici M et al (2005) Advanced glycation end products and bone loss during aging. Ann N Y Acad Sci 1043:710–717
32. Yamamoto M, Yamaguchi T, Yamauchi M, Yano S, Sugimoto T (2008) Serum pentosidine levels are positively associated with the presence of vertebral fractures in postmenopausal women with type 2 diabetes. J Clin Endocrinol Metab 93(3):1013–1019
33. Schwartz AV, Garnero P, Hillier TA, Sellmeyer DE, Strotmeyer ES, Feingold KR et al (2009) Pentosidine and increased fracture risk in older adults with type 2 diabetes. J Clin Endocrinol Metab 94(7):2380–2386
34. Hansma P, Yu H, Schultz D, Rodriguez A, Yurtsev EA, Orr J et al (2009) The tissue diagnostic instrument. Rev Sci Instrum 80(5):054303. doi:10.1063/1.3127602
35. Farr JN, Drake MT, Amin S, Melton LJ 3rd, McCready LK, Khosla S (2014) In vivo assessment of bone quality in postmenopausal women with type 2 diabetes. J Bone Miner Res 29(4):787–795. doi:10.1002/jbmr.2106
36. Yamamoto M, Yamaguchi T, Nawata K, Yamauchi M, Sugimoto T (2012) Decreased PTH levels accompanied by low bone formation are associated with vertebral fractures in postmenopausal women with type 2 diabetes. J Clin Endocrinol Metab 97(4):1277–1284. doi:10.1210/jc.2011-2537
37. Dobnig H, Piswanger-Solkner JC, Roth M, Obermayer-Pietsch B, Tiran A, Strele A et al (2006) Type 2 diabetes mellitus in nursing home patients: effects on bone turnover, bone mass, and fracture risk. J Clin Endocrinol Metab 91(9):3355–3363. doi:10.1210/jc.2006-0460, doi:jc.2006-0460 [pii]
38. Kanazawa I, Yamaguchi T, Yamamoto M, Yamauchi M, Yano S, Sugimoto T (2009) Serum osteocalcin/bone-specific alkaline phosphatase ratio is a predictor for the presence of vertebral fractures in men with type 2 diabetes. Calcif Tissue Int 85(3):228–234. doi:10.1007/s00223-009-9272-4
39. Zhang M, Xuan S, Bouxsein ML, von Stechow D, Akeno N, Faugere MC et al (2002) Osteoblast-specific knockout of the insulin-like growth factor (IGF) receptor gene reveals an essential role of IGF signaling in bone matrix mineralization. J Biol Chem 277 (46):44005–44012. doi:10.1074/jbc.M208265200
40. Mohan S (1993) Insulin-like growth factor binding proteins in bone cell regulation. Growth Regul 3(1):67–70
41. Chen J, Wu A, Sun H, Drakas R, Garofalo C, Cascio S et al (2005) Functional significance of type 1 insulin-like growth factor-mediated nuclear translocation of the insulin receptor substrate-1 and beta-catenin. J Biol Chem 280(33):29912–29920. doi:10.1074/jbc.M504516200
42. Ardawi MS, Akhbar DH, Alshaikh A, Ahmed MM, Qari MH, Rouzi AA et al (2013) Increased serum sclerostin and decreased serum IGF-1 are associated with vertebral fractures among postmenopausal women with type-2 diabetes. Bone 56(2):355–362. doi:10.1016/j.bone.2013.06.029
43. Kanazawa I, Yamaguchi T, Sugimoto T (2011) Serum insulin-like growth factor-I is a marker for assessing the severity of vertebral fractures in postmenopausal women with type 2 diabetes mellitus. Osteoporos Int 22(4):1191–1198. doi:10.1007/s00198-010-1310-6
44. Yamamoto M, Yamauchi M, Sugimoto T (2013) Elevated sclerostin levels are associated with vertebral fractures in patients with type 2 diabetes mellitus. J Clin Endocrinol Metab 98 (10):4030–4037. doi:10.1210/jc.2013-2143
45. Kislinger T, Fu C, Huber B, Qu W, Taguchi A, Du Yan S et al (1999) N(epsilon)-(carboxymethyl)lysine adducts of proteins are ligands for receptor for advanced glycation end products that activate cell signaling pathways and modulate gene expression. J Biol Chem 274(44):31740–31749

46. Yamamoto Y, Kato I, Doi T, Yonekura H, Ohashi S, Takeuchi M et al (2001) Development and prevention of advanced diabetic nephropathy in RAGE-overexpressing mice. J Clin Invest 108(2):261–268
47. Ogawa N, Yamaguchi T, Yano S, Yamauchi M, Yamamoto M, Sugimoto T (2007) The combination of high glucose and advanced glycation end-products (AGEs) inhibits the mineralization of osteoblastic MC3T3-E1 cells through glucose-induced increase in the receptor for AGEs. Horm Metab Res 39(12):871–875
48. Okazaki K, Yamaguchi T, Tanaka K, Notsu M, Ogawa N, Yano S et al (2012) Advanced Glycation End Products (AGEs), but not high glucose, inhibit the osteoblastic differentiation of mouse stromal ST2 cells through the suppression of osterix expression, and inhibit cell growth and increasing cell apoptosis. Calcif Tissue Int 91(4):286–296. doi:10.1007/s00223-012-9641-2
49. Notsu M, Yamaguchi T, Okazaki K, Tanaka K, Ogawa N, Kanazawa I et al (2014) Advanced glycation end product 3 (AGE3) suppresses the mineralization of mouse stromal ST2 cells and human mesenchymal stem cells by increasing TGF-beta expression and secretion. Endocrinology 155(7):2402–2410. doi:10.1210/en.2013-1818
50. Ding KH, Wang ZZ, Hamrick MW, Deng ZB, Zhou L, Kang B et al (2006) Disordered osteoclast formation in RAGE-deficient mouse establishes an essential role for RAGE in diabetes related bone loss. Biochem Biophys Res Commun 340(4):1091–1097
51. Yonekura H, Yamamoto Y, Sakurai S, Petrova RG, Abedin MJ, Li H et al (2003) Novel splice variants of the receptor for advanced glycation end-products expressed in human vascular endothelial cells and pericytes, and their putative roles in diabetes-induced vascular injury. Biochem J 370(Pt 3):1097–1109
52. Yamamoto M, Yamaguchi T, Yamauchi M, Sugimoto T (2009) Low serum level of the endogenous secretory receptor for advanced glycation end products (esRAGE) is a risk factor for prevalent vertebral fractures independent of bone mineral density in patients with type 2 diabetes. Diabetes Care 32(12):2263–2268. doi:10.2337/dc09-0901, doi:dc09-0901 [pii]
53. Petit MA, Paudel ML, Taylor BC, Hughes JM, Strotmeyer ES, Schwartz AV et al (2010) Bone mass and strength in older men with type 2 diabetes: the osteoporotic fractures in men study. J Bone Miner Res 25(2):285–291. doi:10.1359/jbmr.090725
54. Oei L, Zillikens MC, Dehghan A, Buitendijk GH, Castano-Betancourt MC, Estrada K et al (2013) High bone mineral density and fracture risk in type 2 diabetes as skeletal complications of inadequate glucose control: the Rotterdam study. Diabetes Care 36 (6):1619–1628. doi:10.2337/dc12-1188
55. Burghardt AJ, Issever AS, Schwartz AV, Davis KA, Masharani U, Majumdar S et al (2010) High-resolution peripheral quantitative computed tomographic imaging of cortical and trabecular bone microarchitecture in patients with type 2 diabetes mellitus. J Clin Endocrinol Metab 95(11):5045–5055. doi:10.1210/jc.2010-0226, doi:jc.2010-0226 [pii]
56. Patsch JM, Burghardt AJ, Yap SP, Baum T, Schwartz AV, Joseph GB et al (2013) Increased cortical porosity in type 2 diabetic postmenopausal women with fragility fractures. J Bone Miner Res 28(2):313–324. doi:10.1002/jbmr.1763
57. Leslie WD, Aubry-Rozier B, Lamy O, Hans D, Manitoba Bone Density P (2013) TBS (trabecular bone score) and diabetes-related fracture risk. J Clin Endocrinol Metab 98 (2):602–609. doi:10.1210/jc.2012-3118
58. Okazaki R, Totsuka Y, Hamano K, Ajima M, Miura M, Hirota Y et al (1997) Metabolic improvement of poorly controlled noninsulin-dependent diabetes mellitus decreases bone turnover. J Clin Endocrinol Metab 82(9):2915–2920
59. Kanazawa I, Yamaguchi T, Yamauchi M, Yamamoto M, Kurioka S, Yano S et al (2009) Adiponectin is associated with changes in bone markers during glycemic control in type 2 diabetes mellitus. J Clin Endocrinol Metab 94(8):3031–3037. doi:10.1210/jc.2008-2187, doi:jc.2008-2187 [pii]
60. Vestergaard P, Rejnmark L, Mosekilde L (2005) Relative fracture risk in patients with diabetes mellitus, and the impact of insulin and oral antidiabetic medication on relative fracture risk. Diabetologia 48(7):1292–1299

61. Monami M, Cresci B, Colombini A, Pala L, Balzi D, Gori F et al (2008) Bone fractures and hypoglycemic treatment in type 2 diabetic patients: a case-control study. Diabetes Care 31 (2):199–203. doi:10.2337/dc07-1736, doi:dc07-1736 [pii]
62. Melton LJ 3rd, Leibson CL, Achenbach SJ, Therneau TM, Khosla S (2008) Fracture risk in type 2 diabetes: update of a population-based study. J Bone Miner Res 23(8):1334–1342. doi:10.1359/jbmr.080323
63. Kanazawa I, Yamaguchi T, Yamamoto M, Sugimoto T (2010) Relationship between treatments with insulin and oral hypoglycemic agents versus the presence of vertebral fractures in type 2 diabetes mellitus. J Bone Miner Metab 28(5):554–560. doi:10.1007/s00774-010-0160-9
64. Kim JH, Jung MH, Lee JM, Son HS, Cha BY, Chang SA (2012) Diabetic peripheral neuropathy is highly associated with nontraumatic fractures in Korean patients with type 2 diabetes mellitus. Clin Endocrinol (Oxf) 77(1):51–55. doi:10.1111/j.1365-2265.2011.04222.x
65. Napoli N, Strotmeyer ES, Ensrud KE, Sellmeyer DE, Bauer DC, Hoffman AR et al (2014) Fracture risk in diabetic elderly men: the MrOS study. Diabetologia. doi:10.1007/s00125-014-3289-6
66. Xie D, Cheng H, Hamrick M, Zhong Q, Ding KH, Correa D et al (2005) Glucose-dependent insulinotropic polypeptide receptor knockout mice have altered bone turnover. Bone 37 (6):759–769. doi:10.1016/j.bone.2005.06.021
67. Tsukiyama K, Yamada Y, Yamada C, Harada N, Kawasaki Y, Ogura M et al (2006) Gastric inhibitory polypeptide as an endogenous factor promoting new bone formation after food ingestion. Mol Endocrinol 20(7):1644–1651. doi:10.1210/me.2005-0187
68. Yamada C, Yamada Y, Tsukiyama K, Yamada K, Udagawa N, Takahashi N et al (2008) The murine glucagon-like peptide-1 receptor is essential for control of bone resorption. Endocrinology 149(2):574–579. doi:10.1210/en.2007-1292
69. Nuche-Berenguer B, Moreno P, Portal-Nunez S, Dapia S, Esbrit P, Villanueva-Penacarrillo ML (2010) Exendin-4 exerts osteogenic actions in insulin-resistant and type 2 diabetic states. Regul Pept 159(1–3):61–66. doi:10.1016/j.regpep.2009.06.010, doi:S0167-0115(09)00148-7 [pii]
70. Monami M, Dicembrini I, Antenore A, Mannucci E (2011) Dipeptidyl peptidase-4 inhibitors and bone fractures: a meta-analysis of randomized clinical trials. Diabetes Care 34 (11):2474–2476. doi:10.2337/dc11-1099
71. Hirshberg B, Parker A, Edelberg H, Donovan M, Iqbal N (2014) Safety of saxagliptin: events of special interest in 9156 patients with type 2 diabetes mellitus. Diabetes Metab Res Rev 30 (7):556–569. doi:10.1002/dmrr.2502
72. Mabilleau G, Mieczkowska A, Chappard D (2014) Use of glucagon-like peptide-1 receptor agonists and bone fractures: a meta-analysis of randomized clinical trials. J Diabetes 6 (3):260–266. doi:10.1111/1753-0407.12102
73. Bolinder J, Ljunggren O, Johansson L, Wilding J, Langkilde AM, Sjostrom CD et al (2013) Dapagliflozin maintains glycaemic control while reducing weight and body fat mass over 2 years in patients with type 2 diabetes mellitus inadequately controlled on metformin. Diabetes Obes Metab. doi:10.1111/dom.12189
74. Loke YK, Singh S, Furberg CD (2009) Long-term use of thiazolidinediones and fractures in type 2 diabetes: a meta-analysis. CMAJ 180(1):32–39. doi:10.1503/cmaj.080486, doi: cmaj.080486 [pii]
75. Yaturu S, Bryant B, Jain SK (2007) Thiazolidinedione treatment decreases bone mineral density in type 2 diabetic men. Diabetes Care 30(6):1574–1576
76. Colhoun HM, Livingstone SJ, Looker HC, Morris AD, Wild SH, Lindsay RS et al (2012) Hospitalised hip fracture risk with rosiglitazone and pioglitazone use compared with other glucose-lowering drugs. Diabetologia 55(11):2929–2937. doi:10.1007/s00125-012-2668-0
77. Bazelier MT, de Vries F, Vestergaard P, Herings RM, Gallagher AM, Leufkens HG et al (2013) Risk of fracture with thiazolidinediones: an individual patient data meta-analysis. Front Endocrinol 4:11. doi:10.3389/fendo.2013.00011

78. Johnell O, Kanis JA, Black DM, Balogh A, Poor G, Sarkar S et al (2004) Associations between baseline risk factors and vertebral fracture risk in the Multiple Outcomes of Raloxifene Evaluation (MORE) study. J Bone Miner Res 19(5):764–772. doi:10.1359/JBMR.040211
79. Saito M, Marumo K, Soshi S, Kida Y, Ushiku C, Shinohara A (2010) Raloxifene ameliorates detrimental enzymatic and nonenzymatic collagen cross-links and bone strength in rabbits with hyperhomocysteinemia. Osteoporos Int 21(4):655–666. doi:10.1007/s00198-009-0980-4
80. Saito M, Marumo K, Kida Y, Ushiku C, Kato S, Takao-Kawabata R et al (2011) Changes in the contents of enzymatic immature, mature, and non-enzymatic senescent cross-links of collagen after once-weekly treatment with human parathyroid hormone (1–34) for 18 months contribute to improvement of bone strength in ovariectomized monkeys. Osteoporos Int 22 (8):2373–2383. doi:10.1007/s00198-010-1454-4
81. Keegan TH, Schwartz AV, Bauer DC, Sellmeyer DE, Kelsey JL (2004) Effect of alendronate on bone mineral density and biochemical markers of bone turnover in type 2 diabetic women: the fracture intervention trial. Diabetes Care 27(7):1547–1553

Chapter 4
Mechanism for the Development of Bone Disease in Diabetes: Abnormal Glucose Metabolism

Ryo Okazaki and Daisuke Inoue

Abstract Osteoporosis is now generally considered as a complication of diabetes mellitus (DM). Higher HbA1c level and presence of diabetic vascular complications and insulin use are associated with higher risk of fractures, indicating detrimental effects of chronic hyperglycemia on bone. Because bone mineral density does not seem to be affected by glycemic control, this chapter reviews the influence of abnormal glucose metabolism on bone and diabetes-associated factors causing impaired bone strength mainly from clinical studies. Results of human histomorphometrical studies and longitudinal metabolic bone marker studies indicate that bone turnover may not be generally suppressed in DM. With hyperglycemia bone resorption seems to be stimulated, whereas bone formation may be suppressed. Vitamin D deficiency is common in DM, which may or may not be associated with secondary hyperparathyroidism, could not account for such changes in bone turnover. Animal and in vitro studies support this concept. Hyperglycemia per se or via the accumulation of advanced glycation end products (AGEs) appears to stimulate osteoclasts while suppressing osteoblasts, and perhaps mesenchymal stem cells as well as osteocytes. AGE accumulation in bone matrix also compromises mechanical strength. More clinical longitudinal studies would be needed to further elucidate the influence of hyperglycemia in the development of osteoporosis associated with DM.

Keywords Glycemic control • Bone turnover • Metabolic bone markers • Vitamin D • Advanced glycation end products

R. Okazaki (✉) • D. Inoue
Third Department of Medicine, Teikyo University Chiba Medical Center, Anesaki 3426-3, Ichihara, Chiba 299-0111, Japan
e-mail: rokazaki@med.teikyo-u.ac.jp

M. Inaba (ed.), *Musculoskeletal Disease Associated with Diabetes Mellitus*,
DOI 10.1007/978-4-431-55720-3_4

4.1 Mechanism for the Development of Bone Disease in Diabetes: Abnormal Glucose Metabolism

Osteoporosis is a common complication both in type 1 and type 2 DM. As with other diabetic complications, exact mechanisms that result in bone fragility in diabetes are not yet known. In type 1 DM, BMD is low, whereas in type 2DM, BMD is high compared with nondiabetic controls [1]. Thus, between type 1 and type 2 DM, there are some different mechanisms leading to bone fragility. However, both types of DM are associated with high risk of fractures, higher than that estimated from BMD values. This suggests that chronic hyperglycemia per se and resultant glycosuria and various other metabolic changes contribute to bone fragility independent of BMD in DM. This chapter reviews the influence of abnormal glucose metabolism on bone and diabetes-associated factors causing impaired bone strength mainly from clinical studies.

4.2 Influence of Glycemic Control on Bone and Fracture

It is now established that good glycemic control is the key to prevent major diabetic microvascular and macrovascular complications. However, it took a long time for this concept to be established. The importance of good glycemic control was generally accepted only in 1990s after publications from DCCT trial for type 1 diabetes [2] and UKPDS trial for type 2 diabetes [3]. As for diabetic bone complication, however, influence of glycemic control has not yet been well established. Until around 2000, fracture had not been generally accepted as a complication of type 2 DM, as most of the patients have higher BMD than nondiabetic control subjects. Thus, there are very few longitudinal clinical studies on the impact of glycemic control on fracture incidence, BMD, or other bone-related surrogate markers.

4.2.1 Glycemic Control and Fracture Risk

With regard to the relationship between HbA1c and fracture risk, the first large-scale longitudinal study is the Rotterdam study in the Netherlands [4]. In the study, 4,135 participants, of which 420 were diabetics, were followed up to 12.2 years for the occurrence of clinical fracture. The 420 diabetics were subdivided into two groups by HbA1c levels at baseline: 203 subjects with HbA1c less than 7.5 % and 217 subjects with HbA1c $\geq$7.5 %. The latter poorly controlled diabetic subjects at the baseline had higher risk of fracture compared with nondiabetic subjects (HR (hazard ratio) 1.47 [1.12–1.92]) and diabetic subjects with HbA1c $<$7.5 % at the baseline (HR 1.62 [1.09–2.40]). Better-controlled diabetics at the baseline had similar fracture risk with nondiabetics (HR 0.91 [0.67–1.23]). Recently another large-scale retrospective cohort study came out from Taiwan, in which 20,025 type 2 DM subjects over age 65 were followed up for the incidence of hip fracture over an average of 7.4 years and the relationship with the basal HbA1c was analyzed [5]. The authors found significantly higher risk of hip fracture among patients with basal HbA1c 9.0 % or more compared with patients with HbA1c level 6–7 % [5]. These results clearly indicate that poor glycemic control at one time point had deleterious effects on bone in the long term afterward. On the other hand, ACCORD trial, the only prospective randomized study that examined the effects of tight glycemic control on fracture and fall, failed to demonstrate any differences in either event between two groups (median achieved HbA1c 7.5 % vs 6.4 %) [6]. Several explanations are possible for the lack of glycemic control effects on bone in the ACCORD trial. All the ACCORD participants had baseline HbA1c more than 7.5 %, meaning they were all poorly controlled diabetics at the baseline by the criteria in the Rotterdam study. Because the follow-up period was short with only 3.8 years, effects of better glycemic control thereafter could not have been observed. In the ACCORD trial, it is of note that strictly controlled group had significantly higher incidence of hypoglycemia but that this was not associated with higher incidence of fall.

Cross-sectional studies that evaluated the relationship between glycemic control and fracture risk in type 2 DM found conflicting results. An Australian study found that fasting blood glucose level more than 7 mmol/L, diabetes duration more than 10 years, insulin treatment, and the presence of retinopathy were associated with higher fracture risk [7]. A study at the Mayo Clinic [8] did not find any relationship between fracture risk and baseline fasting plasma glucose, but they did find that presence of neuropathy and insulin use was associated with higher fracture risk. Neither study evaluated HbA1c, a better index of glycemic control than blood glucose level. A large Norwegian population study [9] did not find the association between HbA1c >9.5 % and fracture, but did find the association with disease duration >5 years and insulin use. A study in Japanese type 2 diabetic men found that HbA1c >9.0 % and higher BMD were associated with higher risk of prevalent vertebral fracture [10]. An American study of older people found higher fracture risk in DM but not in subjects with impaired fasting glucose, but the authors did not find significant difference in HbA1c level between diabetes patients with and without fractures [11].

In type 1 diabetes, there are even fewer studies looking at the relationship between fracture risk and glycemic control. An observational cross-sectional study demonstrated long-term high HbA1c is associated with higher fracture rate in T1DM [12].

Thus, there are not so many studies looking at the relationship between fracture risk and the glycemic indices such as HbA1c. But relationship between other indications of chronic hyperglycemia and fracture risk have been explored. Many studies have shown that the presence of microvascular complications is associated with fractures [13]. And insulin-use was associated with higher fracture risk in most

[14, 15], but not all [16], studies. All those results indicate that chronic hyperglycemia is a fracture risk.

4.3 Bone Turnover, Metabolic Bone Markers, and Glycemic Control

Bone turnover rate and metabolic bone markers that reflect bone turnover are considered to be a determinant of bone quality in postmenopausal women. Whether the same applies to diabetic subjects is currently unknown. Here again not many studies have looked at their relationship with glycemic control. In many reviews, bone turnover in diabetes, both in type 1 and type 2, has been described low. However, this is mainly based on animal data and cross-sectional studies in human diabetics.

4.3.1 Bone Histomorphometry

Dynamic bone histomorphometry has been accepted as the most authentic method to evaluate bone turnover state. Virtually all type 1 animal models, mostly streptozotocin-induced diabetes in rats or mice, have been reported to have low bone turnover, with decreases in both bone formation and bone resorption parameters [17]. The first histomorphometric study in human type 1 diabetes analyzed only two patients with T1DM together with six T2DM subjects [18]. They reported somewhat decreased bone formation in both types of diabetic patients combined without any changes in bone resorption parameters. However, the only other histomorphometric study in human type 1 diabetes failed to demonstrate any differences in static or dynamic parameters in bone formation or resorption in 18 subjects with T1DM [19] compared with age- and sex-matched controls.

As for human T2DM, only two studies are available for bone histomorphometry [18, 20]. As stated before, Krakauer et al. [18] reported decreased bone formation parameters without changes in bone resorption parameters in eight diabetic patients including six T2DM subjects. Manavalan et al. [20] demonstrated in four T2DM patients that bone formation parameters including bone formation rate, osteoblast surface, mineralizing surface, and osteoid surface are decreased, but none of the resorption parameters, such as eroded surface, adjusted apposition rate, or osteoclast number, were not different from control subjects. Bone characteristics in rodent T2DM models have recently been reviewed [17]. Like human T2DM, most rodent models of T2DM showed decreased bone formation rate [17]. However, bone resorption parameters, notably eroded surface, are increased in most [21–23] but not all [24] rodent models of T2DM.

4.3.2 Metabolic Bone Markers

Many cross-sectional studies have compared the metabolic bone markers between diabetics and controls. Meta-analysis of these results was recently published [25]. They found modest but significant decreases in serum osteocalcin (OC) and C-terminal cross-linked telopeptide (CTX) levels in diabetes but did not find significant differences in any of the other markers including bone formation markers – alkaline phosphatase (ALP), bone-specific alkaline phosphatase (BALP), and procollagen type 1 N-terminal propeptide (P1NP) – or bone resorption markers: urinary N-terminal cross-linked telopeptide of type-I collagen (NTX) and deoxypyridinoline (DPD). It is of note that ALP and NTX levels tended to be higher in diabetics. The meta-analysis also noted high heterogeneity in all the markers. The authors concluded that this heterogeneity may not be caused by glucose per se but be modulated by unknown other factors. Those results suggest that influence of glucose on metabolic bone markers would be better analyzed in longitudinal studies. There are fewer longitudinal studies that have explored the effects of glycemic control on metabolic bone markers in type 2 diabetes. Their results are summarized in Table 4.1.

In 1997, we did the first such study using specific bone markers including urinary DPD, CTX, BALP, as well as OC. Prior to our study, there had been a few longitudinal studies, but they either had not assessed bone resorption markers [26] or used urinary hydroxyproline, a nonspecific collagen degradation product as a bone resorption marker [27, 28]. All three studies [26–28] used OC as a sole bone formation marker and reported conflicting results.

Gregorio et al. [27] reported that in 50 poorly controlled T2DM (basal HbA1c 11.6 %), insulin or oral agents available at that period resulted in a decrease in fasting blood glucose level from around 250 to 130 mg/dl in a month and the improved glycemic control was maintained up to 12 months (HbA1c levels were not reported except at the baseline). This was associated with time-dependent decreases in both OC and HYP. They also reported time-dependent decreases in PTH and urinary Ca along with amelioration of hyperglycosuria. They suggested that osmotic hypercalciuria triggers PTH secretion, which results in high bone turnover state in poorly controlled T2DM, and that glycemic control decreases bone turnover dependent on PTH. Nagasaka et al. [26] also found that glycemic control decreased urinary Ca and PTH, but they reported serum OC was increased rather than decreased. Interestingly they reported total ALP was decreased after glycemic control. They did not assess bone resorption markers. Increase in OC after glycemic control was also reported by Sayinalp et al. [28].

Our study [29] was the first to demonstrate that bone resorption markers, urinary DPD, and urinary CTX were decreased with glycemic control. We found that BALP and ALP were decreased but that OC was increased. Similar to previous studies, glycemic control was associated with a decrease in uCa excretion, but contrary to previous studies, we did not see any change in PTH. We concluded that

Table 4.1 Changes in metabolic bone markers in response to glycemic control

Study, year [ref]	N	Sex	Duration	Design	Intervention	HbA1c, %		Metabolic bone markers						PTH	25(OH)D	IGF-1	Others
		M/F				Baseline	End	CTX	NTX	DPD	BAP	P1NP	OC				
Gregorio, 1994 [27]	50	24/26	12 months	OBS	Various	11.6	NR						↓	↓			Hyp↓ uCa↓
Nagasaka, 1995 [26]	28	13/15	38 days	OBS	Various	11.1	9.3				↓ALP		↑	↓			uCa↓1,25D→
Sayinalp, 1995 [28]	16	NR	NR	OBS	Various	9.8	7.8						↑				Hyp →
Okazaki, 1997 [29]	78	27/49	3 weeks	OBS	Various	9.9	8.7	↓		↓	↓		↑	→			uCa↓1,25D→
Rosato, 1998 [30]	20	12/8	2 months	OBS	Various	10.0	8.1			↑			↑	→	→	↑	PYD↑
Okazaki, 1999 [95]	33	16/17	1 month	OBS	Tro	8.4	8.4	↓		↓	↓		→				
Watanabe, 2003 [96]	25	11/14	1 month	OBS	Tro	8.4	7.6		↓		↓						
			12 months				7.5		→		→						
Capoglu, 2008 [31]	35	17/18	12 months	OBS	Met ± SU	10.6	7.7			↓	↓		↓	→	→		
Kanazawa, 2009 [97]	50	31/19	1 month	OBS	Various	10.0	8.8		→		↓		↑				
Kanazawa, 2011 [32]	50	28/22	6 months	OBS	Various	7.6	6.9		→		↑		→				
Zinman, 2010 [38]	250	F	12 months	RCT	Rosi	7.4	~6.8	↑			↓	↓		↓	↓		E2 ↓
	299	M			Rosi			→			↓	↓		↓	↑		E2 →
	225	F			Met	7.3		→			↓	↓		↓	→		E2 →
	326	M			Met			↓			↓	↓		↓	↓		E2 →
	214	F			Glyburide	7.4		↓			↓	↓		→	↑		E2 →
	291	M			Glyburide			↓			↓	→		→	↓		E2 →

Borges, 2011 [36]	87	43/44	80 weeks	RCT	Met + Rosi	8.6	6.8	↓			↓	↓		→	→		
	87	38/49			Met	8.6	6.6	↓			↓	↓		→	→		
Bilezikian, 2013 [37]	111	F	52 weeks	RCT	Rosi	6.8	6.4	↑			↓	↑		↓	↓	→	
	110	F			Met	6.8	6.3	↓			↓	↓		↓	↓	→	
van Lierop, 2012 [38]	37	M	24 weeks	RCT	Met	7.0	6.3	↓				↓					Scl →
	34	M			Pio	7.1	6.5	↑				→					Scl ↑

OBS observational study, *RCT* randomized control study, *NR* not reported, *Tro* troglitazone, *Met* metformin, *Rosi* rosiglitazone, *CTX* C-terminal cross-linked telopeptide, *NTX* N-terminal cross-linked telopeptide of type-I collagen, *DPD* deoxypyridinoline, *BAP* bone-specific alkaline phosphatase, *ALP* alkaline phosphatase, *P1NP* procollagen type 1 N-terminal propeptide, *OC* Osteocalcin, *Hyp* hydroxyproline, *uCa* urinary Calcium, *1,25D* 1,25(OH)2D, *PYD* pyridinoline, *E2* estradiol, *Scl* sclerostin poor glycemic control in T2DM is associated with increased bone resorption independent of PTH, which would be normalized after short-term glycemic control.

In contrast to our study, Rosato et al. [30] reported that in 20 T2DM patients, glycemic control over a 2-month period (mean HbA1c level, from 10.0 % to 8.1 %) with insulin or various oral hypoglycemic agents (OHA) was associated with significant increase not only in OC but also in uDPD and uPYD. Although details of OHA they used were not described, the use of thiazolidinediones (TZDs) seems unlikely as they were not clinically available at the time. Then this is the only study demonstrating increase in resorption markers after glycemic control with non-TZDs. It is of note that compared with nondiabetic controls, T2DM patients' baseline OC was lower, whereas urinary DPD and PYD were not different. In this study, serum 25(OH)D and PTH did not change significantly, but there was a significant increase in serum IGF-1 level.

The results reported by Capoglu et al. [31] were similar to ours except osteocalcin. They reported that in 35 T2DM patients' urinary DPD and NTX, osteocalcin and BALP were all decreased in the course of 1 year, associated with an improvement in glycemic control from HbA1c level 10.6–7.7 % with metformin and/or sulfonylureas [31]. PTH and 25(OH)D did not change. Kanazawa et al. [32] reported a small but significant increase in BAP after improvement of glycemic control over 6 months, but it is of note that in this study change in HbA1c was positively associated with the change in BAP. On the other hand, OC and NTX did not significantly change, but their changes were negatively associated with the change in HbA1c.

After it became evident that TZDs increase fracture risk, several randomized control studies (RCTs) examined metabolic bone markers in response to TZDs compared with metformin or SUs. The largest RCT is the post hoc analysis of A Diabetes Outcome Progression Trial (ADOPT), in which the effects of rosiglitazone, metformin, and glyburide monotherapy were compared [33–35]. Zinman et al. [33] measured CTX, BALP, and P1NP at the baseline and after 1 year in more than 500 subjects in each monotherapy group. As shown in Table 4.1, all the bone markers were decreased or stable except in female rosiglitazone group showing an increase in CTX. PTH was decreased in rosiglitazone and metformin group but was stable with glyburide. In this post hoc analysis, HbA1c levels were not presented, but in the parental study, basal HbA1c levels were around 7.4 %, which were decreased around 6.8 % after a year [34]. Borges et al. [36] did a RCT comparing effects of rosiglitazone plus metformin versus metformin alone for 80 weeks. Both treatments were associated with decreases in CTX, P1NP, and BALP with improvement in glycemic control with HbA1c level from 8.6 % to around 6.8 %. Another RCT comparing effects of rosiglitazone against metformin reported that similar small improvement in glycemic control (HbA1c 6.8–6.3 %) was associated with decreases in CTX, P1NP, and BALP in metformin but that in rosiglitazone group increases in CTX and P1NP and a decrease in BALP [37]. Finally van Lierop et al. compared the effects of pioglitazone against metformin [38] and reported that 6 months treatment with metformin decreased both CTX and P1NP, whereas pioglitazone increased CTX and had no effect on P1NP.

To summarize all the results, bone resorption markers were decreased in the course of glycemic control with most treatment modalities except TZDs. Among bone formation markers, BALP was also decreased whereas OC was increased at least in some studies. BALP decrease after glycemic control was suggested to be caused by improvement of vitamin D status, but in two studies [33, 37] BALP was decreased despite the decrease in serum 25(OH)D level. P1NP may be also decreased with glycemic control. OC increase after glycemic control may be associated with direct insulin action on osteoblasts, as will be dealt in another chapter.

4.4 Hyperglycemia and Calcium-Regulating Hormones

Bone turnover is controlled by many systemic and local factors. Among the systemic factors, conventional calcium-regulating hormones, PTH and vitamin D, have been studied in relationship with glycemic control. There are little data on other hormones such as sex steroids in the context of bone abnormalities in diabetics.

4.4.1 PTH in Diabetes

It has been often noted that PTH is low in diabetes, especially when associated with overt renal insufficiency [29, 39–43]. However, a recent meta-analysis of PTH level in both type 1 and 2 diabetics revealed no differences compared with nondiabetics [25]. Uncontrolled diabetes with overt glycosuria causes hypercalciuria by osmotic diuresis. Such renal calcium loss would trigger PTH secretion in normal subjects. However, results from longitudinal studies are mixed even at the baseline. Some studies reported high PTH in uncontrolled diabetic state [27, 31], but others reported relatively low PTH despite overt hypercalciuria [26, 29]. PTH responses to the improvement in glycemic control are also variable: decrease, no change, and even increase have been reported (Table 4.1).

The causes of such variations in PTH secretions in diabetics are unknown. As will be discussed later, vitamin D deficiency is common in diabetics, which would stimulate PTH secretion. However, basal serum 25(OH)D levels in those two studies that reported high basal PTH were not very low [27, 31] and comparable to the studies reporting normal PTH at the baseline [33]. Changes in serum 25(OH) D with glycemic control are also mixed, which could not explain variable PTH responses to an improvement of glycemic control (Table 4.1). Serum levels of 1,25 $(OH)_2D$, the most active metabolite of vitamin D, do not significantly change with glycemic improvement [26, 29] (Table 4.1). Thus, vitamin D would affect PTH secretion, but there are likely to be other unknown factors that influence PTH secretion in diabetes. In bovine parathyroid cells, hyperglycemia itself inhibits PTH secretion [44] with unknown mechanisms.

4.4.2 *Vitamin D Deficiency/Insufficiency in DM*

Vitamin D deficiency/insufficiency is very common among diabetics. Indeed, meta-analyses of prospective cohort studies reported that low serum 25(OH)D level is associated with higher incidence of diabetes [45]. Whether this relationship is casual or not remains to be determined. It is of note that obesity with visceral fat deposition is associated with low serum 25(OH)D and high PTH [46]. In obese subjects with or without type 2 diabetes, weight loss by diet and/or exercise, but not by bariatric surgery, is associated with an increase in serum 25(OH)D concentration [47–49]. Furthermore, weight-associated change in serum 25(OH)D concentration is associated with reciprocal change in serum PTH level in nondiabetics [50]. Whether or not such change in PTH is observed in diabetics is not known.

Another factor that results in decreased serum 25(OH)D level in diabetes is diabetic nephropathy. In circulation, most vitamin D metabolites including 25(OH) D are bound to vitamin D-binding protein (DBP). In the kidney, DBP-25(OH)D complex is freely filtered across the glomerulus allowing transport to the proximal tubule. In the proximal tubule, DBP-25(OH)D complex is reabsorbed in a manner dependent on megalin, an endocytic receptor, expressed in polarized epithelial cells including proximal tubule cells [51]. It is a multiligand receptor, with an extensive repertoire of ligands including albumin, lipoproteins, hormones, enzymes, drugs, as well as DBP. Diabetic nephropathy with microalbuminuria or proteinuria causes megalin loss into the urine, which results in a decreased vitamin D reabsorption and aggravates poor vitamin D status [51, 52]. In human type 1 diabetics, it was reported that both albuminuria and urinary megalin levels are associated with low serum 25(OH)D [53]. Similar results have been obtained in both type 2 and type 1 diabetic model rats [52, 54].

4.5 Hyperglycemia and Advanced Glycation End Products (AGEs)

There are several studies examining the direct effects of hyperglycemia on osteoblasts in vitro, with mixed and sometimes conflicting results depending on the cell models and the glucose concentration tested [55, 56]. In human osteoblastic cell line, MG-63, high glucose (49.5 mM) attenuated cell proliferation and responses to PTH and 1,25(OH)2D [57–59], but in mouse osteoblastic MC3T3-E1 cells, high glucose at 15 mM increased proliferation [60]. In primary rat osteoblasts, proliferation was increased at 11 mM whereas inhibited at 22 and 44 mM of glucose

[61]. In MC3T3-E1 cells, high glucose (30 mM) inhibited ALP expression after 24 h [56] but stimulateed ALP expression from 48 h up to 29 days [55]. In primary rat osteoblasts, 11 mM glucose stimulated, whereas 22 and 44 mM glucose inhibited ALP activity [61]. In human osteoblastic cells, 12 mM glucose stimulated, whereas 24 mM glucose inhibited ALP activity after 7 days of culture [62]. It is of note, that in MC3T3-E1 cells, insulin stimulated ALP expression, which was not inhibited rather enhanced by high glucose that markedly inhibited unstimulated ALP expression [56]. With hyperglycemia, osteocalcin expression was enhanced in MC3T3-E1 cells [55] but inhibited in human osteoblasts [62]. In high glucose milieu, RANKL expression was stimulated in both mouse and human cells, whereas OPG was stimulated in mouse but inhibited in human cells [56, 62]. Finally, in vitro mineralization was unchanged [55], stimulated [62, 63], or inhibited [56] with high glucose. To distinguish effects of high glucose from high osmolarity, most studies also tested the effects of the same concentrations of mannitol, and also reported mixed results, indicating some of the effects are through high glucose per se and others through high osmolarity.

One of the consequences of chronic hyperglycemia is accumulation of nonenzymatically glycated proteins known as AGEs in many tissues including bone. Most well-studied AGE accumulation in bone occurs within collagen that accounts for over 90 % of the organic matrix of bone. Under physiological condition, collagen fibers are enzymatically cross-linked, for example, with pyridinoline, which gives bone its toughness. Long-standing hyperglycemia leads to nonenzymatic cross-linking of collagen fibers with AGEs, such as pentosidine. In animal models of diabetes, development of diabetes is associated with decreases in enzymatic cross-links and increases in AGE cross-links [64].

Enzymatic cross-linking of collagen fibers is initiated by the enzyme lysyl oxidase (LOX). LOX is a copper metalloenzyme that requires vitamin B6 (pyridoxal) as a cofactor. Thus, vitamin B6 deficiency results in decreased LOX activity. Among other regulators of LOX activity, IGF-1, vitamin D positively regulates LOX, whereas homocysteine and TNF-α negatively regulate LOX [65, 66]. In animal models of diabetes, before the development of overt diabetes, i.e., at the preclinical stage, decrease in enzymatic cross-links was reported [64], which may be due to vitamin B6 deficiency induced by upregulation of gluconeogenesis [66]. After the onset of overt diabetes, AGEs accumulate and at the same time enzymatic cross-links are decreased. It has been shown that in osteoblastic cells, non-glycated normal collagen itself increases LOX activity, and AGEs attenuate this upregulation of LOX by collagen [67]. Other factors that may contribute are vitamin D deficiency, decreased IGF-1 action, increase in TNF-α, and hyperhomocysteinemia, all of which would be present in diabetic states. Overall changes in bone collagen posttranslational modification, i.e., decreases in normal cross-links and increases in AGE cross-links, result in decreased mechanical strength of bone in diabetic model animals [64] without changes in BMD. Qualitatively similar changes in collagen cross-links in other animal models and human cadaver studies also have been shown to compromise bone strength.

Accumulation of AGEs in bone not only weakens the collagen mechanical properties but also influences bone cells. Non-cross-link types of AGEs, such as carboxymethyllysine as well as cross-link type of AGEs could affect bone cells via the cell surface receptor for AGEs, RAGE. In vitro studies have shown that AGEs impair function of osteoblastic cells. AGEs inhibit differentiation/maturation of osteoblastic cells and inhibit in vitro bone nodule formation [68–71]. AGEs also enhance apoptosis of osteoblasts [70, 72, 73]. These effects of AGEs on osteoblasts are most likely mediated by the changes in the action of many local factors such as IGF-1 [74], sclerostin [75], TNF-α [71], and their signal transduction pathways [76].

AGEs also have influence on osteoblastic precursor mesenchymal stromal cells (MSCs) via RAGE. Kume et al. [77] reported that AGEs attenuate adipocytic as well as chondrocytic differentiation of human MSCs in vitro. Although they did not find any effects of AGEs on ALP induction, generally thought to be an early marker of osteoblastic differentiation, they did find inhibition of bone nodule formation. In mouse stromal ST2 cells, AGEs but not high glucose inhibit ALP induction as well as bone nodule formation [75, 78], which may be mediated by an enhanced endoplasmic reticulum stress [78] and TGF-beta expression [79]. MSCs from STZ rats are less potent in the formation of both total and ALP positive colonies along with AGE accumulation, associated with increased apoptosis and enhanced expression RAGE [80].

AGEs may also affect osteocytes. Tanaka et al. [75] recently reported that AGEs enhance expression of sclerostin, inhibit RANKL expression, and enhance apoptosis of osteocyte-like cells in vitro.

Overall effect of AGEs on bone-forming cells including MSCs, osteoblasts, and osteocytes is inhibitory. In contrast, studies have reported mixed results about the effects of AGEs on bone resorption. In a rat model, AGEs were reported to enhance osteoclastic bone resorption as well as osteoclastogenesis [81, 82]. In contrast, another study reported that human osteoclasts seeded onto bone slices containing pentosidine showed decreased bone resorption and that AGEs inhibited in vitro osteoclastogenesis [83]. The expression of RANKL, one of the most essential local factors for osteoclast generation, survival, and activity, was reported to be enhanced by AGEs in osteoblasts [71, 84], but not in osteocytes [75]. In osteoblasts, AGEs were reported to stimulate expression of cytokines that stimulate osteoclast generation including IL-6 [85] and TNFα [71]. These results suggest that AGEs most likely stimulate osteoclastic bone resorption in the presence of osteoblasts.

A recent study that analyzed the relationship between AGEs and osteoclast activity in human cadaveric bone specimens demonstrated that higher AGEs were associated with an increased number of larger resorption cavities [86]. Furthermore, RAGE-deficient mice showed increased bone mass with decreased number of osteoclasts [87, 88], suggesting RAGE mediates osteoclastic bone resorption. Cathepsin K, the most important collagenolytic enzyme secreted by osteoclasts, was reported to preferentially degrade matured bone matrix characterized by a higher degree of posttranslational modifications, including pentosidine [89]. Thus, overall effect of AGEs on bone resorption appears to be stimulatory.

There are a few clinical studies exploring influence of AGEs on bone, all of which are cross-sectional [90–94]. Yamamoto et al. [90] reported that increased serum pentosidine level was associated with prevalent vertebral fractures in postmenopausal type 2 diabetic women independent of BMD. Similar results were reported in Korean men and women with type 2 diabetes [93]. Schwartz et al. [92] reported that increased urinary pentosidine is associated with clinical fractures in type 2 diabetic men and women over age 70. High serum pentosidine level was also associated with prevalent vertebral fracture in type 1 diabetes [94]. Yamamoto et al. [91] also reported that low serum endogenous secretory RAGE (esRAGE), which binds AGEs extracellularly and reduces the activity of intracellular signaling pathways via RAGE, was associated with higher prevalent vertebral fracture in type 2 diabetes. However, serum esRAGE level did not correlate with prevalent vertebral fracture in type 1 diabetes [94].

4.6 Summary

In this chapter the authors have focused on the influence of glycemic control over various aspects of bone metabolism. Now we have much evidence that chronic hyperglycemia per se, by changing actions of other hormones or cytokines, via accumulation of AGEs, or by unknown mechanisms, affects bone cell functions in favor of stimulating osteoclasts while inhibiting osteoblasts and possibly osteoblast progenitors and osteocytes as well. Chronic hyperglycemia also has detrimental effects on the material property of bone matrix proteins, such as collagen. Many of those changes may not be clinically detected by our current measures such as DXA machines or biochemical bone turnover markers, but high fracture risk in diabetes confirms that the net effect of chronic hyperglycemia is detrimental to bone. Further studies will be needed especially at the clinical level to see the long-term impact of changes in glycemic control, either better or worse, on the various aspects of bone strength.

References

1. Vestergaard P (2007) Discrepancies in bone mineral density and fracture risk in patients with type 1 and type 2 diabetes – a meta-analysis. Osteoporos Int 18(4):427–444 doi:10.1007/s00198-006-0253-4
2. The Diabetes Control and Complications Trial Research Group (1993) The effect of intensive treatment of diabetes on the development and progression of long-term complications in insulin-dependent diabetes mellitus. N Engl J Med 329(14):977–986. doi:10.1056/nejm199309303291401
3. UK Prospective Diabetes Study (UKPDS) Group (1998) Intensive blood-glucose control with sulphonylureas or insulin compared with conventional treatment and risk of complications in patients with type 2 diabetes (UKPDS 33). Lancet 352(9131):837–853
4. Oei L, Zillikens MC, Dehghan A, Buitendijk GH, Castano-Betancourt MC, Estrada K, Stolk L, Oei EH, van Meurs JB, Janssen JA, Hofman A, van Leeuwen JP, Witteman JC, Pols HA,

Uitterlinden AG, Klaver CC, Franco OH, Rivadeneira F (2013) High bone mineral density and fracture risk in type 2 diabetes as skeletal complications of inadequate glucose control: the Rotterdam Study. Diabetes Care 36(6):1619–1628. doi:10.2337/dc12-1188

5. Li CI, Liu CS, Lin WY, Chen CC, Yang SY, Chen HJ, Lin CC, Li TC (2015) Glycated hemoglobin level and risk of hip fracture in older people with type 2 diabetes: a competing risk analysis of Taiwan diabetes cohort study. J Bone Miner Res. doi:10.1002/jbmr.2462
6. Schwartz AV, Margolis KL, Sellmeyer DE, Vittinghoff E, Ambrosius WT, Bonds DE, Josse RG, Schnall AM, Simmons DL, Hue TF, Palermo L, Hamilton BP, Green JB, Atkinson HH, O'Connor PJ, Force RW, Bauer DC (2012) Intensive glycemic control is not associated with fractures or falls in the ACCORD randomized trial. Diabetes Care 35(7):1525–1531. doi:10.2337/dc11-2184
7. Ivers RQ, Cumming RG, Mitchell P, Peduto AJ (2001) Diabetes and risk of fracture: the Blue Mountains eye study. Diabetes Care 24(7):1198–1203
8. Melton LJ 3rd, Leibson CL, Achenbach SJ, Therneau TM, Khosla S (2008) Fracture risk in type 2 diabetes: update of a population-based study. J Bone Miner Res 23(8):1334–1342. doi:10.1359/jbmr.080323
9. Forsen L, Meyer HE, Midthjell K, Edna TH (1999) Diabetes mellitus and the incidence of hip fracture: results from the Nord-Trondelag Health Survey. Diabetologia 42(8):920–925. doi:10.1007/s001250051248
10. Kanazawa I, Yamaguchi T, Yamamoto M, Yamauchi M, Yano S, Sugimoto T (2008) Combination of obesity with hyperglycemia is a risk factor for the presence of vertebral fractures in type 2 diabetic men. Calcif Tissue Int 83(5):324–331. doi:10.1007/s00223-008-9178-6
11. Strotmeyer ES, Cauley JA, Schwartz AV, Nevitt MC, Resnick HE, Bauer DC, Tylavsky FA, de Rekeneire N, Harris TB, Newman AB (2005) Nontraumatic fracture risk with diabetes mellitus and impaired fasting glucose in older white and black adults: the health, aging, and body composition study. Arch Intern Med 165(14):1612–1617. doi:10.1001/archinte.165.14.1612
12. Neumann T, Samann A, Lodes S, Kastner B, Franke S, Kiehntopf M, Hemmelmann C, Lehmann T, Muller UA, Hein G, Wolf G (2011) Glycemic control is positively associated with prevalent fractures but not with bone mineral density in patients with Type 1 diabetes. Diabet Med 28(7):872–875. doi:10.1111/j.1464-5491.2011.03286.x
13. Vestergaard P, Rejnmark L, Mosekilde L (2009) Diabetes and its complications and their relationship with risk of fractures in type 1 and 2 diabetes. Calcif Tissue Int 84(1):45–55. doi:10.1007/s00223-008-9195-5
14. Schwartz AV, Sellmeyer DE, Ensrud KE, Cauley JA, Tabor HK, Schreiner PJ, Jamal SA, Black DM, Cummings SR (2001) Older women with diabetes have an increased risk of fracture: a prospective study. J Clin Endocrinol Metab 86(1):32–38. doi:10.1210/jcem.86.1.7139
15. Ahmed LA, Joakimsen RM, Berntsen GK, Fonnebo V, Schirmer H (2006) Diabetes mellitus and the risk of non-vertebral fractures: the Tromso study. Osteoporos Int 17(4):495–500. doi:10.1007/s00198-005-0013-x
16. Vestergaard P, Rejnmark L, Mosekilde L (2005) Relative fracture risk in patients with diabetes mellitus, and the impact of insulin and oral antidiabetic medication on relative fracture risk. Diabetologia 48(7):1292–1299. doi:10.1007/s00125-005-1786-3
17. Fajardo RJ, Karim L, Calley VI, Bouxsein ML (2014) A review of rodent models of type 2 diabetic skeletal fragility. J Bone Miner Res 29(5):1025–1040. doi:10.1002/jbmr.2210
18. Krakauer JC, McKenna MJ, Buderer NF, Rao DS, Whitehouse FW, Parfitt AM (1995) Bone loss and bone turnover in diabetes. Diabetes 44(7):775–782
19. Armas LA, Akhter MP, Drincic A, Recker RR (2012) Trabecular bone histomorphometry in humans with type 1 diabetes mellitus. Bone 50(1):91–96. doi:10.1016/j.bone.2011.09.055
20. Manavalan JS, Cremers S, Dempster DW, Zhou H, Dworakowski E, Kode A, Kousteni S, Rubin MR (2012) Circulating osteogenic precursor cells in type 2 diabetes mellitus. J Clin Endocrinol Metab 97(9):3240–3250. doi:10.1210/jc.2012-1546

21. Baek K, Hwang HR, Park HJ, Kwon A, Qadir AS, Ko SH, Woo KM, Ryoo HM, Kim GS, Baek JH (2014) TNF-alpha upregulates sclerostin expression in obese mice fed a high-fat diet. J Cell Physiol 229(5):640–650. doi:10.1002/jcp.24487
22. Turner RT, Kalra SP, Wong CP, Philbrick KA, Lindenmaier LB, Boghossian S, Iwaniec UT (2013) Peripheral leptin regulates bone formation. J Bone Miner Res 28(1):22–34. doi:10.1002/jbmr.1734
23. Zhang L, Liu Y, Wang D, Zhao X, Qiu Z, Ji H, Rong H (2009) Bone biomechanical and histomorphometrical investment in type 2 diabetic Goto-Kakizaki rats. Acta Diabetol 46 (2):119–126. doi:10.1007/s00592-008-0068-1
24. Fujii H, Hamada Y, Fukagawa M (2008) Bone formation in spontaneously diabetic Torii-newly established model of non-obese type 2 diabetes rats. Bone 42(2):372–379. doi:10.1016/j.bone.2007.10.007
25. Starup-Linde J, Eriksen SA, Lykkeboe S, Handberg A, Vestergaard P (2014) Biochemical markers of bone turnover in diabetes patients – a meta-analysis, and a methodological study on the effects of glucose on bone markers. Osteoporos Int 25(6):1697–1708. doi:10.1007/s00198-014-2676-7
26. Nagasaka S, Murakami T, Uchikawa T, Ishikawa SE, Saito T (1995) Effect of glycemic control on calcium and phosphorus handling and parathyroid hormone level in patients with non-insulin-dependent diabetes mellitus. Endocr J 42(3):377–383
27. Gregorio F, Cristallini S, Santeusanio F, Filipponi P, Fumelli P (1994) Osteopenia associated with non-insulin-dependent diabetes mellitus: what are the causes? Diabetes Res Clin Pract 23 (1):43–54
28. Sayinalp S, Gedik O, Koray Z (1995) Increasing serum osteocalcin after glycemic control in diabetic men. Calcif Tissue Int 57(6):422–425
29. Okazaki R, Totsuka Y, Hamano K, Ajima M, Miura M, Hirota Y, Hata K, Fukumoto S, Matsumoto T (1997) Metabolic improvement of poorly controlled non-insulin-dependent diabetes mellitus decreases bone turnover. J Clin Endocrinol Metab 82(9):2915–2920. doi:10.1210/jcem.82.9.4258
30. Rosato MT, Schneider SH, Shapses SA (1998) Bone turnover and insulin-like growth factor I levels increase after improved glycemic control in non-insulin-dependent diabetes mellitus. Calcif Tissue Int 63(2):107–111
31. Capoglu I, Ozkan A, Ozkan B, Umudum Z (2008) Bone turnover markers in patients with type 2 diabetes and their correlation with glycosylated hemoglobin levels. J Int Med Res 36 (6):1392–1398
32. Kanazawa I, Yamaguchi T, Sugimoto T (2011) Relationship between bone biochemical markers versus glucose/lipid metabolism and atherosclerosis; a longitudinal study in type 2 diabetes mellitus. Diabetes Res Clin Pract 92(3):393–399. doi:10.1016/j.diabres.2011.03.015
33. Zinman B, Haffner SM, Herman WH, Holman RR, Lachin JM, Kravitz BG, Paul G, Jones NP, Aftring RP, Viberti G, Kahn SE (2010) Effect of rosiglitazone, metformin, and glyburide on bone biomarkers in patients with type 2 diabetes. J Clin Endocrinol Metab 95(1):134–142. doi:10.1210/jc.2009-0572
34. Kahn SE, Haffner SM, Heise MA, Herman WH, Holman RR, Jones NP, Kravitz BG, Lachin JM, O'Neill MC, Zinman B, Viberti G (2006) Glycemic durability of rosiglitazone, metformin, or glyburide monotherapy. N Engl J Med 355(23):2427–2443. doi:10.1056/NEJMoa066224
35. Kahn SE, Zinman B, Lachin JM, Haffner SM, Herman WH, Holman RR, Kravitz BG, Yu D, Heise MA, Aftring RP, Viberti G (2008) Rosiglitazone-associated fractures in type 2 diabetes: an Analysis from A Diabetes Outcome Progression Trial (ADOPT). Diabetes Care 31 (5):845–851. doi:10.2337/dc07-2270
36. Borges JL, Bilezikian JP, Jones-Leone AR, Acusta AP, Ambery PD, Nino AJ, Grosse M, Fitzpatrick LA, Cobitz AR (2011) A randomized, parallel group, double-blind, multicentre study comparing the efficacy and safety of Avandamet (rosiglitazone/metformin) and metformin on long-term glycemic control and bone mineral density after 80 weeks of treatment in

drug-naive type 2 diabetes mellitus patients. Diabetes Obes Metab 13(11):1036–1046. doi:10.1111/j.1463-1326.2011.01461.x

37. Bilezikian JP, Josse RG, Eastell R, Lewiecki EM, Miller CG, Wooddell M, Northcutt AR, Kravitz BG, Paul G, Cobitz AR, Nino AJ, Fitzpatrick LA (2013) Rosiglitazone decreases bone mineral density and increases bone turnover in postmenopausal women with type 2 diabetes mellitus. J Clin Endocrinol Metab 98(4):1519–1528. doi:10.1210/jc.2012-4018
38. van Lierop AH, Hamdy NA, van der Meer RW, Jonker JT, Lamb HJ, Rijzewijk LJ, Diamant M, Romijn JA, Smit JW, Papapoulos SE (2012) Distinct effects of pioglitazone and metformin on circulating sclerostin and biochemical markers of bone turnover in men with type 2 diabetes mellitus. Eur J Endocrinol/Eur Fed Endocrinol Soc 166(4):711–716. doi:10.1530/eje-11-1061
39. McNair P, Christensen MS, Madsbad S, Christiansen C, Transbol I (1981) Hypoparathyroidism in diabetes mellitus. Acta Endocrinol (Copenh) 96(1):81–86
40. McNair P (1988) Bone mineral metabolism in human type 1 (insulin dependent) diabetes mellitus. Dan Med Bull 35(2):109–121
41. Ishida H, Suzuki K, Someya Y, Nishimura M, Sugimoto C, Goto M, Taguchi Y, Kasahara H, Kadowaki S, Imura H et al (1993) Possible compensatory role of parathyroid hormone-related peptide on maintenance of calcium homeostasis in patients with non-insulin-dependent diabetes mellitus. Acta Endocrinol (Copenh) 129(6):519–524
42. Thalassinos NC, Hadjiyanni P, Tzanela M, Alevizaki C, Philokiprou D (1993) Calcium metabolism in diabetes mellitus: effect of improved blood glucose control. Diabet Med 10 (4):341–344
43. Akizawa T, Kinugasa E, Akiba T, Tsukamoto Y, Kurokawa K (1997) Incidence and clinical characteristics of hypoparathyroidism in dialysis patients. Kidney Int Suppl 62:S72–S74
44. Sugimoto T, Ritter C, Morrissey J, Hayes C, Slatopolsky E (1990) Effects of high concentrations of glucose on PTH secretion in parathyroid cells. Kidney Int 37(6):1522–1527
45. Afzal S, Bojesen SE, Nordestgaard BG (2013) Low 25-hydroxyvitamin D and risk of type 2 diabetes: a prospective cohort study and metaanalysis. Clin Chem 59(2):381–391. doi:10.1373/clinchem.2012.193003
46. Valina-Toth AL, Lai Z, Yoo W, Abou-Samra A, Gadegbeku CA, Flack JM (2010) Relationship of vitamin D and parathyroid hormone with obesity and body composition in African Americans. Clin Endocrinol 72(5):595–603. doi:10.1111/j.1365-2265.2009.03676.x
47. Ibero-Baraibar I, Navas-Carretero S, Abete I, Martinez JA, Zulet MA (2014) Increases in plasma 25(OH)D levels are related to improvements in body composition and blood pressure in middle-aged subjects after a weight loss intervention: longitudinal study. Clin Nutr (Edinb Scotl). doi:10.1016/j.clnu.2014.11.004
48. Rock CL, Emond JA, Flatt SW, Heath DD, Karanja N, Pakiz B, Sherwood NE, Thomson CA (2012) Weight loss is associated with increased serum 25-hydroxyvitamin D in overweight or obese women. Obesity (Silver Spring Md) 20(11):2296–2301. doi:10.1038/oby.2012.57
49. Tzotzas T, Papadopoulou FG, Tziomalos K, Karras S, Gastaris K, Perros P, Krassas GE (2010) Rising serum 25-hydroxy-vitamin D levels after weight loss in obese women correlate with improvement in insulin resistance. J Clin Endocrinol Metab 95(9):4251–4257. doi:10.1210/jc.2010-0757
50. Hinton PS, LeCheminant JD, Smith BK, Rector RS, Donnelly JE (2009) Weight loss-induced alterations in serum markers of bone turnover persist during weight maintenance in obese men and women. J Am Coll Nutr 28(5):565–573
51. Nykjaer A, Dragun D, Walther D, Vorum H, Jacobsen C, Herz J, Melsen F, Christensen EI, Willnow TE (1999) An endocytic pathway essential for renal uptake and activation of the steroid 25-(OH) vitamin D3. Cell 96(4):507–515
52. Fowlkes JL, Bunn RC, Cockrell GE, Clark LM, Wahl EC, Lumpkin CK, Thrailkill KM (2011) Dysregulation of the intrarenal vitamin D endocytic pathway in a nephropathy-prone mouse model of type 1 diabetes. Exp Diabetes Res 2011:269378. doi:10.1155/2011/269378

53. Thrailkill KM, Jo CH, Cockrell GE, Moreau CS, Fowlkes JL (2011) Enhanced excretion of vitamin D binding protein in type 1 diabetes: a role in vitamin D deficiency? J Clin Endocrinol Metab 96(1):142–149. doi:10.1210/jc.2010-0980
54. Anderson RL, Ternes SB, Strand KA, Rowling MJ (2010) Vitamin D homeostasis is compromised due to increased urinary excretion of the 25-hydroxycholecalciferol-vitamin D-binding protein complex in the Zucker diabetic fatty rat. Am J Physiol Endocrinol Metab 299(6):E959–E967. doi:10.1152/ajpendo.00218.2010
55. Botolin S, McCabe LR (2006) Chronic hyperglycemia modulates osteoblast gene expression through osmotic and non-osmotic pathways. J Cell Biochem 99(2):411–424. doi:10.1002/jcb.20842
56. Cunha JS, Ferreira VM, Maquigussa E, Naves MA, Boim MA (2014) Effects of high glucose and high insulin concentrations on osteoblast function in vitro. Cell Tissue Res 358(1):249–256. doi:10.1007/s00441-014-1913-x
57. Inaba M, Terada M, Koyama H, Yoshida O, Ishimura E, Kawagishi T, Okuno Y, Nishizawa Y, Otani S, Morii H (1995) Influence of high glucose on 1,25-dihydroxyvitamin D3-induced effect on human osteoblast-like MG-63 cells. J Bone Miner Res 10(7):1050–1056. doi:10.1002/jbmr.5650100709
58. Terada M, Inaba M, Yano Y, Hasuma T, Nishizawa Y, Morii H, Otani S (1998) Growth-inhibitory effect of a high glucose concentration on osteoblast-like cells. Bone 22(1):17–23
59. Yoshida O, Inaba M, Terada M, Shioi A, Nishizawa Y, Otani S, Morii H (1995) Impaired response of human osteosarcoma (MG-63) cells to human parathyroid hormone induced by sustained exposure to high glucose. Miner Electrolyte Metab 21(1-3):201–204
60. Balint E, Szabo P, Marshall CF, Sprague SM (2001) Glucose-induced inhibition of in vitro bone mineralization. Bone 28(1):21–28
61. Zhen D, Chen Y, Tang X (2010) Metformin reverses the deleterious effects of high glucose on osteoblast function. J Diabetes Complicat 24(5):334–344. doi:10.1016/j.jdiacomp.2009.05.002
62. Garcia-Hernandez A, Arzate H, Gil-Chavarria I, Rojo R, Moreno-Fierros L (2012) High glucose concentrations alter the biomineralization process in human osteoblastic cells. Bone 50(1):276–288. doi:10.1016/j.bone.2011.10.032
63. Li YM, Schilling T, Benisch P, Zeck S, Meissner-Weigl J, Schneider D, Limbert C, Seufert J, Kassem M, Schutze N, Jakob F, Ebert R (2007) Effects of high glucose on mesenchymal stem cell proliferation and differentiation. Biochem Biophys Res Commun 363(1):209–215. doi:10.1016/j.bbrc.2007.08.161
64. Saito M, Fujii K, Mori Y, Marumo K (2006) Role of collagen enzymatic and glycation induced cross-links as a determinant of bone quality in spontaneously diabetic WBN/Kob rats. Osteoporos Int 17(10):1514–1523. doi:10.1007/s00198-006-0155-5
65. Garnero P (2012) The contribution of collagen crosslinks to bone strength. Bone Key Rep 1:182. doi:10.1038/bonekey.2012.182
66. Saito M, Kida Y, Kato S, Marumo K (2014) Diabetes, collagen, and bone quality. Curr Osteoporos Rep 12(2):181–188. doi:10.1007/s11914-014-0202-7
67. Khosravi R, Sodek KL, Faibish M, Trackman PC (2014) Collagen advanced glycation inhibits its Discoidin Domain Receptor 2 (DDR2)-mediated induction of lysyl oxidase in osteoblasts. Bone 58:33–41. doi:10.1016/j.bone.2013.10.001
68. Katayama Y, Akatsu T, Yamamoto M, Kugai N, Nagata N (1996) Role of nonenzymatic glycosylation of type I collagen in diabetic osteopenia. J Bone Miner Res 11(7):931–937. doi:10.1002/jbmr.5650110709
69. Sanguineti R, Storace D, Monacelli F, Federici A, Odetti P (2008) Pentosidine effects on human osteoblasts in vitro. Ann N Y Acad Sci 1126:166–172. doi:10.1196/annals.1433.044
70. Gangoiti MV, Cortizo AM, Arnol V, Felice JI, McCarthy AD (2008) Opposing effects of bisphosphonates and advanced glycation end products on osteoblastic cells. Eur J Pharmacol 600(1–3):140–147. doi:10.1016/j.ejphar.2008.10.031

71. Franke S, Ruster C, Pester J, Hofmann G, Oelzner P, Wolf G (2011) Advanced glycation end products affect growth and function of osteoblasts. Clin Exp Rheumatol 29(4):650–660
72. Alikhani M, Alikhani Z, Boyd C, MacLellan CM, Raptis M, Liu R, Pischon N, Trackman PC, Gerstenfeld L, Graves DT (2007) Advanced glycation end products stimulate osteoblast apoptosis via the MAP kinase and cytosolic apoptotic pathways. Bone 40(2):345–353. doi:10.1016/j.bone.2006.09.011
73. Mercer N, Ahmed H, Etcheverry SB, Vasta GR, Cortizo AM (2007) Regulation of advanced glycation end product (AGE) receptors and apoptosis by AGEs in osteoblast-like cells. Mol Cell Biochem 306(1-2):87–94. doi:10.1007/s11010-007-9557-8
74. McCarthy AD, Etcheverry SB, Cortizo AM (2001) Effect of advanced glycation end products on the secretion of insulin-like growth factor-I and its binding proteins: role in osteoblast development. Acta Diabetol 38(3):113–122
75. Tanaka KI, Yamaguchi T, Kanazawa I, Sugimoto T (2015) Effects of high glucose and advanced glycation end products on the expressions of sclerostin and RANKL as well as apoptosis in osteocyte-like MLO-Y4-A2 cells. Biochem Biophys Res Commun. doi:10.1016/j.bbrc.2015.02.091
76. Cortizo AM, Lettieri MG, Barrio DA, Mercer N, Etcheverry SB, McCarthy AD (2003) Advanced glycation end products (AGEs) induce concerted changes in the osteoblastic expression of their receptor RAGE and in the activation of extracellular signal-regulated kinases (ERK). Mol Cell Biochem 250(1-2):1–10
77. Kume S, Kato S, Yamagishi S, Inagaki Y, Ueda S, Arima N, Okawa T, Kojiro M, Nagata K (2005) Advanced glycation end products attenuate human mesenchymal stem cells and prevent cognate differentiation into adipose tissue, cartilage, and bone. J Bone Miner Res 20(9):1647–1658. doi:10.1359/jbmr.050514
78. Okazaki K, Yamaguchi T, Tanaka K, Notsu M, Ogawa N, Yano S, Sugimoto T (2012) Advanced glycation end products (AGEs), but not high glucose, inhibit the osteoblastic differentiation of mouse stromal ST2 cells through the suppression of osterix expression, and inhibit cell growth and increasing cell apoptosis. Calcif Tissue Int 91(4):286–296. doi:10.1007/s00223-012-9641-2
79. Notsu M, Yamaguchi T, Okazaki K, Tanaka K, Ogawa N, Kanazawa I, Sugimoto T (2014) Advanced glycation end product 3 (AGE3) suppresses the mineralization of mouse stromal ST2 cells and human mesenchymal stem cells by increasing TGF-beta expression and secretion. Endocrinology 155(7):2402–2410. doi:10.1210/en.2013-1818
80. Stolzing A, Sellers D, Llewelyn O, Scutt A (2010) Diabetes induced changes in rat mesenchymal stem cells. Cells Tissues Organs 191(6):453–465. doi:10.1159/000281826
81. Miyata T, Kawai R, Taketomi S, Sprague SM (1996) Possible involvement of advanced glycation end products in bone resorption. Nephrol Dial Transplant 11(Suppl 5):54–57
82. Miyata T, Notoya K, Yoshida K, Horie K, Maeda K, Kurokawa K, Taketomi S (1997) Advanced glycation end products enhance osteoclast-induced bone resorption in cultured mouse unfractionated bone cells and in rats implanted subcutaneously with devitalized bone particles. J Am Soc Nephrol 8(2):260–270
83. Valcourt U, Merle B, Gineyts E, Viguet-Carrin S, Delmas PD, Garnero P (2007) Non-enzymatic glycation of bone collagen modifies osteoclastic activity and differentiation. J Biol Chem 282(8):5691–5703. doi:10.1074/jbc.M610536200
84. Franke S, Siggelkow H, Wolf G, Hein G (2007) Advanced glycation end products influence the mRNA expression of RAGE, RANKL and various osteoblastic genes in human osteoblasts. Arch Physiol Biochem 113(3):154–161. doi:10.1080/13813450701602523
85. Takagi M, Kasayama S, Yamamoto T, Motomura T, Hashimoto K, Yamamoto H, Sato B, Okada S, Kishimoto T (1997) Advanced glycation end products stimulate interleukin-6 production by human bone-derived cells. J Bone Miner Res Off J Am Soc Bone Miner Res 12(3):439–446. doi:10.1359/jbmr.1997.12.3.439

86. Dong XN, Qin A, Xu J, Wang X (2011) In situ accumulation of advanced glycation end products (AGEs) in bone matrix and its correlation with osteoclastic bone resorption. Bone 49 (2):174–183. doi:10.1016/j.bone.2011.04.009
87. Zhou Z, Immel D, Xi CX, Bierhaus A, Feng X, Mei L, Nawroth P, Stern DM, Xiong WC (2006) Regulation of osteoclast function and bone mass by RAGE. J Exp Med 203 (4):1067–1080. doi:10.1084/jem.20051947
88. Ding KH, Wang ZZ, Hamrick MW, Deng ZB, Zhou L, Kang B, Yan SL, She JX, Stern DM, Isales CM, Mi QS (2006) Disordered osteoclast formation in RAGE-deficient mouse establishes an essential role for RAGE in diabetes related bone loss. Biochem Biophys Res Commun 340(4):1091–1097. doi:10.1016/j.bbrc.2005.12.107
89. Borel O, Gineyts E, Bertholon C, Garnero P (2012) Cathepsin K preferentially solubilizes matured bone matrix. Calcif Tissue Int 91(1):32–39. doi:10.1007/s00223-012-9604-7
90. Yamamoto M, Yamaguchi T, Yamauchi M, Yano S, Sugimoto T (2008) Serum pentosidine levels are positively associated with the presence of vertebral fractures in postmenopausal women with type 2 diabetes. J Clin Endocrinol Metab 93(3):1013–1019. doi:10.1210/jc.2007-1270
91. Yamamoto M, Yamaguchi T, Yamauchi M, Sugimoto T (2009) Low serum level of the endogenous secretory receptor for advanced glycation end products (esRAGE) is a risk factor for prevalent vertebral fractures independent of bone mineral density in patients with type 2 diabetes. Diabetes Care 32(12):2263–2268. doi:10.2337/dc09-0901
92. Schwartz AV, Garnero P, Hillier TA, Sellmeyer DE, Strotmeyer ES, Feingold KR, Resnick HE, Tylavsky FA, Black DM, Cummings SR, Harris TB, Bauer DC (2009) Pentosidine and increased fracture risk in older adults with type 2 diabetes. J Clin Endocrinol Metab 94 (7):2380–2386. doi:10.1210/jc.2008-2498
93. Lee CH, Lee MK, Han HJ, Kim TH, Lee JH, and Kim SH (2012). The association between serum endogenous secretory receptor for advanced glycation end products and vertebral fractures in type 2 diabetes (Endocrinol Metab 27:289–94, Cheol Ho Lee et al.). Endocrinol Metab (Seoul, Korea) 27 (1):289–294. doi:10.3803/EnM.2013.28.1.78
94. Neumann T, Lodes S, Kastner B, Franke S, Kiehntopf M, Lehmann T, Muller UA, Wolf G, Samann A (2014) High serum pentosidine but not esRAGE is associated with prevalent fractures in type 1 diabetes independent of bone mineral density and glycemic control. Osteoporos Int 25(5):1527–1533. doi:10.1007/s00198-014-2631-7
95. Okazaki R, Miura M, Toriumi M, Taguchi M, Hirota Y, Fukumoto S, Fujita T, Tanaka K, Takeuchi A (1999) Short-term treatment with troglitazone decreases bone turnover in patients with type 2 diabetes mellitus. Endocr J 46(6):795–801
96. Watanabe S, Takeuchi Y, Fukumoto S, Fujita H, Nakano T, Fujita T (2003) Decrease in serum leptin by troglitazone is associated with preventing bone loss in type 2 diabetic patients. J Bone Miner Metab 21(3):166–171. doi:10.1007/s007740300026
97. Kanazawa I, Yamaguchi T, Yamauchi M, Yamamoto M, Kurioka S, Yano S, Sugimoto T (2009) Adiponectin is associated with changes in bone markers during glycemic control in type 2 diabetes mellitus. J Clin Endocrinol Metab 94(8):3031–3037

Chapter 5
Mechanism for the Development of Bone Disease in Diabetes: Increased Oxidative Stress and Advanced Glycation End Products

Sho-ichi Yamagishi

Abstract The prevalence and incidence of osteoporosis is high in diabetic patients. There is a growing body of evidence that advanced glycation end products (AGEs), senescent macroprotein derivatives formed at an accelerated rate under hyperglycemic and oxidative stress conditions, play a central role in osteoporosis and bone fractures in diabetes. Indeed, accumulation of AGE-modified cross-links of collagen alters bone strength and impairs its biomechanical properties. Further, AGE-modified proteins in the bone have been shown to disturb physiological function of osteoblasts and osteoclasts via oxidative stress generation through the interaction with the receptor for AGEs (RAGE). Therefore, activation of the AGE-RAGE system in the bone not only decreases bone mineral density but also impairs bone quality in patients with diabetes. In this review, I discuss the molecular mechanism for osteoporosis in diabetes, especially focusing on the AGE-RAGE-induced oxidative stress axis.

Keywords AGEs • Osteoporosis • Oxidative stress • RAGE • Diabetes

5.1 Introduction

Osteoporosis is a systemic skeletal disorder characterized by reduced bone mineral density (BMD) and quality, which could compromise bone strength and subsequently increase the risk of bone fractures [1]. The prevalence and cumulative incidence of osteoporosis is high in postmenopausal women, which increases with age. About 40 % of white postmenopausal women are suffering from osteoporosis [2]. Osteoporotic fractures, particularly vertebral and hip fractures, extremely reduce the quality of life in patients [2]. Further, several papers have shown that

S.-i. Yamagishi (✉)
Department of Pathophysiology and Therapeutics of Diabetic Vascular Complications, Kurume University School of Medicine, 67 Asahi-machi, Kurume-shi, Fukuoka 830-0011, Japan
e-mail: shoichi@med.kurume-u.ac.jp

M. Inaba (ed.), *Musculoskeletal Disease Associated with Diabetes Mellitus*,
DOI 10.1007/978-4-431-55720-3_5

osteoporotic bone fractures are also associated with the increased risk of morbidity and mortality [1–4]. Indeed, hip fracture was independently associated with a greater risk for future event of acute myocardial infarction in a large, nationwide cohort study [3]. Increased risk of all-cause mortality persisted till 5 years after hip fracture; men with hip fracture had higher risk for deaths from stroke and cancer up to 1 year post fracture, whereas women from coronary artery disease for 5 years after fracture [4]. Therefore, to identify modifiable risk factors that could influence the bone health and treat osteoporosis would be helpful to prevent its devastating complications.

5.2 Diabetes and Osteoporosis

The risk of osteoporosis-related bone fractures is also increased in both type 1 and type 2 diabetic patients [5–8]. Although accumulating evidence has shown that bone mineral density (BMD) is decreased in patients with type 1 diabetes, increased risk of osteoporotic bone fractures in diabetes is not entirely explained by low BMD because BMD is increased *rather than* decreased in type 2 diabetes [8–11]. Furthermore, a meta-analysis revealed that the relative risk of hip fracture in type 1 diabetic subjects was 6.9, which was much higher than that calculated based on BMD (relative risk 1.4) [8]. The Rotterdam study showed that bone fracture risk was higher only in already established and treated type 2 diabetic patients, but not in subjects with newly diagnosed diabetes compared with nondiabetic individuals [12]. So, cumulative diabetic exposure could be involved in the pathogenesis of osteoporosis and increased risk for bone fractures in diabetes. In addition, subjects with impaired glucose tolerance had a lower risk of nonvertebral fracture, thus indicating that hyperinsulinemia and/or obesity might be protective against osteoporotic bone fractures [6]. These observations suggest that the increased risk of bone fractures in diabetic subjects could be partly ascribed to the impairment of bone quality, whose deterioration was enhanced by long-term history of diabetes.

5.3 Advanced Glycation End Products (AGEs)

Sugars, including glucose and fructose, can react nonenzymatically with the amino groups of proteins, lipids, and nucleic acids to form reversible Schiff bases and then Amadori products [13–16]. These early glycation products undergo further complex reactions such as rearrangement, dehydration, and condensation to become irreversibly cross-linked, heterogeneous fluorescent derivatives called "advanced glycation end products (AGEs)" [13–16]. The process of nonenzymatic glycation is also known as the Maillard reaction, and formation and accumulation of AGEs in various tissues have progressed at a physiological normal aging and at an extremely accelerated rate under hyperglycemic and/or oxidative stress conditions [13–16]. Cross-linking modification of the organic bone matrix proteins such as collagen by AGEs has been known to adversely affect bone strength and subsequently impair bone quality, thereby reducing the fracture resistance of bone [17–19]. Furthermore, there is a growing body of evidence that engagement of AGEs with their receptor (RAGE) elicits oxidative stress generation and evokes inflammatory reactions in a variety of cells, including osteoblasts and osteoclasts, thus disturbing the physiological interaction between the two cell types [17–25]. These observations suggest that activation of the AGE-RAGE axis could influence both quantity and quality of bone and resultantly increase the risk of osteoporosis in diabetic subjects, especially with a long history of diabetes or elderly patients. In this review, I describe the pathophysiological role of the AGE-RAGE-oxidative stress system in decreased BMD, impaired bone quality, and increased bone fragility in diabetes. I also discuss here the potential therapeutic interventions of the AGE-RAGE axis for improving the quality of bone and preventing osteoporotic bone fractures in diabetes.

5.4 AGE-RAGE Axis and Osteoblasts

AGE-modified albumin up-regulated RAGE expression, increased intracellular reactive oxygen species (ROS) generation, and subsequently induced apoptotic cell death of two different osteoblast-like cell lines, rat osteosarcoma UMR 106 and mouse nontransformed MC3T3E1 cells via activation of capase-3, a key enzyme in the execution of apoptosis [26, 27]. Further, apoptotic cell death signals of AGEs were mediated via RAGE-induced mitogen-activated protein kinases (MAPKs) activation because *N*-carboxymethyllysine (CML)-modified collagen increased p38 and c-Jun N-terminal kinase (JNK) activity and induced apoptotic cell death of primary human-cultured osteoblasts, which was blocked by anti-RAGE antibody, inhibitors of p38, or JNK [28]. Although AGEs increased the activities of caspase-3, caspase-8, and caspase-9 in human osteoblasts, an inhibitor of caspase-8 blocked the AGE-induced caspase-3 activation and osteoblasts apoptosis more effectively than that of caspase-9, thus suggesting that cytoplasmic (caspase-8-dependent) pathway might be relatively more important than mitochondrial (caspase-9) pathway for the apoptotic signals of AGEs in osteoblasts [28].

Methylglyoxal is a reactive dicarbonyl compound produced by glycolytic pathway and a precursor of AGEs [29–31]. Methylglyoxal has been reported to induce MC3T3E1 cell damage and impair the osteoblastic differentiation by increasing the intracellular ROS generations via reducing mitochondrial membrane potential and intracellular ATP levels [28]. Methylglyoxal also inactivates glyoxalase I and further potentiates the formation of methylglyoxal-derived AGEs in MC3T3E1 cells [29, 30]. Further, these deleterious effects of methylglyoxal on osteoblastic MC3T3E1 cells were significantly blocked by the pretreatment with aminoguanidine, an inhibitor of AGEs formation; Trolox, an antioxidant; and apocynin, an inhibitor of NADPH oxidase [29–31].

AGEs formed on type 1 collagen, a predominant matrix protein of bone, could also play a role in reduced BMD in diabetes [32, 33]. Indeed, when rat osteoblastic cells were cultured on AGE-modified type 1 collagen, alkaline phosphatase (ALP) activity and osteocalcin secretion were decreased and nodule formation was dramatically impaired [32, 33]. Accelerated accumulation of AGEs was observed in the bone collagen of streptozotocin-induced diabetic rats, which was associated with reduced BMD in the diabetic animals [32]. AGE-modified type 1 collagen decreased adhesion of UMR 106 and inhibited cellular proliferation, spreading, and ALP activity through intracellular ROS production as well [34]. AGE modification of type 1 collagen may impair the integrin-mediated adhesion of osteoblastic cells to the matrix [35]. Further, recently, the AGE-RAGE interaction has been shown to inhibit the osteoblast proliferation via suppression of Wnt signaling in MC3T3E1 cells [36]. Pentosidine, a well-characterized glycoxidative end product, also hampered the formation of bone nodules of human osteoblasts [37]. Taken together, these findings suggest that the AGE-RAGE interaction could not only induce apoptosis, but also inhibit the proliferation and differentiation of osteoblasts, thereby being involved in reduced BMD in diabetes. In addition, nonenzymatic glycation of ALP was reported to alter its biological activity as well [38] (Fig. 5.1).

5.5 AGE-RAGE Axis and Osteoclasts

There is some controversy about the pathological role of AGEs in osteoclast function in osteoporosis. Miyata et al. reported that when mouse unfractionated bone cells containing osteoclasts were cultured on dentin slices, AGE-modified proteins increased the number of resorption pits formed by osteoclasts [39]. Moreover, bone resorption was augmented when unfractionated bone cells were cultured on AGE-modified dentin slices [39]. They also showed that AGE-modified bone particles implanted subcutaneously in rats were resorbed to a much greater extent than nonglycated control bone particles [39]. Since AGEs did not increase the

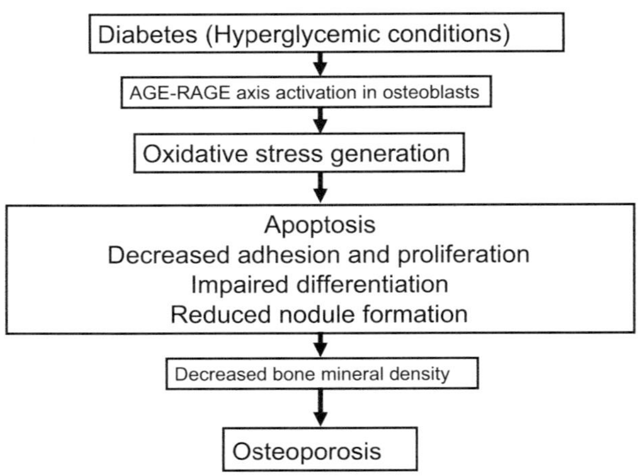

Fig. 5.1 Effects of the AGE-RAGE axis on osteoblasts

number of newly formed osteoclasts, AGEs could not promote the differentiation of osteoclasts but may activate osteoclasts or alter microenvironments favorable for bone resorption by osteoclasts. In addition, human AGE-rich cortical bone specimens were reported to increase bone resorption activities of osteoclasts [40]. These observations suggest the pathological role of AGEs in osteoclast activation in osteoporosis, which might lead to increased bone resorption and bone loss in diabetes. However, Valcourt et al. reported that when mature osteoclasts were seeded on AGE-modified bone and ivory slices, bone resorption was inhibited *rather than* increased due to decreased solubility of AGE-modified type 1 collagen molecules [41]. Further, they found that AGE-modified proteins inhibited osteoclastogenesis partly by blocking the osteoclastic differentiation process. So, they finally concluded that bone remodeling could be impaired in diabetes.

There is accumulating evidence that RAGE plays an important role in osteoporosis [32–47] (Fig. 5.2). Mice lacking RAGE had increased BMD and bone biomechanical strength and decreased number of osteoclasts and its bone resorptive activity in vivo [42, 43]. In vitro-differentiated RAGE-deficient osteoclasts exhibited disrupted actin ring and sealing zone structures, impaired maturation, and reduced bone resorptive activity [42]. These observations suggest that RAGE is involved in osteoclast actin reorganization, adhesion, and activation, thereby contributing to reduced bone mass in diabetes. AGEs increased mRNA levels of RAGE and receptor activator of nuclear factor-κB ligand (RANKL) in osteoblasts [44]. RANKL is an essential cytokine for osteoclastogenesis, and osteoblasts express RANKL in response to bone-resorbing factors, thus further suggesting the active participation of RAGE in osteoclastogenesis [45]. Moreover, high-mobility group box 1 (HMGB1), a nonhistone nuclear protein and one of the ligands of RAGE, has been shown to enhance RANKL-induced osteoclastogenesis both in cell culture and animal model [46].

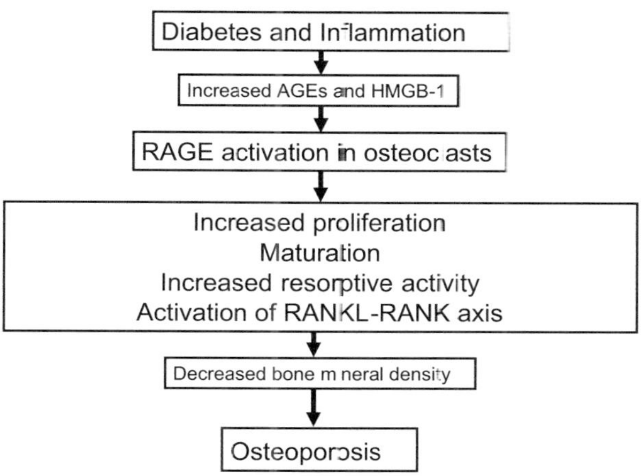

Fig. 5.2 Role of RAGE in osteoclast dysfunction

5.6 AGE-RAGE Axis and Mesenchymal Stem Cells (MSCs)

AGE-modified albumin induced generation of ROS through the interaction with RAGE and inhibited proliferation and migration of bone marrow MSCs [48]. AGEs stimulated expression and secretion of chemokines and cytokines including CC chemokine ligand (Ccl) 2, Ccl3, Ccl4, and interleukin-1β via activation of p38, which could exert the inhibitory effects on MSCs growth and migration, thereby impairing bone repair in diabetes [48]. MSCs from rats with streptozotocin-induced diabetes were more likely to become senescent, and their ability to proliferate and differentiate to the bone was reduced compared with those from control rats [49]. Glyoxal, a highly reactive dicarbonyl and one of the precursors of AGEs, which is produced by auto-oxidation of glucose, also induced senescence in bone marrow-derived telomerase-immortalized MSCs that were accompanied by increased extent of DNA breaks and AGEs accumulation [50]. Glyoxal also impaired the differentiation of MSCs determined by decreased ALP activity and reduced mineralized matrix formation as well [50]. In addition, AGEs not only inhibited the osteoblastic differentiation and growth but also induced apoptosis of mouse stromal ST2 cells [51]. Furthermore, methylglyoxal suppressed the expression of osteotrophic Wnt-targeted genes, including osteoprotegerin, a decoy receptor of RANKL via oxidative stress generation, thus causing low-turnover osteoporosis in diabetes [52]. Levels of AGEs, RAGE, ROS, and apoptosis in diabetic MSCs were increased, and extensive loss of trabecular bone in the tibiae was observed in diabetic animals [49]. AGEs inhibited the proliferation, self-renewal, and osteogenic differentiation of MSCs in vitro [49]. We also found that AGEs increased RAGE induction, ROS generation, and apoptosis and consequently inhibited mineralization and mature bone nodule formation of MSCs [53].

Up-regulation of heme oxygenase 1 (HO-1) expression and increased HO activity stimulated the differentiation of MSCs in favor of the osteoblast lineage by decreasing peroxisome proliferator-activated receptor-γ and increasing osteogenic markers such as ALP and bone morphogenetic protein-2 [54].

Taken together, these findings suggest that the AGE-RAGE-oxidative stress system could contribute to exhaustion of MSCs and loss of their differentiation potential to bone, thereby increasing the risk for osteoporosis in diabetes (Fig. 5.3).

5.7 AGE-RAGE Axis and Bone Quality

In vitro glycation of human tibial cancellous bone cores increased the microdamage and reduced the fracture resistance [55]. AGE-modified collagen impaired lysyl oxidase enzyme-dependent physiological collagen cross-links both in primary nondifferentiated and in differentiating mouse and rat osteoblast cells via blocking the binding of collagen to discoidin domain receptor-2 [56]. AGEs accumulation in

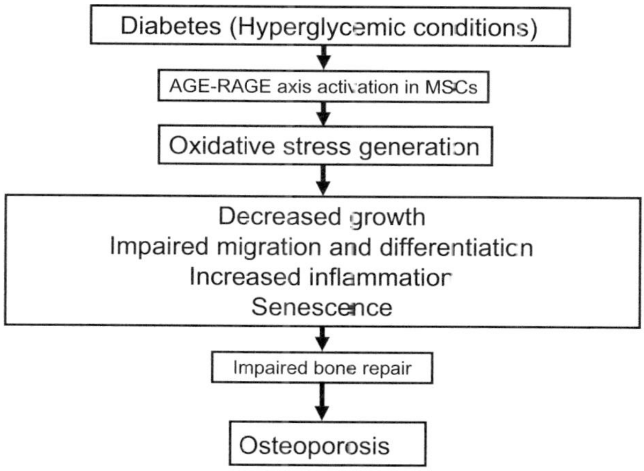

Fig. 5.3 Effects of the AGE-RAGE axis on MSCs

the bone also suppressed lysyl oxidase and induced bone collagen degradation in a rat model of renal osteodystrophy [57]. Further, in other animal models, despite the lack of reduction in BMD, bone mechanical properties were impaired in spontaneously diabetic WBN/Kob rats, which were coincided with decreased enzymatic cross-link formation and increased pentosidine level in the bone collagen [58]. Using a high-resolution nonlinear finite element model that incorporates cohesive elements and micro-computed tomography-based 3D meshes, Tang et al. reported that age-related increase in bone porosity and AGEs resulted in an 88 % reduction in propagation toughness [59]. Moreover, trabecular pentosidine in human vertebrae was significantly associated with whole bone strength [60]. In addition, the intensity of staining of AGEs in bone specimens of osteoporotic subjects was correlated with patient age and inversely associated with the percentage of bone surface covered with osteoblasts [61]. Vitamin C transporter expression in the type 1 diabetic mouse bone and bone marrow was suppressed which was accompanied with decreased bone formation and lower bone quality in these animals [62]. These observations suggest that mechanical integrity of the collagen network in the bone might deteriorate with diabetes and/or age due to enhanced accumulation of bone AGEs and increased oxidative stress, being involved in osteoporosis in these subjects.

5.8 Serum and Urinary Level of AGEs as a Biomarker of Osteoporosis

Serum pentosidine level was significantly increased in postmenopausal type 2 diabetic women with vertebral fractures compared with those without fractures [63]. In the same study, serum pentosidine level was also associated with the presence of vertebral fractures independent of BMD, risk factors for osteoporosis, diabetic status, and renal function [63]. Hein et al. have reported that the osteoporosis group has significantly higher serum concentrations of pentosidine and CML than healthy subjects [64]. In subgroups characterized by increased bone resorption, serum pentosidine was correlated significantly with histomorphometric marker reflecting osteoclast activity and bone resorption [64]. Shiraki et al. showed that urinary pentosidine level was correlated with time-dependent incidence of vertebral fractures in elder women who were not receiving any drug treatment for osteoporosis, whose association was totally independent of the traditional risk factors for osteoporosis [65]. When examining the relationship between baseline characteristics and incident vertebral fracture in Japanese osteoporosis patients undergoing bisphosphonate treatment, they also found that patients who developed incident vertebral fractures were older and had lower lumbar spine BMD, a higher prevalent vertebral fracture number, and higher urinary pentosidine level than patients who did not develop vertebral fractures [66]. In the Cox's proportional hazard model, higher baseline urinary excretion level of pentosidine was one of the independent predictors of the incident vertebral fracture in these subjects [66]. Moreover, Schwartz et al. reported that elevation in urinary pentosidine level was independently associated with both increased clinical fracture incidence and vertebral fracture prevalence in elderly patients with type 2 diabetes [67].

Serum level of endogenous secretory RAGE (esRAGE)-to-pentosidine ratio in type 2 diabetic patients with vertebral fractures was significantly lower than in those without vertebral fractures [68]. Multivariate logistic regression analysis adjusted for age, serum creatinine, duration of diabetes, therapeutic agents, osteoporotic risk factors, and lumbar BMD showed that both low serum level of esRAGE and decreased esRAGE-to-pentosidine ratio were independently associated with the prevalence of vertebral fractures in patients with type 2 diabetes as well [68]. These findings suggest that serum esRAGE level and esRAGE-to-pentosidine ratio might be a more useful biomarker than BMD for assessing the risk of vertebral fractures in type 2 diabetic patients. Bone quality is more important than BMD in defining the increased risk for osteoporotic bone fractures in type 2 diabetic patients [17–19]. Furthermore, since the AGE-RAGE system plays a role in impaired bone quality in type 2 diabetic subjects [47], the authors speculated that an insufficient amount of esRAGE to counteract AGEs could intensify the binding of AGEs to RAGE and resultantly exert harmful effects on bones, thereby being involved in the increased risk of vertebral fractures in their patients. However, soluble form of RAGE (sRAGE) can be generated both from proteolytic cleavage of cell membrane surface full-length RAGE by sheddase and novel splice variants of RAGE [69, 70]. Circulating sRAGE in humans is mainly derived from the cleavage of membrane-bound RAGE, whereas esRAGE is one of the C-truncated splice isoforms of RAGE and only constitutes small part of endogenous sRAGE [69, 70]. Moreover, since interaction of RAGE with the ligands such as AGEs and HMGB1 promotes the RAGE shedding [70], it is conceivable that sRAGE level could correlate with high levels of ongoing inflammation in diabetes. Therefore, although exogenously administered high amounts of sRAGE were shown to block the harmful effects of AGEs in animals by acting as a decoy receptor [71, 72], it is questionable that esRAGE may also exert the same biological effects in humans. Serum concentration of esRAGE in humans is about 5,000 times lower than needed for the binding to and efficiently eliminating circulating AGEs [69, 73]. Taken together, decreased level of esRAGE may be associated with the prevalence of vertebral fractures in type 2 diabetes in unknown mechanisms other than working as a decoy receptor for AGEs. Since we and others have recently found that sRAGE levels are independently and inversely associated with HMGB1 level in an apparently healthy population and that sRAGE is absent and HMGB1 level is higher in diabetic RAGE$^{-/-}$/apoE$^{-/-}$ mice [74, 75], esRAGE might protect against vertebral fractures by working as a decoy receptor for circulating HMGB1. Binding affinity of HMGB1 to RAGE is ten times higher than that of AGEs, whereas serum concentration of HMGB1 is 1,000 times less than that of AGEs [69, 74, 75], thus supporting the concept that circulating HMGB1 *but not* AGEs might be a molecular target for esRAGE in diabetic patients with osteoporosis.

In a cross-sectional study, 128 men and premenopausal women with type 1 diabetes, individuals with bone fractures had higher pentosidine level compared to those without fractures, while there was no significant difference of CML and esRAGE values between the two groups [76]. Moreover, multivariate logistic regression analysis revealed that the pentosidine level but not BMD was independently associated with prevalent fractures [76]. These findings suggest that osteoporotic bone fractures could result from impaired bone quality due to accumulation of pentosidine in the bone, which was unrelated with decreased esRAGE levels.

5.9 Other Biomarkers

As discussed above, oxidative stress or low levels of antioxidants are supposed to reduce BMD and cause osteoporosis in diabetic patients. An imbalance between natural antioxidative and oxidative markers was observed in patients with osteoporosis [77, 78]. Plasma total homocysteine level was higher in postmenopausal diabetes women with osteoporosis than those without osteoporosis [77]. BMD was closely correlated with homocysteine value in these subjects [78]. Homocysteine level was also shown to be inversely correlated with BMD and with both dietary intake and serum concentration of folate in Japanese type 2 diabetic patients, thus suggesting that nutritional status of folate might affect the homocysteine level, a putative risk factor for osteoporosis [78]. Furthermore, Kuyumcu et al. reported that higher serum uric acid and albumin levels were associated with a lower prevalence of osteoporosis, whereas higher homocysteine level was correlated with lower BMD and higher osteoporosis prevalence [79]. Increased uric acid levels were also associated with higher lumbar spine BMD in peri- and postmenopausal Japanese women [80].

5.10 Bisphosphonates

Bisphosphonates are a potent inhibitor of bone resorption and are one of the most widely used drugs for treatment of osteoporosis [81]. Farnesyl pyrophosphate synthase has been shown to be as a molecular target of nitrogen-containing bisphosphonates, and inhibition of posttranslational prenylation of small molecular weight G proteins is likely involved in their antiresorptive activity on osteoclasts [82, 83]. Since AGEs exert various biological actions on a variety of cells through RAGE-mediated, NADPH oxidase-induced ROS generation and subsequent NF-κB activation via Ras-MAPK pathway [84–86], it is conceivable that nitrogen-containing bisphosphonates might have pleiotropic properties by blocking farnesylation of small G proteins, which serve as lipid attachments for a variety of intracellular signaling molecules. Indeed, we have previously found that minodronate, a nitrogen-containing bisphosphonate, inhibits the AGE-induced vascular cell adhesion molecule-1 expression in endothelial cells by suppressing ROS generation via suppression of geranylgeranylation of Rac, a component of endothelial NADPH oxidase [86]. Incadronate also reverted the angiogenic activity of AGEs in endothelial cells by suppressing the RAGE-downstream signaling [85]. Moreover, AGEs significantly decreased osteoblast proliferation, ALP activity, and type 1 collagen production while increasing osteoblastic apoptosis and ROS production, all of which were completely reverted by low doses of bisphosphonates [87]. Bisphosphonates may block the deleterious actions of AGEs on osteoblastic cells via Ca(2+) influx, because the L-type calcium channel blocker, nifedipine, has been shown to inhibit the effects of bisphosphonates on AGE-exposed osteoblasts [87]. These findings could suggest a novel beneficial aspect of bisphosphonates on osteoporosis; bisphosphonates could protect against the AGE-induced bone loss partly by suppressing the RAGE-downstream signaling pathways in osteoblasts via inhibition of NADPH oxidase-mediated ROS generation.

However, it should be mentioned that 1 year of high-dose bisphosphonate therapy in dogs allowed the increased accumulation of AGEs and reduced postyield work-to-fracture of the cortical bone matrix [88]. Furthermore, pentosidine contents were increased following 3-year treatment with incadronate in dogs [89]. These observations suggest that long-term use of bisphosphonates might impair physiological bone remodeling, which could lead to an increase in nonenzymatic cross-linking in the bone, thereby altering bone matrix quality and being involved in bisphosphonate-related atypical femoral fractures [90]. AGEs disrupted the osteoblastic actin cytoskeleton and altered the cell morphology with a decrease in cell-substratum interactions, thereby causing apoptotic cell death of osteoblasts, all of which was deteriorated by the treatment with high concentration of alendronate [91].

5.11 Selective Estrogen Receptor Modulator (SERM)

Raloxifene, one of the widely used SERMs, which has estrogen-like effects on bone and "antiestrogen effects" on other tissues, has been in development for osteoporosis prevention and treatment in postmenopausal women [92]. Raloxifene has been shown to ameliorate detrimental enzymatic and nonenzymatic collagen cross-links and bone strength in rabbits with hyperhomocysteinemia [93]. ROS-activated FoxOs in early mesenchymal progenitor cells inhibited the Wnt signaling pathways, thereby impairing the osteoblastogenesis, which was prevented by estrogen [94]. Further, we have very recently found that bazedoxifene could inhibit the AGE-RAGE-induced endothelial cell damage through its antioxidative properties (unpublished data). Pullerits et al. reported that postmenopausal rheumatoid arthritis patients receiving hormone replacement therapy (estradiol plus norethisterone acetate) displayed significantly decreased serum level of sRAGE, which was associated with the elevation in serum estradiol [95]. They also found that sRAGE level at baseline was correlated with bone/cartilage turnover markers. The decrease of sRAGE level after hormone replacement therapy paralleled with diminished concentration of the markers and was correlated with an increase in total BMD in these subjects [95]. These findings further support the concept that sRAGE might be a biomarker that could reflect tissue RAGE expression in the bone and that hormone replacement therapy could exert beneficial effects on bone metabolism in postmenopausal rheumatoid arthritis patients by inhibiting the AGE-RAGE-oxidative stress axis in the bone.

5.12 Parathyroid Hormone (PTH)

Panuccio et al. reported that plasma pentosidine level was inversely related with circulating PTH and bone ALP value in hemodialysis patients [96]. The observations could suggest that AGEs accumulation may be a factor involved in low bone turnover in dialysis patients. Human PTH(1–34) treatments for 18 months were shown to increase bone volume and trabecular thickness and to decrease pentosidine level in an ovariectomized primate model [97]. Administration of human PTH(1–34) is a promising strategy for the treatment of osteoporosis; it not only increases BMD but also may improve bone quality by reducing the accumulation of AGEs in the bone of postmenopausal women.

5.13 Vitamin D

AGEs suppressed the differentiation osteoblasts via osteoglycin production from the myoblasts, which was prevented by 1α-25-dihydroxyvitamin D3 [98].

5.14 Conclusions

Inhibition of the AGEs formation in the bone matrix and blockade of the AGE-RAGE-oxidative stress system among osteoblasts, osteoclasts, and MSCs may be novel therapeutic strategies for preventing osteoporotic bone fractures in diabetes.

Acknowledgments This work was supported in part by Grants-in-Aid for Scientific Research (B) from the Ministry of Education, Culture, Sports, Science, and Technology of Japan. No potential conflicts of interest relevant to this article were reported.

References

1. Osteoporosis Prevention, Diagnosis and Therapy: NIH Consensus Statement (2000)17:1–36. http://consensus.nih.gov/2000/2000Osteoporosis111html.htm
2. Rachner TD, Khosla S, Hofbauer LC (2011) Osteoporosis: now and the future. Lancet 377:1276–1287
3. Chiang CH, Liu CJ, Chen PJ, Huang CC, Hsu CY, Chen ZY, Chan WL, Huang PH, Chen TJ, Chung CM, Lin SJ, Chen JW, Leu HB (2013) Hip fracture and risk of acute myocardial infarction: a nationwide study. J Bone Miner Res 28:404–411
4. Koh GC, Tai BC, Ang LW, Heng D, Yuan JM, Koh WP (2013) All-cause and cause-specific mortality after hip fracture among Chinese women and men: the Singapore Chinese health study. Osteoporos Int 24:1981–1989
5. Drake MT, Murad MH, Mauck KF, Lane MA, Undavalli C, Elraiyah T, Stuart LM, Prasad C, Shahrour A, Mullan RJ, Hazem A, Erwin PJ, Montori VM (2012) Clinical review. Risk factors for low bone mass-related fractures in men: a systematic review and meta-analysis. J Clin Endocrinol Metab 97:1861–1870
6. Merlotti D, Gennari L, Dotta F, Lauro D, Nuti R (2010) Mechanisms of impaired bone strength in type 1 and 2 diabetes. Nutr Metab Cardiovasc Dis 20:683–690
7. Kurra S, Siris E (2011) Diabetes and bone health: the relationship between diabetes and osteoporosis-associated fractures. Diabetes Metab Res Rev 27:430–435
8. Vestergaard P (2007) Discrepancies in bone mineral density and fracture risk in patients with type 1 and type 2 diabetes – a meta-analysis. Osteoporos Int 18:427–444
9. Hofbauer LC, Brueck CC, Singh SK, Dobnig H (2007) Osteoporosis in patients with diabetes mellitus. J Bone Miner Res 22:1317–1328
10. Pietschmann P, Patsch JM, Schernthaner G (2010) Diabetes and bone. Horm Metab Res 42:763–768
11. Isidro ML, Ruano B (2010) Bone disease in diabetes. Curr Diabetes Rev 6:144–155
12. De Liefde II, van der Klift M, de Laet CE, van Daele PL, Hofman A, Pols HA (2005) Bone mineral density and fracture risk in type-2 diabetes mellitus: the Rotterdam study. Osteoporos Int 16:1713–1720
13. Brownlee M, Cerami A, Vlassara H (1988) Advanced glycosylation end products in tissue and the biochemical basis of diabetic complications. N Engl J Med 318:1315–1321
14. Vlassara H, Palace MR (2002) Diabetes and advanced glycation endproducts. J Intern Med 251:87–101
15. Yamagishi S, Imaizumi T (2005) Diabetic vascular complications: pathophysiology, biochemical basis and potential therapeutic strategy. Curr Pharm Des 11:2279–2299
16. Dyer DG, Blackledge JA, Thorpe SR, Baynes JW (1991) Formation of pentosidine during nonenzymatic browning of proteins by glucose. Identification of glucose and other carbohydrates as possible precursors of pentosidine in vivo. J Biol Chem 266:11654–11660

17. Hein GE (2006) Glycation endproducts in osteoporosis – is there a pathophysiologic importance? Clin Chim Acta 371:32–36
18. Odetti P, Rossi S, Monacelli F, Poggi A, Cirnigliaro M, Federici M, Federici A (2005) Advanced glycation end products and bone loss during aging. Ann N Y Acad Sci 1043:710–717
19. Saito M, Marumo K (2010) Collagen cross-links as a determinant of bone quality: a possible explanation for bone fragility in aging, osteoporosis, and diabetes mellitus. Osteoporos Int 21:195–214
20. Yamagishi S (2011) Role of advanced glycation end products (AGEs) and receptor for AGEs (RAGE) in vascular damage in diabetes. Exp Gerontol 46:217–224
21. Stern D, Yan SD, Yan SF, Schmidt AM (2002) Receptor for advanced glycation endproducts: a multiligand receptor magnifying cell stress in diverse pathologic settings. Adv Drug Deliv Rev 54:1615–1625
22. Bierhaus A, Hofmann MA, Ziegler R, Nawroth PP (1998) AGEs and their interaction with AGE-receptors in vascular disease and diabetes mellitus. I. The AGE concept. Cardiovasc Res 37:586–600
23. Yamagishi S, Matsui T (2010) Smooth muscle cell pathophysiology and advanced glycation end products (AGEs). Curr Drug Targets 11:875–881
24. Yamagishi S (2012) Potential clinical utility of advanced glycation end product cross-link breakers in age- and diabetes-associated disorders. Rejuvenation Res 15:564–572
25. Yamagishi S, Nakamura K, Inoue H (2005) Possible participation of advanced glycation end products in the pathogenesis of osteoporosis in diabetic patients. Med Hypotheses 65:1013–1015
26. Mercer N, Ahmed H, Etcheverry SB, Vasta GR, Cortizo AM (2007) Regulation of advanced glycation end product (AGE) receptors and apoptosis by AGEs in osteoblast-like cells. Mol Cell Biochem 306:87–94
27. Schurman L, McCarthy AD, Sedlinsky C, Gangoiti MV, Arnol V, Bruzzone L, Cortizo AM (2008) Metformin reverts deleterious effects of advanced glycation end-products (AGEs) on osteoblastic cells. Exp Clin Endocrinol Diabetes 116:333–340
28. Alikhani M, Alikhani Z, Boyd C, MacLellan CM, Raptis M, Liu R, Pischon N, Trackman PC, Gerstenfeld L, Graves DT (2007) Advanced glycation end products stimulate osteoblast apoptosis via the MAP kinase and cytosolic apoptotic pathways. Bone 40:345–353
29. Suh KS, Choi EM, Rhee SY, Kim YS (2014) Methylglyoxal induces oxidative stress and mitochondrial dysfunction in osteoblastic MC3T3-E1 cells. Free Radic Res 48:206–217
30. Choi EM, Suh KS, Rhee SY, Kim YS (2014) Sciadopitysin alleviates methylglyoxal-mediated glycation in osteoblastic MC3T3-E1 cells by enhancing glyoxalase system and mitochondrial biogenesis. Free Radic Res 48:729–739
31. Suh KS, Rhee SY, Kim YS, Choi EM (2014) Inhibitory effect of apocynin on methylglyoxal-mediated glycation in osteoblastic MC3T3-E1 cells. J Appl Toxicol. doi:10.1002/jat.3016
32. Katayama Y, Akatsu T, Yamamoto M, Kugai N, Nagata N (1996) Role of nonenzymatic glycosylation of type I collagen in diabetic osteopenia. J Bone Miner Res 11:931–937
33. Katayama Y, Celic S, Nagata N, Martin TJ, Findlay DM (1997) Nonenzymatic glycation of type I collagen modifies interaction with UMR 201-10B preosteoblastic cells. Bone 21:237–242
34. McCarthy AD, Etcheverry SB, Bruzzone L, Lettieri G, Barrio DA, Cortizo AM (2001) Non-enzymatic glycosylation of a type I collagen matrix: effects on osteoblastic development and oxidative stress. BMC Cell Biol 2:16
35. McCarthy AD, Uemura T, Etcheverry SB, Cortizo AM (2004) Advanced glycation endproducts interefere with integrin-mediated osteoblastic attachment to a type-I collagen matrix. Int J Biochem Cell Biol 36:840–848
36. Li G, Xu J, Li Z (2012) Receptor for advanced glycation end products inhibits proliferation in osteoblast through suppression of Wnt, PI3K and ERK signaling. Biochem Biophys Res Commun 423:684–689

37. Sanguineti R, Storace D, Monacelli F, Federici A, Odetti P (2008) Pentosidine effects on human osteoblasts in vitro. Ann N Y Acad Sci 1126:166–172
38. McCarthy AD, Cortizo AM, Giménez Segura G, Bruzzone L, Etcheverry SB (1998) Non-enzymatic glycosylation of alkaline phosphatase alters its biological properties. Mol Cell Biochem 181:63–69
39. Miyata T, Notoya K, Yoshida K, Horie K, Maeda K, Kurokawa K, Taketomi S (1997) Advanced glycation end products enhance osteoclast-induced bone resorption in cultured mouse unfractionated bone cells and in rats implanted subcutaneously with devitalized bone particles. J Am Soc Nephrol 8:260–270
40. Dong XN, Qin A, Xu J, Wang X (2011) In situ accumulation of advanced glycation endproducts (AGEs) in bone matrix and its correlation with osteoclastic bone resorption. Bone 49:174–183
41. Valcourt U, Merle B, Gineyts E, Viguet-Carrin S, Delmas PD, Garnero P (2007) Non-enzymatic glycation of bone collagen modifies osteoclastic activity and differentiation. J Biol Chem 282:5691–5703
42. Zhou Z, Immel D, Xi CX, Bierhaus A, Feng X, Mei L, Nawroth P, Stern DM, Xiong WC (2006) Regulation of osteoclast function and bone mass by RAGE. J Exp Med 203:1067–1080
43. Ding KH, Wang ZZ, Hamrick MW, Deng ZB, Zhou L, Kang B, Yan SL, She JX, Stern DM, Isales CM, Mi QS (2006) Disordered osteoclast formation in RAGE-deficient mouse establishes an essential role for RAGE in diabetes related bone loss. Biochem Biophys Res Commun 340:1091–1097
44. Franke S, Siggelkow H, Wolf G, Hein G (2007) Advanced glycation endproducts influence the mRNA expression of RAGE, RANKL and various osteoblastic genes in human osteoblasts. Arch Physiol Biochem 113:154–161
45. Kobayashi Y, Udagawa N, Takahashi N (2009) Action of RANKL and OPG for osteoclastogenesis. Crit Rev Eukaryot Gene Expr 19:61–72
46. Zhou Z, Han JY, Xi CX, Xie JX, Feng X, Wang CY, Mei L, Xiong WC (2008) HMGB1 regulates RANKL-induced osteoclastogenesis in a manner dependent on RAGE. J Bone Miner Res 23:1084–1096
47. Yamagishi S (2011) Role of advanced glycation end products (AGEs) in osteoporosis in diabetes. Curr Drug Targets 12:2096–2102
48. Yang K, Wang XQ, He YS, Lu L, Chen QJ, Liu J, Shen WF (2010) Advanced glycation end products induce chemokine/cytokine production via activation of p38 pathway and inhibit proliferation and migration of bone marrow mesenchymal stem cells. Cardiovasc Diabetol 9:66
49. Stolzing A, Sellers D, Llewelyn O, Scutt A (2010) Diabetes induced changes in rat mesenchymal stem cells. Cells Tissues Organs 191:453–465
50. Larsen SA, Kassem M, Rattan SI (2012) Glucose metabolite glyoxal induces senescence in telomerase-immortalized human mesenchymal stem cells. Chem Cent J 6:18
51. Okazaki K, Yamaguchi T, Tanaka K, Notsu M, Ogawa N, Yano S, Sugimoto T (2012) Advanced glycation end products (AGEs), but not high glucose, inhibit the osteoblastic differentiation of mouse stromal ST2 cells through the suppression of osterix expression, and inhibit cell growth and increasing cell apoptosis. Calcif Tissue Int 91:286–296
52. Mori K, Kitazawa R, Kondo T, Mori M, Hamada Y, Nishida M, Minami Y, Haraguchi R, Takahashi Y, Kitazawa S (2014) Diabetic osteopenia by decreased β-catenin signaling is partly induced by epigenetic derepression of sFRP-4 gene. PLoS One 9:e102797
53. Kume S, Kato S, Yamagishi S et al (2005) Advanced glycation end-products attenuate human mesenchymal stem cells and prevent cognate differentiation into adipose tissue, cartilage, and bone. J Bone Miner Res 20:1647–1658
54. Vanella L, Sanford C Jr, Kim DH, Abraham NG, Ebraheim N (2012) Oxidative stress and heme oxygenase-1 regulated human mesenchymal stem cells differentiation. Int J Hypertens 2012:890671

55. Tang SY, Vashishth D (2010) Non-enzymatic glycation alters microdamage formation in human cancellous bone. Bone 46:148–154
56. Khosravi R, Sodek KL, Faibish M, Trackman PC (2014) Collagen advanced glycation inhibits its discoidin domain receptor 2 (DDR2)-mediated induction of lysyl oxidase in osteoblasts. Bone 58:33–41
57. Aoki C, Uto K, Honda K, Kato Y, Oda H (2013) Advanced glycation end products suppress lysyl oxidase and induce bone collagen degradation in a rat model of renal osteodystrophy. Lab Invest 93:1170–1183
58. Saito M, Fujii K, Mori Y, Marumo K (2006) Role of collagen enzymatic and glycation induced cross-links as a determinant of bone quality in spontaneously diabetic WBN/Kob rats. Osteoporos Int 17:1514–1523
59. Tang SY, Vashishth D (2011) The relative contributions of non-enzymatic glycation and cortical porosity on the fracture toughness of aging bone. J Biomech 44:330–336
60. Viguet-Carrin S, Roux JP, Arlot ME, Merabet Z, Leeming DJ, Byrjalsen I, Delmas PD, Bouxsein ML (2006) Contribution of the advanced glycation end product pentosidine and of maturation of type I collagen to compressive biomechanical properties of human lumbar vertebrae. Bone 39:1073–1079
61. Hein G, Weiss C, Lehmann G, Niwa T, Stein G, Franke S (2006) Advanced glycation end product modification of bone proteins and bone remodelling: hypothesis and preliminary immunohistochemical findings. Ann Rheum Dis 65:101–104
62. Sangani R, Naime M, Zakhary I, Ahmad S, Chutkan N, Zhu A, Ha Y, Hamrick M, Isales C, Elsalanty M, Smith S, Liou GI, Fulzele S (2013) Regulation of vitamin C transporter in the type 1 diabetic mouse bone and bone marrow. Exp Mol Pathol 95:298–306
63. Yamamoto M, Yamaguchi T, Yamauchi M, Yano S, Sugimoto T (2008) Serum pentosidine levels are positively associated with the presence of vertebral fractures in postmenopausal women with type 2 diabetes. J Clin Endocrinol Metab 93:1013–1019
64. Hein G, Wiegand R, Lehmann G, Stein G, Franke S (2003) Advanced glycation end-products pentosidine and N epsilon-carboxymethyllysine are elevated in serum of patients with osteoporosis. Rheumatology (Oxford) 42:1242–1246
65. Shiraki M, Kuroda T, Tanaka S, Saito M, Fukunaga M, Nakamura T (2008) Nonenzymatic collagen cross-links induced by glycoxidation (pentosidine) predicts vertebral fractures. J Bone Miner Metab 26:93–100
66. Shiraki M, Kuroda T, Shiraki Y, Tanaka S, Higuchi T, Saito M (2011) Urinary pentosidine and plasma homocysteine levels at baseline predict future fractures in osteoporosis patients under bisphosphonate treatment. J Bone Miner Metab 29:62–70
67. Schwartz AV, Garnero P, Hillier TA, Sellmeyer DE, Strotmeyer ES, Feingold KR, Resnick HE, Tylavsky FA, Black DM, Cummings SR, Harris TB, Bauer DC (2009) Health, aging, and body composition study. Pentosidine and increased fracture risk in older adults with type 2 diabetes. J Clin Endocrinol Metab 94:2380–2386
68. Yamamoto M, Yamaguchi T, Yamauchi M, Sugimoto T (2009) Low serum level of the endogenous secretory receptor for advanced glycation end products (esRAGE) is a risk factor for prevalent vertebral fractures independent of bone mineral density in patients with type 2 diabetes. Diabetes Care 32:2263–2268
69. Yamagishi S, Matsui T, Nakamura K (2007) Kinetics, role and therapeutic implications of endogenous soluble form of receptor for advanced glycation end products (sRAGE) in diabetes. Curr Drug Targets 8:1138–1143
70. Raucci A, Cugusi S, Antonelli A, Barabino SM, Monti L, Bierhaus A, Reiss K, Saftig P, Bianchi ME (2008) A soluble form of the receptor for advanced glycation endproducts (RAGE) is produced by proteolytic cleavage of the membrane-bound form by the sheddase a disintegrin and metalloprotease 10 (ADAM10). FASEB J 22:3716–3727
71. Park L, Raman KG, Lee KJ, Lu Y, Ferran LJ Jr, Chow WS Stern D, Schmidt AM (1998) Suppression of accelerated diabetic atherosclerosis by the soluble receptor for advanced glycation endproducts. Nat Med 4:1025–1031

72. Bucciarelli LG, Wendt T, Qu W, Lu Y, Lalla E, Rong LL, Goova MT, Moser B, Kislinger T, Lee DC, Kashyap Y, Stern DM, Schmidt AM (2002) RAGE blockade stabilizes established atherosclerosis in diabetic apolipoprotein E-null mice. Circulation 106:2827–2835
73. Humpert PM, Djuric Z, Kopf S, Rudofsky G, Morcos M, Nawroth PP, Bierhaus A (2007) Soluble RAGE but not endogenous secretory RAGE is associated with albuminuria in patients with type 2 diabetes. Cardiovasc Diabetol 6:9
74. Fukami A, Adachi H, Yamagishi S, Matsui T, Ueda S, Nakamura K, Enomoto M, Otsuka M, Kumagae S, Nanjo Y, Kumagai E, Esaki E, Murayama K, Hirai Y, Imaizumi T (2009) Factors associated with serum high mobility group box 1 (HMGB1) levels in a general population. Metabolism 58:1688–1693
75. Soro-Paavonen A, Watson AM, Li J, Paavonen K, Koitka A, Calkin AC, Barit D, Coughlan MT, Drew BG, Lancaster GI, Thomas M, Forbes JM, Nawroth PP, Bierhaus A, Cooper ME, Jandeleit-Dahm KA (2008) Receptor for advanced glycation end products (RAGE) deficiency attenuates the development of atherosclerosis in diabetes. Diabetes 57:2461–2469
76. Neumann T, Lodes S, Kästner B, Franke S, Kiehntopf M, Lehmann T, Müller UA, Wolf G, Sämann A (2014) High serum pentosidine but not esRAGE is associated with prevalent fractures in type 1 diabetes independent of bone mineral density and glycaemic control. Osteoporos Int 25:1527–1533
77. Jianbo L, Zhang H, Yan L, Xie M, Mei Y, Jiawei C (2013) Homocysteine, an additional factor, is linked to osteoporosis in postmenopausal women with type 2 diabetes. J Bone Miner Metab. doi:10.1007/s00774-013-0548-4
78. Yamada C, Fujimoto S, Ikeda K, Nomura Y, Matsubara A, Kanno M, Shide K, Tanaka K, Imai E, Fukuwatari T, Shibata K, Inagaki N (2011) Relationship of homocysteine and homocysteine-related vitamins to bone mineral density in Japanese patients with type 2 diabetes. J Diabetes Invest 2:233–239
79. Kuyumcu ME, Yesil Y, Oztürk ZA, Cınar E, Kızılarslanoglu C, Halil M, Ulger Z, Yesil NK, Cankurtaran M, Arıoğul S (2012) The association between homocysteine (hcy) and serum natural antioxidants in elderly bone mineral densitometry (BMD). Arch Gerontol Geriatr 55:739–743
80. Ishii S, Miyao M, Mizuno Y, Tanaka-Ishikawa M, Akishita M, Ouchi Y (2014) Association between serum uric acid and lumbar spine bone mineral density in peri- and postmenopausal Japanese women. Osteoporos Int 25:1099–1105
81. Brown DL, Robbins R (1999) Developments in the therapeutic applications of bisphosphonates. J Clin Pharmacol 39:651–660
82. Van Beek E, Pieterman E, Cohen L, Lowik C, Papapoulos S (1999) Farnesyl pyrophosphate synthase is the molecular target of nitrogen-containing bisphosphonates. Biochem Biophys Res Commun 264:108–111
83. Yamagishi S, Abe R, Inagaki Y (2004) Minodronate, a newly developed nitrogen-containing bisphosphonate, suppresses melanoma growth and improves survival in nude mice by blocking vascular endothelial growth factor signaling. Am J Pathol 165:1865–1874
84. Okamoto T, Yamagishi S, Inagaki Y, Amano S, Koga K, Abe R, Takeuchi M, Ohno S, Yoshimura A, Makita Z (2002) Angiogenesis induced by advanced glycation end products and its prevention by cerivastatin. FASEB J 16:1928–1930
85. Okamoto T, Yamagishi S, Inagaki Y, Amano S, Takeuchi M, Kikuchi S, Ohno S, Yoshimura A (2002) Incadronate disodium inhibits advanced glycation end products-induced angiogenesis in vitro. Biochem Biophys Res Commun 297:419–424
86. Yamagishi S, Matsui T, Nakamura K, Takeuchi M (2005) Minodronate, a nitrogen-containing bisphosphonate, inhibits advanced glycation end product-induced vascular cell adhesion molecule-1 expression in endothelial cells by suppressing reactive oxygen species generation. Int J Tissue React 27:189–195
87. Gangoiti MV, Cortizo AM, Arnol V, Felice JI, McCarthy AD (2008) Opposing effects of bisphosphonates and advanced glycation end-products on osteoblastic cells. Eur J Pharmacol 600:140–147

88. Tang SY, Allen MR, Phipps R, Burr DB, Vashishth D (2009) Changes in non-enzymatic glycation and its association with altered mechanical properties following 1-year treatment with risedronate or alendronate. Osteoporos Int 20:887–894
89. Saito M, Mori S, Mashiba T, Komatsubara S, Marumo K (2008) Collagen maturity, glycation induced-pentosidine, and mineralization are increased following 3-year treatment with incadronate in dogs. Osteoporos Int 19:1343–1354
90. Shane E, Burr D, Ebeling PR, Abrahamsen B, Adler RA, Brown TD, Cheung AM, Cosman F, Curtis JR, Dell R, Dempster D, Einhorn TA, Genant HK, Geusens P, Klaushofer K, Koval K, Lane JM, McKiernan F, McKinney R, Ng A, Nieves J, O'Keefe R, Papapoulos S, Sen HT, van der Meulen MC, Weinstein RS, Whyte M, American Society for Bone and Mineral Research (2010) Atypical subtrochanteric and diaphyseal femoral fractures: report of a task force of the American Society for Bone and Mineral Research. J Bone Miner Res 25:2267–2294
91. Gangoiti MV, Anbinder PS, Cortizo AM, McCarthy AD (2013) Morphological changes induced by advanced glycation endproducts in osteoblastic cells: effects of co-incubation with alendronate. Acta Histochem 115:649–657
92. Silverman SL (2010) New selective estrogen receptor modulators (SERMs) in development. Curr Osteoporos Rep 8:151–153
93. Magnolagas SC (2010) From estrogen-centric to aging and oxidative stress: a revised perspective of the pathogenesis of osteoporosis. Endocr Rev 31:266–300
94. Saito M, Marumo K, Soshi S, Kida Y, Ushiku C, Shinohara A (2010) Raloxifene ameliorates detrimental enzymatic and nonenzymatic collagen cross-links and bone strength in rabbits with hyperhomocysteinemia. Osteoporos Int 21:655–666
95. Pullerits R, d'Elia HF, Tarkowski A, Carlsten H (2009) The decrease of soluble RAGE levels in rheumatoid arthritis patients following hormone replacement therapy is associated with increased bone mineral density and diminished bone/cartilage turnover: a randomized controlled trial. Rheumatology (Oxford) 48:785–790
96. Panuccio V, Mallamaci F, Tripepi G, Parlongo S, Cutrupi S, Asahi K, Miyata T, Zoccali C (2002) Low parathyroid hormone and pentosidine in hemodialysis patients. Am J Kidney Dis 40:810–815
97. Saito M, Marumo K, Kida Y, Ushiku C, Kato S, Takao-Kawabata R, Kuroda T (2011) Changes in the contents of enzymatic immature, mature, and non-enzymatic senescent cross-links of collagen after once-weekly treatment with human parathyroid hormone (1–34) for 18 months contribute to improvement of bone strength in ovariectomized monkeys. Osteoporos Int 22:2373–2383
98. Tanaka K, Kanazawa I, Yamaguchi T, Yano S, Kaji H, Sugimoto T (2014) Active vitamin D possesses beneficial effects on the interaction between muscle and bone. Biochem Biophys Res Commun 450:482–487

Chapter 6
Mechanism for the Development of Bone Disease in Diabetes: Renal Bone Disease

Yasuo Imanishi and Masaaki Inaba

Abstract Bone fragility is caused by chronic kidney disease (CKD). Renal osteodystrophy induced by secondary hyperparathyroidism of uremia is considered the main factor for the bone disease. Meanwhile, studies on degeneration of bone quality in CKD have recently advanced, and development of diagnostic and treatment methods is awaited.

Keywords Osteoporosis • Chronic kidney disease (CKD) • Chronic kidney disease-mineral and bone disease (CKD-MBD) • Bone quality

6.1 Introduction

Fragility fracture in osteoporosis may impair the patient's activities of daily living or lead to a bedridden state. As a result, not only is the patient's quality of life substantially lowered, but the patient's life prognosis may also be threatened. At the 2001 Consensus Meeting of the National Institutes of Health in the United States, osteoporosis was defined as a skeletal disorder characterized by compromised bone strength predisposing to an increased risk of fracture [1]. Bone fragility is worsened, and the fracture risk is increased in osteoporosis due to reduced bone mass and lowered bone quality associated with bone microstructure.

In chronic kidney disease-mineral and bone disorder (CKD-MBD), serum calcium (Ca) and phosphate (P) concentrations are important factors in determining prognosis [2]. Regulation of Ca and P concentrations is related to bone fragility caused by secondary hyperparathyroidism of uremia (SHPT) [3] and to cardiovascular death [4].

Diagnosis and management of osteoporosis in patients with CKD stages 1–3 and patients without CKD are similar, but diagnosis and management decisions differ greatly once patients have CKD stages 4–5 [5]. Accordingly, the impaired bone quality as well as CKD-MBD, in addition to the lowered bone density, must be understood and controlled in order to deal with osteoporosis in CKD.

Y. Imanishi, M.D., Ph.D. (✉) • M. Inaba, M.D., Ph.D.
Department of Metabolism, Endocrinology, and Molecular Medicine, Osaka City University Graduate School of Medicine, 1-4-3 Asahi-machi, Abeno-ku, Osaka 545-8585, Japan
e-mail: imanishi@med.osaka-cu.ac.jp

M. Inaba (ed.), *Musculoskeletal Disease Associated with Diabetes Mellitus*,
DOI 10.1007/978-4-431-55720-3_6

6.2 Bone Fragility in Chronic Renal Disease

In addition to osteoporosis, fragility fracture-associated metabolic bone diseases include osteomalacia, osteogenesis imperfecta, fibrocystic osteitis, bone metastasis of malignant tumor, osteopetrosis, and Paget's disease of bone. Renal osteodystrophy (ROD) in CKD-MBD is important because of the large number of patients with ROD.

6.2.1 Renal Osteodystrophy

ROD is a collective term for different bone diseases observed in CKD-MBD. Not only osteoporosis but also fibrocystic osteitis, osteomalacia, aplastic bone disease (aluminum bone disease included), and amyloid bone disease are included in ROD-related diseases that induce bone fragility. Therefore, in cases of advanced CKD, a bone biopsy is sometimes required to confirm the histological type [6]. Bone morphometry-based bone turnover, mineralization, and volume (TMV) classification (Table 6.1) has recently been used for histological classification of ROD and is an important assessment method for ROD [6].

6.2.2 Bone Mineral Density in CKD

According to a survey of 2174 Japanese men age 65 or older, bone density of lumbar spine and femur was negatively correlated to renal function [7]. Furthermore, a meta-analysis of the patients with end-stage renal failure (CKD stage 5) showed that bone density was low in the patients who had previously experienced bone fractures [8], suggesting that bone density measurement may be useful for fracture risk assessment in CKD stage 5. However, the prevalence of fracture in the proximal femur is higher in patients on maintenance hemodialysis (CKD stage 5D), regardless of age or sex, compared with the general public [9], indicating that CKD itself is a factor for bone fragility.

Table 6.1 TMV classification system for renal osteodystrophy [6]

Turnover	Mineralization	Volume
High	Normal	High
Normal	Abnormal	Normal
Low		Low

TMV bone turnover, mineralization, and volume

6.2.3 Residual Renal Function and Bone Fragility

Even in CKD stages 1–3 with mild renal dysfunction, lower renal function has been shown to be a risk for fracture in the proximal femur, after correction for bone density [10]. Accordingly, bone density alone has a limitation in assessing bone fragility in CKD as in the case of diabetes [11].

Fracture prevalence is particularly high in CKD patients with a glomerular filtration rate (GFR) <60 mL/min, and their prevalence has been reported as 2.12 times that of the patients with GFR ≥60 mL/min [12]. Furthermore, as already mentioned (Sect. 6.2.2), maintenance hemodialysis patients with advanced renal dysfunction (CKD stage 5D) have a higher prevalence of proximal femur fracture than the general population, regardless of age or sex [9]. Even in the CKD stage 5D patients on hemodialysis for less than 1 year, their prevalence of proximal femur fracture is higher compared with non-CKD patients, a trend that continues over a long time [13] (Fig. 6.1).

6.2.4 SHPT and Bone Fragility

In CKD stage 5D patients, the prevalence of SHPT associated with a marked increase of parathyroid hormone (PTH) is still high, which is a risk factor for

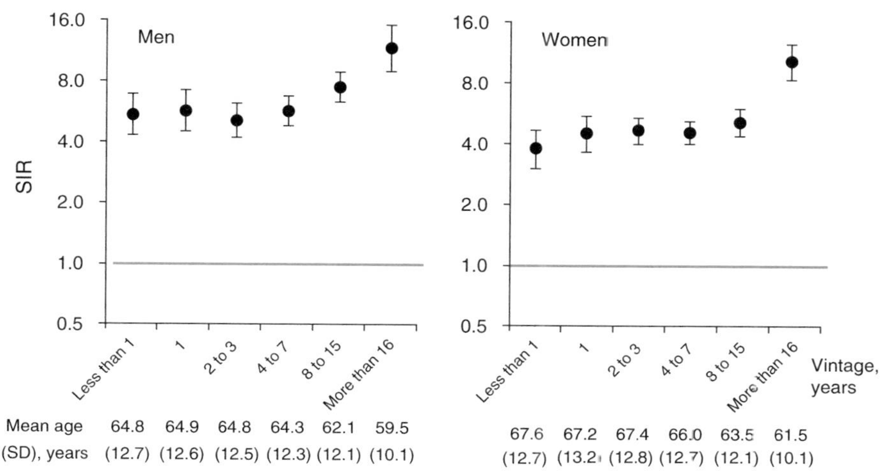

Fig. 6.1 Incidence of proximal femur fracture after introduction of hemodialysis [13]. Standardized incidence ratios (SIRs) stratified by vintage for men and women and standardized for age. *Error bars* indicate 95 % confidence intervals. Less than 1 year after introduction of hemodialysis, SIR was already substantially higher than that of the general public (*horizontal line* set as 1.0 on the y-axis), a trend that continued for 15 years after hemodialysis introduction. At 16 years and beyond, SIRs rapidly increased

fracture. An excessive increase of PTH in SHPT worsens ROD, particularly osteitis fibrosa, increasing the fracture risk [3].

Increased bone turnover in SHPT is considered a factor for bone fragility in CKD [14]. According to a report on cross-sectional examination of bone biopsy specimens of CKD stage 5D patients, bone turnover markers, namely, osteon activation frequency and bone formation rate, are negatively correlated with serum sclerostin and positively correlated with serum intact PTH [15], and this finding is one piece of the evidence for PTH's acceleration of bone turnover.

6.2.5 Bone Quality in CKD

In CKD, only a weak correlation is found between bone density and fracture rate, compared with primary osteoporosis [16]. Therefore, decreased bone quality, rather than decreased bone density, is suspected as a factor for fragility fracture in CKD. Bone quality deteriorates due to advancement of hyperhomocysteinemia in association with progression of CKD [17], thereby increasing formation of pentosidine cross-links, which are nonphysiological cross-links for type 1 collagen in bone tissue, and bone fragility develops [18]. According to a study on iliac biopsies of CKD stage 5D patients with advanced SHPT, mature cross-links decreased and immature cross-links increased in bone tissue [19]. The content of pentosidine increased substantially in the bone tissue of CKD stage 5D patients compared with that of healthy people, and bone formation rate per bone volume and mineral apposition (bone calcification) rate were inversely proportional. Based on the above, the increase in advanced glycation end-product cross-links such as pentosidine cross-links is strongly related to abnormal bone metabolism in CKD stage 5D patients.

Bone density cannot accurately assess fracture risk because of technological problems with bone densitometry measured by dual-energy X-ray absorptiometry (DXA). High-resolution peripheral quantitative computed tomography (HR-pQCT) for peripheral bones produces images of minute bone tissues and therefore is more reliable than DXA for evaluation of osteoporosis [20]. HR-pQCT is particularly good for evaluating cortical bone. In CKD patients, cortical bone becomes osteoporotic due to SHPT and acceleration of bone metabolic turnover [21]. Because osteoporosis of cortical bone cannot be captured by a traditional DXA, it is considered an aspect of bone quality.

6.2.6 Other Factors Affecting Bone Fragility in CKD

In a retrospective cohort study of 144 patients with CKD stage 5D using the onset of fragility fracture as the outcome [22], sex (female), fracture history, decreased radial bone density, relative hypoparathyroidism, and vitamin D deficiency were

Table 6.2 Correlates of bone fracture in prevalent hemodialysis patients

	OR	*P*	95 % CI
Sex (female)	18.092	0.026	1.406–232.937
Fracture before HD	73.786	0.001	6.143–886.217
Previous transplantation	0.462	0.541	0.039–5.508
Duration of RRT	0.998	0.740	0.986–1.010
iPTH <100 pg/mL	37.774	0.022	1.694–842.189
iPTH >300 pg/mL	1.981	0.499	0.273–14.372
Kt/V	0.023	0.154	0.000–4.141
Radius Z-score (1-SD decrease)	2.691	0.006	1.327–5.459
25-OHD <20 nmol/L	11.215	0.026	1.326–94.813

In a multivariate logistic regression model, Hosmer-Lemeshow χ^2 $P=0.811$ [22]
OR odds ratio, *CI* confidence interval, *HD* hemodialysis, *RRT* renal replacement therapy, *iPTH* intact parathyroid hormone, *Kt/V* efficiency of hemodialysis, *SD* standard deviation, *25-OHD* 25-hydroxyvitamin D

found to be independent risk factors for fragility fracture (Table 6.2). Even in healthy people without reduced kidney function, the level of vitamin D sufficiency and prevalence of proximal femur fracture are correlated [23]. In patients on CKD stage 5D, attention should be paid not only to the decrease of serum 1,25-dihydroxyvitamin D (1,25-$(OH)_2$D) but also to the level of nutritional vitamin D sufficiency or serum 25-hydroxyvitamin D (25-OHD) level.

In the present study, relative hypoparathyroidism was demonstrated as a significant risk factor for fragility fracture [22] (Table 6.2). Excessive suppression of bone metabolism may delay the repair of bone microdamage, leading to the onset of fragility fracture.

6.3 Chronic Kidney Disease-Mineral and Bone Disease

With progression of CKD, calcium and phosphate homeostasis collapses and risk of death and cardiovascular events increases [2]. In CKD, bone diseases and ectopic calcification develop concurrently. Therefore, the term "chronic kidney disease-mineral and bone disorder (CKD-MBD)" has been recommended to represent the concept of bone mineral metabolism disorder [6].

6.3.1 Calcium and Phosphate Homeostasis

Homeostasis for calcium (Ca) and phosphate (P) concentrations in serum involves three hormones: PTH, 1,25-$(OH)_2$D, and fibroblast growth factor 23 (FGF-23). PTH, 1,25-$(OH)_2$D, and FGF-23 form a feedback loop with Ca and P [24] (Fig. 6.2).

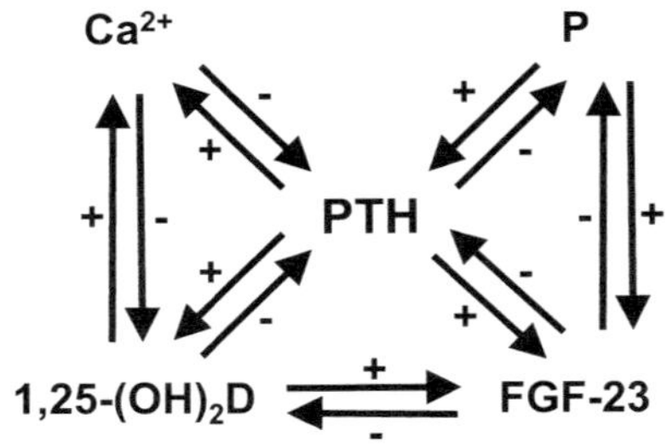

Fig. 6.2 Feedback loops in calcium and phosphate homeostasis [24]. Calcium and phosphate homeostasis is regulated by three hormones: parathyroid hormone (PTH), 1,25-dihydroxyvitamin D (1,25-$(OH)_2$D), and fibroblast growth factor 23 (FGF-23). A feedback loop is formed between respective factors, playing an important role in serum Ca-P homeostasis

Table 6.3 Receptors in parathyroid cells affecting PTH secretion [25]

Receptor	Location
VDR	Cell nucleus
CaSR	Cell membrane
FGFR-Klotho complex	Cell membrane

VDR vitamin D receptor
CaSR calcium-sensing receptor
FGFR fibroblast growth factor receptor

Furthermore, PTH, 1,25-$(OH)_2$D, and FGF-23 form feedback loops among each other. These hormones play an important role in serum Ca-P homeostasis.

PTH, produced from the parathyroid gland, is important for the minute-to-minute regulation of serum Ca concentration. In the parathyroid gland, there are vitamin D receptors (VDRs), calcium-sensing receptors (CaSRs), and fibroblast growth factor receptor (FGFR)-Klotho complexes [25] (Table 6.3), which transmit to parathyroid cells information regarding the 1,25-$(OH)_2$D, Ca, and FGF-23 concentrations in the blood, respectively, thus modulating PTH secretion.

CaSR, in particular, has an important role in regulating serum Ca concentration. CaSR is a seven-transmembrane receptor in the parathyroid cell membrane. PTH is a hormone with high responsiveness for maintaining the serum Ca concentration. The parathyroid cell is highly sensitive to the changes in extracellular Ca concentration and regulates PTH secretion accordingly [25] (Fig. 6.3). Cinacalcet and other CaSR agonists modulate CaSR allosterically and make the parathyroid cell behave in a way as if the extracellular Ca concentration were high. In addition to the regulation of PTH release from the secretory granules in the parathyroid cell [26], cinacalcet is involved in PTH gene transcription and posttranscriptional regulation [27]. Furthermore, cinacalcet is involved in the regulation of parathyroid cell growth [28] and also contributes to the PTH secretion regulatory mechanism.

FGF-23 is produced from bone and can regulate serum phosphate concentration without causing much change in the serum Ca concentration. Secretion of FGF-23 from osteocytes is regulated by dietary phosphorus loading, 1,25-$(OH)_2$D, and PTH [24] (Fig. 6.2). The FGFR-Klotho complex is a receptor for FGF-23. In Klotho-mutant mice, the function of Klotho (part of the receptor) is deficient, and

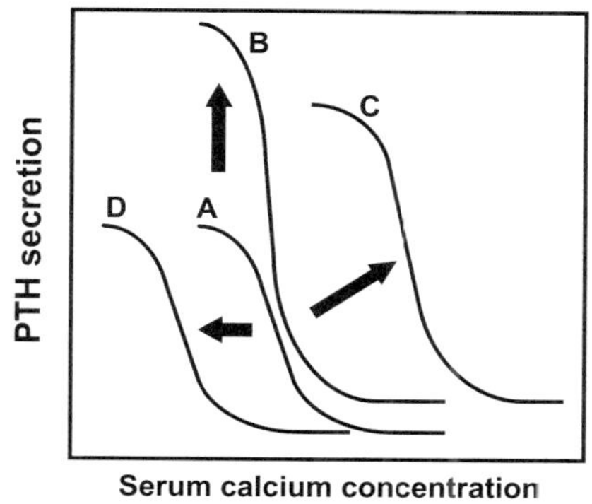

Fig. 6.3 Extracellular calcium-induced changes in the parathyroid hormone (PTH) secretion-regulating mechanism and changes in pathological condition [25]. (**a**) Normal PTH-Ca sigmoid curve. In accordance with the changes in serum calcium, PTH is produced. The serum calcium concentration corresponding to the midpoint PTH value between maximal and minimal PTH secretion is called the set point, which is used to evaluate parathyroid sensitivity to serum calcium concentration. The increase of the set point indicates a reduction of sensitivity to serum calcium, suggesting decreased calcium-sensing receptor (CaSR) expression in the parathyroid. (**b**) The case where only the number of secretory cells increases with no set-point abnormality. The PTH-Ca sigmoid curve only moves upward with no rightward shift and no hypercalcemia. (**c**) In primary hyperparathyroidism or severe secondary hyperparathyroidism, the number of secretory cells increases, and the PTH-Ca sigmoid curve moves upward, thus reducing CaSR expression in the parathyroid, with elevation of the set point and a rightward shift of the PTH-Ca sigmoid curve. In such a condition, hypercalcemia and excessive PTH concentration in the blood may coexist. (**d**) In autosomal dominant hypocalcemia induced by an activating mutation of the CaSR, parathyroid sensitivity to serum Ca increases, with a leftward shift of the PTH-Ca sigmoid curve due to the lowered set point. Calcimimetic CaSR agonists such as cinacalcet also lower the set point

acceleration of aging and ectopic calcification have been reported [29]. The phosphorus metabolism regulatory system controlled by the FGF-23 signaling has an important role in Ca-P homeostasis in the blood, particularly in suppression of ectopic calcification.

6.3.2 *Pathogenesis of SHPT*

In the initial stage of CKD, the serum Klotho concentration decreases first and then the serum FGF-23 concentration increases [30] (Fig. 6.4). With progression of CKD, the elevation of serum phosphorus concentration cannot be suppressed by only the increased FGF-23, leading to an increase of PTH. When FGF-23 and PTH finally fail to regulate phosphorus metabolism, the serum phosphorus concentration rises.

Acceleration of PTH synthesis/secretion, parathyroid cell growth, and parathyroid hyperplasia occur due to hyperphosphatemia-induced relative hypocalcemia, a

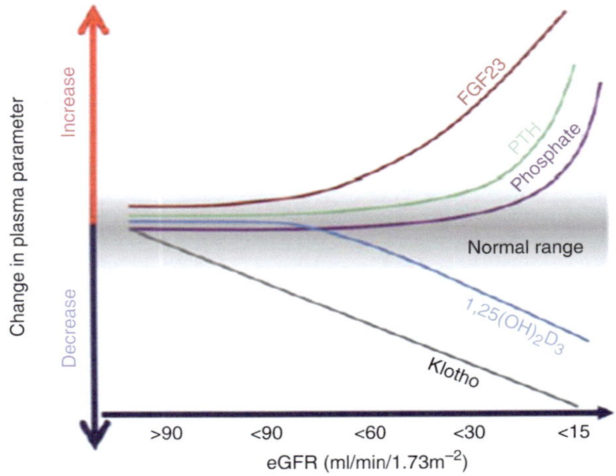

Fig. 6.4 Time profile of changes in plasma fibroblast growth factor 23 (FGF-23), Klotho, active vitamin D, and phosphate levels as chronic kidney disease (CKD) progresses [30]. With progression of CKD, the serum Klotho concentration decreases and the serum FGF-23 concentration increases, thereby suppressing the elevation of serum P concentration. However, with further deterioration of renal function, the 1,25-dihydroxyvitamin D_3 (1,25-$(OH)_2D_3$) concentration decreases, and the serum parathyroid hormone (PTH) concentration increases in order to maintain the serum P concentration, but the serum P concentration goes up due to substantial progression of CKD. *eGFR* estimated glomerular filtration rate

direct effect of hyperphosphatemia on the parathyroid, and vitamin D activation disorder. In such conditions, PTH activity becomes excessive, transferring phosphorus from bone to blood and further aggravating the hyperphosphatemia, leading to progression of CKD. Even if hemodialysis or peritoneal dialysis is introduced, its capacity to remove phosphorus is limited, and hyperphosphatemia persists, resulting in aggravation of SHPT.

According to the analysis of uremia-associated parathyroid tumors removed by parathyroidectomy (PTX) in the patients with medically refractory SHPT, many of these tumors were found to be monoclonal tumors (produced from a single cell) with somatic mutations [31]. The parathyroid initially demonstrates diffuse hyperplasia due to polyclonal growth but undergoes somatic mutation by a persistent proliferative stimulus and finally progresses to monoclonal nodular hyperplasia originating in a single cell [24] (Fig. 6.5). In such uremia-associated parathyroid tumors, decreased expression of VDR and CaSR is observed [32, 33].

Reduction of CaSR expression in the cellular membrane induces an abnormality in the extracellular Ca-sensing mechanism. The mechanism of regulating PTH secretion according to the serum Ca concentration is then impaired, and the PTH-Ca sigmoid curve is shifted to the right [24] (Fig. 6.3), indicating that a higher concentration of extracellular Ca is required to suppress PTH secretion. When the sigmoid curve is shifted substantially to the right due to progression of SHPT, the

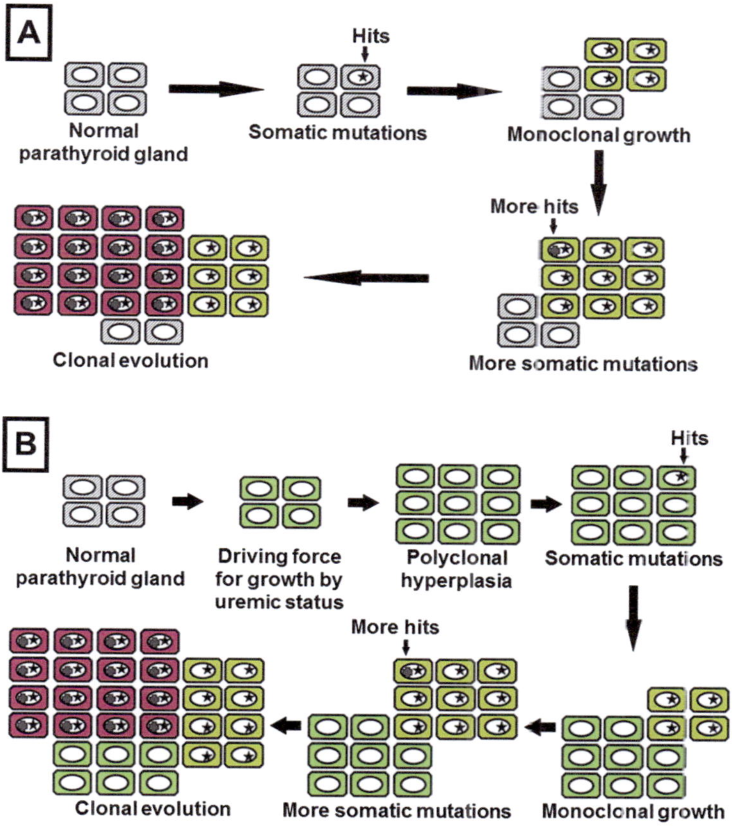

Fig. 6.5 Formation of uremia-associated parathyroid tumors (modification of reference [24]). (**a**) In primary hyperparathyroidism (parathyroid adenoma), a sequence of somatic mutations occurs and provides the cells with proliferative predominance. In such cells with increased proliferative potency, additional somatic mutations are likely to occur. Eventually, monoclonal tumors are formed. (**b**) With progression of chronic kidney disease (CKD), polyclonal parathyroid tumors are formed by growth stimulation on parathyroid gland. The actively dividing cells are likely to induce somatic mutations. As a result of proliferative predominance through somatic mutation, monoclonal uremia-associated parathyroid tumors are formed

serum Ca concentration may sometimes exceed the normal level to induce hypercalcemia.

Due to progression of CKD and hyperphosphatemia, the activity of 1-α-hydroxylase in kidney tubules decreases, and the serum 1,25-$(OH)_2D$ concentration is reduced. In the parathyroid, expression of VDR, one of the nuclear receptors, is reduced [32]. The PTH secretion-suppressing activity via 1,25-$(OH)_2D$ and parathyroid cell proliferation-suppressing activity are disturbed, resulting in further progression of SHPT.

In the physiological state, FGF-23 has phosphaturic activity as well as PTH secretion-suppressing activity. In the patients on maintenance hemodialysis (CKD5D), despite a substantial increase of the FGF-23 concentration in blood, FGF-23 is positively correlated with PTH. Even a high concentration of FGF-23 cannot sufficiently suppress PTH secretion [34], possibly because reduction of Klotho and FGFR expression in the parathyroid gland [35] impairs the FGF-23 signal transmission to parathyroid cells via the FGFR-Klotho complex, leading to the failure to suppress PTH secretion.

As discussed above, PTH secretion and parathyroid cell proliferation increase due to hyperphosphatemia, impaired vitamin D activation, and dysfunctions of various receptors in the parathyroid gland (CaSR, VDR, and FGFR-Klotho complex) (Table 6.3), finally resulting in the substantial collapse of Ca-P homeostasis in serum [25].

6.3.3 Role of FGF-23 in Bone Fragility

In Swedish-elderly males who participated in the multicenter prospective MrOS study, a positive correlation was demonstrated between serum FGF-23 concentration and fracture [36]. After correction for renal function, correlations were found between FGF-23 concentration and the total fracture risk (age-corrected hazard ratio 1.20 [95 % confidence interval 1.03–1.40]) and vertebral facture risk (age-corrected hazard ratio 1.33 [95 % confidence interval 1.02–1.75]). In this study, whether FGF-23 itself induced bone fragility could not be determined, but FGF-23 was shown to be a prognostic factor for fracture risks.

When phosphaturia is likely to occur without much impairment of renal function, excessive FGF-23 may cause bone calcification disorder due to hypophosphatemia and vitamin D activation disorder induced by accelerated phosphaturia [37]. However, in CKD, there is no or a very limited incidence of phosphaturia, and the state of hypophosphatemia does not emerge, which raises the question of whether or not the bone tissue would be directly affected by excessive FGF-23 levels in the blood of CKD patients.

In a cellular experimental system (in vitro), excessive FGF-23 has been reported to suppress osteoblast differentiation and matrix calcification, via FGFR1 [38], indicating a direct effect of FGF-23 on bone tissue. However, in a model mouse of primary hyperparathyroidism with accelerated bone turnover, FGF-23 gene expression increased in bone tissue [39]. Increased FGF-23 in fracture patients may be caused by accelerated bone turnover. The question of a direct effect, or not, of FGF-23 on bone will have to be further studied.

6.4 Treatment for Bone Fragility in CKD

ROD classification-based treatment is recommended for the patients with advanced CKD, when lower bone density or bone fragility is observed, and a bone biopsy is sometimes required to confirm the histological type [6]. However, a bone biopsy is not always carried out before treatment, and treatment may be started by guesswork regarding histological type based on metabolism markers and other serological test results. Treatment of bone in CKD is usually carried out with three types of agents: antiresorptive agents such as bisphosphonate, denosumab, and selective estrogen receptor modulators (SERMs); osteoporosis drugs such as bone-forming agents (e.g., teriparatide); and drugs used to treat CKD-MBD.

6.4.1 *Bisphosphonates*

In nine clinical studies including 8,996 women with CKD (stages 1–3) and post-menopausal osteoporosis, risedronate was found to reduce the fracture rate [40], even in a group with significant renal dysfunction (median GFR $\leq$30 mL/min). In the Fracture Intervention Trial (FIT), alendronate lowered the fracture rate, regardless of renal function at the start of the trial [8]. However, in a 6-month placebo-controlled study in CKD5D patients, alendronate significantly, although modestly, suppressed the decrease of femoral bone density [41]. Therefore, the usefulness of bisphosphonates in CKD5D will have to be further examined. Although the use of bisphosphonates in CKD is an interesting subject, awareness is needed in advanced CKD that it may result in adynamic bone formation.

6.4.2 *Denosumab*

In mild to moderate CKD, the efficacy of denosumab has been demonstrated [42]. However, hypocalcemia has been reported to develop in some patients with kidney failure requiring hemodialysis [43]. Therefore, denosumab must be cautiously administered in advanced CKD patients.

6.4.3 *Selective Estrogen Receptor Modulators*

Aiming to elucidate the fracture-preventing activity of raloxifene, a large-scale clinical study (Multiple Outcomes of Raloxifene Evaluation [MORE] study) was carried out in 180 centers of 25 countries. The subjects were 7705 osteoporotic women at least 2 years away from menopause. Whether or not they had fractures

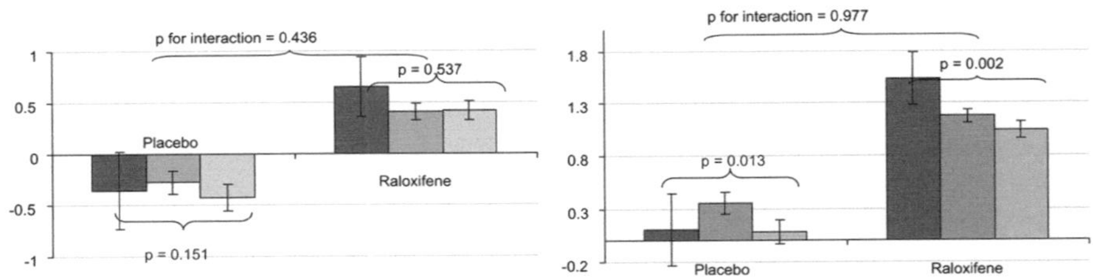

Fig. 6.6 Effect of raloxifene to increase bone density [45]. From among 7,705 participants in the MORE study, 7,316 patients (chronic kidney disease stages 1–3) whose serum creatinine had been determined at the time of study initiation were reanalyzed. Analysis was made of three groups divided by estimated glomerular filtration rate calculated by the modification of diet in renal disease (MDRD) method: ≤45, 45–59, and ≥60 mL/min. In all of the groups, raloxifene increased lumbar and vertebral density and reduced the rate of vertebral compression fracture. No effects were found on the nonvertebral fracture rate

previously, the onset of new vertebral fracture was prevented [44]. From among the MORE study participants, 7316 patients whose serum creatinine had been measured at the time of study initiation were reanalyzed. Regardless of the level of renal function, raloxifene increased femoral bone density and vertebral bone density. It further reduced the vertebral compression fracture rate [45] (Fig. 6.6). Bazedoxifene, an SERM, lowered bone metabolism marker levels, regardless of renal function before treatment, and improved lumbar and femoral density [46]. Furthermore, no serious adverse reactions were reported in association with renal dysfunction.

In a study of CKD5D, raloxifene increased vertebral density [47]. Furthermore, administration of raloxifene for 1 year improved calcaneal density and bone metabolism marker levels in diabetic as well as nondiabetic CKD5D patients [48]. Based on these findings, SERMs are considered useful in improving bone fragility of CKD patients including CKD5D patients.

6.4.4 *Teriparatide*

Although the efficacy of teriparatide was demonstrated in mild to moderate CKD [49], it is considered a contraindication for patients with SHPT [50]. Some people recommend teriparatide for CKD with adynamic bone disease [51]. However, a report suggested that the bone of CKD patients is less responsive to PTH [52], and therefore, further investigation is required in this area.

6.4.5 Therapy for CKD-MBD

Dietary therapy is first conducted to sufficiently control the serum P level. However, in the case of insufficient control, a phosphate binder should be orally administered. In the past, calcium-based phosphate binders (e.g., calcium carbonate) were used, but the concurrent use of VDR agonists (VDRAs) easily induced hypercalcemia or increased the calcium-phosphate product, and therefore, non-calcium-based phosphate binders such as sevelamer hydrochloride and lanthanum carbonate have been more frequently used.

In the parathyroid gland, VDRAs suppress PTH gene transcription and PTH secretion as well as proliferation of parathyroid cells. However, in the uremia-associated parathyroid tumors, the expression of VDR, the target molecule for VDRAs, is reduced, and therefore, the effect of the VDRA is limited. Furthermore, VDRAs accelerate calcium absorption in the small intestine, inducing hypercalcemia depending upon the dose level. Accordingly, the dosage level is restricted, and serum PTH cannot be fully suppressed in many cases.

CaSR agonists (calcimimetics) allosterically act on the CaSR in the parathyroid gland and suppress PTH secretion [26, 53], thus reducing the serum calcium-phosphate product. Furthermore, the calcimimetics inhibit parathyroid cell proliferation [28]. The effect of calcimimetics is maintained to a certain level even in parathyroid tumors where expression of the target CaSR is reduced [54].

According to the results of a combined analysis of four studies on cinacalcet in maintenance hemodialysis patients, the risks for PTX-, fracture-, and cardiovascular event-related hospitalization were significantly reduced by cinacalcet [55]. Furthermore, in maintenance hemodialysis patients in the EVOLVE trial, cinacalcet significantly reduced the incidence of fracture with a hazard ratio of 0.84 by intention-to-treat analysis after correction for fracture risk factors (history of fracture, age, smoking, etc.) [56].

PTX is recommended for SHPT that is refractory to medical treatment. In a matched cohort study to monitor the long-term effect of PTX, PTX reduced the occurrence of femoral fracture by 32 % and the combined rate of fracture in femur, vertebra, and distal forearm by 31 % [57]. However, sometimes there are five or more parathyroid glands, and ectopic parathyroid tumors may be found in the mediastinum or thyroid. Therefore, the parathyroid should be fully observed before and during surgery. Subtotal resection, total resection, and autograft after total resection are recommended as surgical procedures.

6.5 Conclusion

CKD stages 1–3 patients can be treated by the same drug therapy as osteoporotic patients with normal renal function. However, the treatment of CKD-MBD is the central therapy for CKD stages 4, 5, and 5D. SHPT control, in particular, can reduce cardiovascular events and prevent fragility fracture in CKD-MBD.

In CKD patients, decreased bone quality due to deterioration of the collagen bridge is another cause of bone fragility. Improvement of bone quality by SERM treatment is expected to reduce the fracture rate. Progression of osteoporosis in cortical bone is also considered to reduce bone quality in CKD. However, it is still difficult to evaluate bone quality in the clinical setting. Further advancement in this area is expected for the future.

References

1. NIH Consensus Development Panel on Osteoporosis Prevention D, Therapy (2001) Osteoporosis prevention, diagnosis, and therapy. JAMA 285(6):785–795
2. Go AS, Chertow GM, Fan D, McCulloch CE, Hsu CY (2004) Chronic kidney disease and the risks of death, cardiovascular events, and hospitalization. N Engl J Med 351(13):1296–1305. doi:10.1056/NEJMoa041031
3. Goldsmith D, Kothawala P, Chalian A, Bernal M, Robbins S, Covic A (2009) Systematic review of the evidence underlying the association between mineral metabolism disturbances and risk of fracture and need for parathyroidectomy in CKD. Am J Kidney Dis 53 (6):1002–1013. doi:10.1053/j.ajkd.2009.02.010
4. Covic A, Kothawala P, Bernal M, Robbins S, Chalian A, Goldsmith D (2009) Systematic review of the evidence underlying the association between mineral metabolism disturbances and risk of all-cause mortality, cardiovascular mortality and cardiovascular events in chronic kidney disease. Nephrol Dial Transplant 24(5):1506–1523. doi:10.1093/ndt/gfn613
5. Miller PD (2014) Bone disease in CKD: a focus on osteoporosis diagnosis and management. Am J Kidney Dis 64(2):290–304. doi:10.1053/j.ajkd.2013.12.018
6. Moe S, Drueke T, Cunningham J, Goodman W, Martin K, Olgaard K, Ott S, Sprague S, Lameire N, Eknoyan G, Kidney Disease: Improving Global Outcomes (2006) Definition, evaluation, and classification of renal osteodystrophy: a position statement from Kidney Disease: Improving Global Outcomes (KDIGO). Kidney Int 69(11):1945–1953. doi:10.1038/sj.ki.5000414
7. Fujita Y, Iki M, Tamaki J, Kouda K, Yura A, Kadowaki E, Sato Y, Moon JS, Tomioka K, Okamoto N, Kurumatani N (2013) Renal function and bone mineral density in community-dwelling elderly Japanese men: the Fujiwara-kyo Osteoporosis Risk in Men (FORMEN) Study. Bone 56(1):61–66. doi:10.1016/j.bone.2013.05.004
8. Jamal SA, Bauer DC, Ensrud KE, Cauley JA, Hochberg M, Ishani A, Cummings SR (2007) Alendronate treatment in women with normal to severely impaired renal function: an analysis of the fracture intervention trial. J Bone Miner Res 22(4):503–508. doi:10.1359/jbmr.070112
9. Alem AM, Sherrard DJ, Gillen DL, Weiss NS, Beresford SA, Heckbert SR, Wong C, Stehman-Breen C (2000) Increased risk of hip fracture among patients with end-stage renal disease. Kidney Int 58(1):396–399. doi:10.1046/j.1523-1755.2000.00178.x
10. Ensrud KE, Lui LY, Taylor BC, Ishani A, Shlipak MG, Stone KL, Cauley JA, Jamal SA, Antoniucci DM, Cummings SR, Osteoporotic Fractures Research G (2007) Renal function and

risk of hip and vertebral fractures in older women. Arch Intern Med 167(2):133–139. doi:10.1001/archinte.167.2.133

11. Schwartz AV, Vittinghoff E, Bauer DC, Hillier TA, Strotmeyer ES, Ensrud KE, Donaldson MG, Cauley JA, Harris TB, Koster A, Womack CR, Palermo L, Black DM, Study of Osteoporotic Fractures Research Group, Osteoporotic Fractures in Men Research Group, Health Aging and Body Composition Research Group (2011) Association of BMD and FRAX score with risk of fracture in older adults with type 2 diabetes. JAMA 305 (21):2184–2192. doi:10.1001/jama.2011.715
12. Nickolas TL, McMahon DJ, Shane E (2006) Relationship between moderate to severe kidney disease and hip fracture in the United States. J Am Soc Nephrol 17(11):3223–3232. doi:10.1681/ASN.2005111194
13. Wakasugi M, Kazama JJ, Taniguchi M, Wada A, Iseki K, Tsubakihara Y, Narita I (2013) Increased risk of hip fracture among Japanese hemodialysis patients. J Bone Miner Metab 31 (3):315–321. doi:10.1007/s00774-012-0411-z
14. Cunningham J, Sprague SM, Cannata-Andia J, Coco M, Cohen-Solal M, Fitzpatrick L, Goltzmann D, Lafage-Proust MH, Leonard M, Ott S, Rodriguez M, Stehman-Breen C, Stern P, Weisinger J, Osteoporosis Work G (2004) Osteoporosis in chronic kidney disease. Am J Kidney Dis 43(3):566–571
15. Cejka D, Herberth J, Branscum AJ, Fardo DW, Monier-Faugere MC, Diarra D, Haas M, Malluche HH (2011) Sclerostin and Dickkopf-1 in renal osteodystrophy. Clin J Am Soc Nephrol 6(4):877–882. doi:10.2215/CJN.06550810
16. Kidney Disease: Improving Global Outcomes (KDIGO) CKD-MBD Work Group (2009) KDIGO clinical practice guideline for the diagnosis, evaluation, prevention, and treatment of Chronic Kidney Disease-Mineral and Bone Disorder (CKD-MBD). Kidney Int Suppl (113): S1–130
17. Saito M, Marumo K (2010) Collagen cross-links as a determinant of bone quality: a possible explanation for bone fragility in aging, osteoporosis, and diabetes mellitus. Osteoporos Int 21 (2):195–214. doi:10.1007/s00198-009-1066-z
18. Saito M, Marumo K, Soshi S, Kida Y, Ushiku C, Shinohara A (2010) Raloxifene ameliorates detrimental enzymatic and nonenzymatic collagen cross-links and bone strength in rabbits with hyperhomocysteinemia. Osteoporos Int 21(4):655–666. doi:10.1007/s00198-009-0980-4
19. Mitome J, Yamamoto H, Saito M, Yokoyama K, Marumo K, Hosoya T (2011) Nonenzymatic cross-linking pentosidine increase in bone collagen and are associated with disorders of bone mineralization in dialysis patients. Calcif Tissue Int 88(6):521–529. doi:10.1007/s00223-011-9488-y
20. Patsch JM, Burghardt AJ, Yap SP, Baum T, Schwartz AV, Joseph GB, Link TM (2013) Increased cortical porosity in type 2 diabetic postmenopausal women with fragility fractures. J Bone Miner Res 28(2):313–324. doi:10.1002/jbmr.1763
21. Nickolas TL, Stein EM, Dworakowski E, Nishiyama KK, Komandah-Kosseh M, Zhang CA, McMahon DJ, Liu XS, Boutroy S, Cremers S, Shane E (2013) Rapid cortical bone loss in patients with chronic kidney disease. J Bone Miner Res 28(8) 1811–1820. doi:10.1002/jbmr.1916
22. Ambrus C, Almasi C, Berta K, Deak G, Marton A, Molnar MZ, Nemeth Z, Horvath C, Lakatos P, Szathmari M, Mucsi I (2011) Vitamin D insufficiency and bone fractures in patients on maintenance hemodialysis. Int Urol Nephrol 43(2):475–482. doi:10.1007/s11255-010-9723-x
23. Looker AC, Mussolino ME (2008) Serum 25-hydroxyvitamin D and hip fracture risk in older U.S. white adults. J Bone Miner Res 23(1):143–150. doi:10.1359/jbmr.071003
24. Imanishi Y, Inaba M, Kawata T, Nishizawa Y (2009) Animal models of hyperfunctioning parathyroid diseases for drug development. Expert Opin Drug Discov 4(7):727–740
25. Imanishi Y, Nishizawa Y, Inaba M (2013) Chapter 5: Pathogenesis and treatment of chronic kidney disease-mineral and bone disorder. In: Suzuki H (ed) Hemodialysis. InTech, Rijeka, pp 81–100

26. Kawata T, Imanishi Y, Kobayashi K, Onoda N, Okuno S, Takemoto Y, Komo T, Tahara H, Wada M, Nagano N, Ishimura E, Miki T, Ishikawa T, Inaba M, Nishizawa Y (2006) Direct *in vitro* evidence of the suppressive effect of cinacalcet HCl on parathyroid hormone secretion in human parathyroid cells with pathologically reduced calcium-sensing receptor levels. J Bone Miner Metab 24(4):300–306. doi:10.1007/s00774-006-0687-y
27. Nechama M, Ben-Dov IZ, Silver J, Naveh-Many T (2009) Regulation of PTH mRNA stability by the calcimimetic R568 and the phosphorus binder lanthanum carbonate in CKD. Am J Physiol Ren Physiol 296(4):F795–F800. doi:10.1152/ajprenal.90625.2008
28. Imanishi Y, Kawata T, Kenko T, Wada M, Nagano N, Miki T, Arnold A, Inaba M (2011) Cinacalcet HCl suppresses Cyclin D1 oncogene-derived parathyroid cell proliferation in a murine model for primary hyperparathyroidism. Calcif Tissue Int 89(1):29–35. doi:10.1007/s00223-011-9490-4
29. Kuro-o M, Matsumura Y, Aizawa H, Kawaguchi H, Suga T, Utsugi T, Ohyama Y, Kurabayashi M, Kaname T, Kume E, Iwasaki H, Iida A, Shiraki-Iida T, Nishikawa S, Nagai R, Nabeshima YI (1997) Mutation of the mouse klotho gene leads to a syndrome resembling aging. Nature 390(6655):45–51. doi:10.1038/36285
30. Kim HR, Nam BY, Kim DW, Kang MW, Han JH, Lee MJ, Shin DH, Doh FM, Koo HM, Ko KI, Kim CH, Oh HJ, Yoo TH, Kang SW, Han DS, Han SH (2013) Circulating alpha-klotho levels in CKD and relationship to progression. Am J Kidney Dis 61(6):899–909. doi:10.1053/j.ajkd.2013.01.024
31. Imanishi Y, Tahara H, Palanisamy N, Spitalny S, Salusky IB, Goodman W, Brandi ML, Drueke TB, Sarfati E, Urena P, Chaganti RS, Arnold A (2002) Clonal chromosomal defects in the molecular pathogenesis of refractory hyperparathyroidism of uremia. J Am Soc Nephrol 13(6):1490–1498
32. Tokumoto M, Tsuruya K, Fukuda K, Kanai H, Kuroki S, Hirakata H (2002) Reduced p21, p27 and vitamin D receptor in the nodular hyperplasia in patients with advanced secondary hyperparathyroidism. Kidney Int 62(4):1196–1207. doi:10.1111/j.1523-1755.2002.kid585.x
33. Gogusev J, Duchambon P, Hory B, Giovannini M, Goureau Y, Sarfati E, Drueke TB (1997) Depressed expression of calcium receptor in parathyroid gland tissue of patients with hyperparathyroidism. Kidney Int 51(1):328–336
34. Imanishi Y, Inaba M, Nakatsuka K, Nagasue K, Okuno S, Yoshihara A, Miura M, Miyauchi A, Kobayashi K, Miki T, Shoji T, Ishimura E, Nishizawa Y (2004) FGF-23 in patients with end-stage renal disease on hemodialysis. Kidney Int 65(5):1943–1946. doi:10.1111/j.1523-1755.2004.00604.x
35. Komaba H, Goto S, Fujii H, Hamada Y, Kobayashi A, Shibuya K, Tominaga Y, Otsuki N, Nibu K, Nakagawa K, Tsugawa N, Okano T, Kitazawa R, Fukagawa M, Kita T (2010) Depressed expression of Klotho and FGF receptor 1 in hyperplastic parathyroid glands from uremic patients. Kidney Int 77(3):232–238. doi:10.1038/ki.2009.414
36. Mirza MA, Karlsson MK, Mellstrom D, Orwoll E, Ohlsson C, Ljunggren O, Larsson TE (2011) Serum fibroblast growth factor 23 (FGF-23) and fracture risk in elderly men. J Bone Miner Res 26(4):857–864. doi:10.1002/jbmr.263
37. Jonsson KB, Zahradnik R, Larsson T, White KE, Sugimoto T, Imanishi Y, Yamamoto T, Hampson G, Koshiyama H, Ljunggren O, Oba K, Yang IM, Miyauchi A, Econs MJ, Lavigne J, Juppner H (2003) Fibroblast growth factor 23 in oncogenic osteomalacia and X-linked hypophosphatemia. N Engl J Med 348(17):1656–1663. doi:10.1056/NEJMoa020881
38. Wang H, Yoshiko Y, Yamamoto R, Minamizaki T, Kozai K, Tanne K, Aubin JE, Maeda N (2008) Overexpression of fibroblast growth factor 23 suppresses osteoblast differentiation and matrix mineralization in vitro. J Bone Miner Res 23(6):939–948. doi:10.1359/jbmr.080220
39. Kawata T, Imanishi Y, Kobayashi K, Miki T, Arnold A, Inaba M, Nishizawa Y (2007) Parathyroid hormone regulates fibroblast growth factor-23 in a mouse model of primary hyperparathyroidism. J Am Soc Nephrol 18(10):2683–2688. doi:10.1681/ASN.2006070783
40. Miller PD, Roux C, Boonen S, Barton IP, Dunlap LE, Burgio DE (2005) Safety and efficacy of risedronate in patients with age-related reduced renal function as estimated by the Cockcroft

and Gault method: a pooled analysis of nine clinical trials. J Bone Miner Res 20 (12):2105–2115. doi:10.1359/JBMR.050817
41. Wetmore JB, Benet LZ, Kleinstuck D, Frassetto L (2005) Effects of short-term alendronate on bone mineral density in hemodialysis patients. Nephrology 10(4):393–399. doi:10.1111/j.1440-1797.2005.00436.x
42. Jamal SA, Ljunggren O, Stehman-Breen C, Cummings SR, McClung MR, Goemaere S, Ebeling PR, Franek E, Yang YC, Egbuna OI, Boonen S, Miller PD (2011) Effects of denosumab on fracture and bone mineral density by level of kidney function. J Bone Miner Res 26(8):1829–1835. doi:10.1002/jbmr.403
43. Block GA, Bone HG, Fang L, Lee E, Padhi D (2012) A single-dose study of denosumab in patients with various degrees of renal impairment. J Bone Miner Res 27(7):1471–1479. doi:10.1002/jbmr.1613
44. Delmas PD, Ensrud KE, Adachi JD, Harper KD, Sarkar S, Gennari C, Reginster JY, Pols HA, Recker RR, Harris ST, Wu W, Genant HK, Black DM, Eastell R, Mulitple Outcomes of Raloxifene Evaluation I (2002) Efficacy of raloxifene on vertebral fracture risk reduction in postmenopausal women with osteoporosis: four-year results from a randomized clinical trial. J Clin Endocrinol Metab 87(8):3609–3617
45. Ishani A, Blackwell T, Jamal SA, Cummings SR, Ensrud KE, Investigators M (2008) The effect of raloxifene treatment in postmenopausal women with CKD. J Am Soc Nephrol 19 (7):1430–1438. doi:10.1681/ASN.2007050555
46. Adami S, Palacios S, Rizzoli R, Levine AB, Sutradhar S, Chines AA (2014) The efficacy and safety of bazedoxifene in postmenopausal women by baseline kidney function status. Climacteric 17(3):273–284. doi:10.3109/13697137.2013.830605
47. Hernandez E, Valera R, Alonzo E, Bajares-Lilue M, Carlini R, Capriles F, Martinis R, Bellorin-Font E, Weisinger JR (2003) Effects of raloxifene on bone metabolism and serum lipids in postmenopausal women on chronic hemodialysis. Kidney Int 63(6):2269–2274. doi:10.1046/j.1523-1755.2003.00005.x
48. Saito O, Saito T, Asakura S, Akimoto T, Inoue M, Ando Y, Muto S, Kusano E (2012) Effects of raloxifene on bone metabolism in hemodialysis patients with type 2 diabetes. Int J Endocrinol Metab 10(2):464–469. doi:10.5812/ijem.3794
49. Miller PD, Schwartz EN, Chen P, Misurski DA, Krege JH (2007) Teriparatide in postmenopausal women with osteoporosis and mild or moderate renal impairment. Osteoporos Int 18 (1):59–68. doi:10.1007/s00198-006-0189-8
50. Gordon PL, Frassetto LA (2010) Management of osteoporosis in CKD Stages 3 to 5. Am J Kidney Dis 55(5):941–956. doi:10.1053/j.ajkd.2010.02.338
51. Cejka D, Haas M (2011) Should teriparatide ever be used for adynamic bone disease? Semin Dial 24(4):431–433. doi:10.1111/j.1525-139X.2011.00911.x
52. Goto S, Fujii H, Hamada Y, Yoshiya K, Fukagawa M (2010) Association between indoxyl sulfate and skeletal resistance in hemodialysis patients. Ther Apher Dial 14(4):417–423. doi:10.1111/j.1744-9987.2010.00813.x
53. Hammerland LG, Garrett JE, Hung BC, Levinthal C, Nemeth EF (1998) Allosteric activation of the Ca^{2+} receptor expressed in *Xenopus laevis* oocytes by NPS 467 or NPS 568. Mol Pharmacol 53(6):1083–1088
54. Kawata T, Imanishi Y, Kobayashi K, Kenko T, Wada M, Ishimura E, Miki T, Nagano N, Inaba M, Arnold A, Nishizawa Y (2005) Relationship between parathyroid calcium-sensing receptor expression and potency of the calcimimetic, cinacalcet, in suppressing parathyroid hormone secretion in an *in vivo* murine model of primary hyperparathyroidism. Eur J Endocrinol 153(4):587–594. doi:10.1530/eje.1.02007
55. Cunningham J, Danese M, Olson K, Klassen P, Chertow GM (2005) Effects of the calcimimetic cinacalcet HCl on cardiovascular disease, fracture, and health-related quality of life in secondary hyperparathyroidism. Kidney Int 68(4):1793–1800. doi:10.1111/j.1523-1755.2005.00596

56. Moe SM, Abdalla S, Chertow GM, Parfrey PS, Block GA, Correa-Rotter R, Floege J, Herzog CA, London GM, Mahaffey KW, Wheeler DC, Dehmel B, Goodman WG, Drueke TB, for the Evaluation of Cinacalcet HTtL CETI (2015) Effects of cinacalcet on fracture events in patients receiving hemodialysis: the EVOLVE Trial. J Am Soc Nephrol. doi:10.1681/ASN.2014040414
57. Rudser KD, de Boer IH, Dooley A, Young B, Kestenbaum B (2007) Fracture risk after parathyroidectomy among chronic hemodialysis patients. J Am Soc Nephrol 18(8):2401–2407. doi:10.1681/ASN.2007010022

Chapter 7
Impaired Parathyroid Function and Bone Formation: A Risk for Development of Adynamic Bone Disease to Enhance Vascular Calcification

Shinsuke Yamada

Abstract The prognosis of diabetes mellitus (DM) patients on hemodialysis (HD) is markedly worse than for non-DM HD patients. One of the causes for poor prognosis in DM HD patients is pointed out: the presence of specific bone metabolic disorders. Bone metabolic abnormalities are closely related to the onset of vascular calcification, and both of these complications are thought to be caused by inappropriate glycemic control. Because osteoblast/osteocyte function is impaired and parathyroid hormone (PTH) secretion ability is suppressed under the sustained hyperglycemic status, bone turnover becomes low and adynamic bone disease (ABD) is exhibited. As a direct result of ABD, cushioning action of serum calcium and phosphorus on the bone is weakened, in addition to vascular calcification.

Meanwhile, both hyperinsulinemia and obesity positively affect bone status. Accordingly, these factors should have been excluded to investigate the influences of glycemic control alone on bone status. We will give an outline into focus on DM HD patients who are not obese and generally have depleted insulin secretion ability.

Keywords Hyperglycemia • Bone turnover • Adynamic bone • Vascular calcification

7.1 Introduction

The population of diabetes mellitus (DM) patients is increasing worldwide every year. The current number of patients also including borderline DM patients is estimated to exceed 400 million people in the world. Plantinga et al. analyzed the medical examination data of 8,188 randomly extracted individuals and found that 39.6 % had impaired glucose tolerance and 41.7 % of whom had a diagnosis of

S. Yamada (✉)
Metabolism, Endocrinology, and Molecular Medicine, Osaka City University Graduate School of Medicine, Asahimachi 1-4-3, Abeno-ku, Osaka 545-8585, Japan
e-mail: m1265626@med.osaka-cu.ac.jp

M. Inaba (ed.), *Musculoskeletal Disease Associated with Diabetes Mellitus*,
DOI 10.1007/978-4-431-55720-3_7

chronic kidney disease (CKD) [1]. Thus, DM is an important risk factor for CKD and it is estimated that many DM patients already are in latent CKD.

Diabetic nephropathy is highly likely to develop into end-stage renal disease. As a reflection of this, approximately one-third (about 600,000 patients) of the estimated two million dialysis patients worldwide has been DM patients on dialysis (HD). In general, prognosis and quality of life (QOL) are markedly worse in DM on hemodialysis (HD) patients than in non-DM HD patients. It may be considered that DM HD patients tend to be older or they often already have cardiovascular disease when HD treatment is newly initiated, but it is a severe medical problem that the 5-year survival rate after initiation of HD treatment is only 60 % in DM HD patients.

One significant reason for poor prognosis in DM HD patients is the high complication rates of bone metabolism disorders and vascular calcification. Not only bone metabolism disorders and vascular calcification share many common risk factors such as aging, lack of exercise, smoking, and alcohol consumption, there is also the relationship called the "bone-vascular axis," whereby each pathophysiology is related as risk factors for the other. In particular, bone metabolism disorders and vascular calcification are closely linked in DM HD patients. This report will focus on DM HD patients who could also be said to be in the terminal stage of DM nephropathy and give an outline of the relationship between bone metabolism disorders and vascular calcification.

7.2 The Present State of Glycemic Control in DM HD Patients

DM HD patients can often have severe hypoglycemia easily for some factors such as serum insulin accumulation accompanying renal dysfunction or serum glucose losing due to HD treatment itself. HbA1c level also decreases in most patients after initiating of HD treatment. Accordingly, the focus of glycemic control in clinical site tends to be placed on prevention of hypoglycemia and it is common for insulin treatment to be discontinued after the initiation of HD treatment.

Since the Diabetes Control and Complications Trial (DCCT; [2]), HbA1c has become the standard clinical indicator for glycemic control in DM patients in Japan. However, HbA1c has often exhibited false low values compared to glycoalbumin (GA) in DM HD patients, because lifespan of red blood cell is shortened due to the increasing immature erythrocyte by erythropoietin use or blood loss by the HD treatment itself [3, 4]. The simultaneous measurement of actual HbA1c and GA levels in 538 randomly selected DM HD patients revealed significant dissociation of patient distribution between HbA1c and GA levels, indicating that HbA1c levels lead to overestimation of glycemic control (Table 7.1) [4]. Lately, it has been reported that only GA but not HbA1c is a glycemic control index related to

Table 7.1 HbA1c, GA patient distribution in 538 DM HD patients

Glycemic control	HbA1C	GA
Excellent (HbA1C≤6 %, GA≤18 %)	307 (57.1 %)	152 (28.3 %)
Good (6 %<HbA1C≤7 %, 18 %<GA≤21 %)	128 (23.7 %)	106 (19.7 %)
Good (7 %<HbA1C≤8 %, 21 %<GA≤24 %)	65 (12.1 %)	84 (15.6 %)
Poor (8 %<HbA1C, 24 %<GA)	38 (7.1 %)	196 (36.4 %)

Cited from reference Inaba et al. [4]/partially revised
Simultaneous measurement of HbA1c and GA in 538 DM HD patients shows how much HbA1c overestimates the state of glycemic control

mortality risk [5], and the "Diabetes Treatment Guidelines for Dialysis Patients" in Japan in 2012 recommend using GA, rather than HbA1c for glycemic control.

Accordingly, this means that glycemic control of DM HD patients is being less strictly managed than is optimal – a key point in understanding the high rates of bone metabolism disorders and vascular calcification in DM HD patients.

7.3 Low-Turnover Bone Loss in DM Patients

Because osteoblasts contain insulin and insulin growing factor (IGF)-1 receptor, the lack of these factors impairs osteoblast function, leading to low-turnover bone loss. Accordingly, most of type 1 DM patients with absolute insulin deficiency exhibit bone loss, because type 1 DM develops before reaching bone peak mass around the age of 20 years [6–8].

Meanwhile, type 2 DM patients are known to exhibit decreased osteoblast function with worse glycemic control [9]. Therefore, in a sustained hyperglycemic state, the same low-turnover bone loss seen in type 1 DM occurs even without an insulin deficiency. Furthermore, the tumor necrosis factor that is involved in the pathology of type 2 DM impairs osteoblast function and promotes osteoclast function [10]. It has been reported that the bone mass of type 2 DM patients who have had the disease for 5 years or longer is significantly decreased compared to normal individuals [11]. However, in some disease stages of type 2 DM, factors that are favorable for bones such as obesity or hyperinsulinemia may become dominant. Therefore, bone turnover and bone mass are not necessarily decreased in type 2 DM like in type 1 DM.

7.4 High-Turnover Bone Loss in CKD Patients

When vitamin D is absorbed from the intestinal tract, 25-hydroxylation in the liver and 1-alpha- hydroxylation in the kidneys activate the vitamin D (1,25(OH)$_2$D) so that it exhibits effects. However, decreased kidney function lowers the amount of

1-alpha-hydroxylase, therefore leading to a decrease in 1,25(OH)$_2$D. This impairs reabsorption of calcium from the intestinal tract, causing hypocalcemia and promoting the secretion of parathyroid hormones (PTH). Decreased nephron number accompanying decreased kidney function lowers the amount of phosphate excretion in urine, leading to elevated serum phosphate levels. This encourages secretion of fibroblast growth factor (FGF)-23, a bone-derived phosphaturic hormone [12]. Increased serum FGF-23 levels also lower 1,25(OH)$_2$D through decreased 1-alpha-hydroxylase activation, promoting PTH secretion [13]. Through these mechanisms, particularly in stage 3 or higher CKD patients who have GFR of below 60 ml/min/1.73 m^2, decreased GFR lowers serum 1,25(OH)$_2$D levels [14], causing serum PTH levels to rise [15]. Thus, CKD patients develop secondary hyperparathyroidism as their CKD stage progresses. As a result, high-turnover bone metabolism is exhibited, causing decreased bone mass.

7.5 Histological Classification of Renal Osteodystrophy

After tetracycline double labeling, iliac bone biopsy specimens underwent histomorphometry, and measurements including osteoid mass, fibrous tissue mass, and ossification rate, etc. were calculated. Based on these, bone metabolism abnormalities accompanying CKD were classified into the five types shown in Table 7.2 [16]. A general name for this condition is renal osteodystrophy (ROD). Conventionally, osteitis fibrosa (OF) type accompanying secondary hyperparathyroidism was frequent. However, the recent increases in the number of people with DM and overtreatment with calcium or vitamin D preparations have led to an increase in adynamic bone disease (ABD) type.

OF is a type of high-turnover bone metabolism abnormality in which excessive secretion of PTH causes abnormally increased bone turnover. Lamellar bone with normal stratification decreases and is replaced with reticular woven bone, increasing fibrous tissue. In osteomalacia (OM) type, 1,25-dihydroxyvitamin D3 (1,25 (OH)2D3) deficiency and deposition of aluminum and iron in the mineralization front impair calcification, causing abnormal osteoid proliferation. The calcification disorder leads to a lowered ossification rate. Mixed type cases exhibit mixed OF and OM histology, with both increased fiber components and increased osteoids. This pathology is also considered a subtype of secondary hyperparathyroidism. In the mild change type (MIL), bone state is almost normal.

ABD cases initially appear to exhibit histology results identical to MIL cases. However, they can be distinguished by the fact that there is hardly any uptake of the tetracycline labeled prior to the biopsy. Therefore, it can be considered to be a low-turnover bone metabolism disorder in which bone turnover is extremely decreased. Risk factors for ABD onset include decreased PTH secretion due to aging or after total parathyroidectomy, excessive doses of calcium or vitamin D preparations, or relative deficiency accompanying decreased PTH responsiveness of bone due to accumulation of aluminum or iron. In DM patients, direct effects on

Table 7.2 ROD histological classifications

	Osteoid mass (%)		Fibrous tissue mass (%)	Ossification rate (%)	
	OV/BV	OV/TV	Tb. V/TV	BFR/BV	PTH concentration
OF	<15 %	<3 %	>0.5 %	Accelerated	High
MIX	>15 %	>3 %	>0.5 %	Normal–low	Mildly elevated
OM	>15 %	>3 %	<0.5 %	Low	Normal–mildly elevated
MIL	<15 %	<3 %	<0.5 %	Normal	Normal–mildly elevated
ABD	<15 %	<3 %	<0.5 %	Low	Low

Cited from reference Sherrard et al. [16]/partially revised
ROD histological classifications
OF osteitis fibrosa, *MIX* mixed type, *OM* osteomalacia, *MIL* mild change, *ABD* adynamic bone disease, *OV* osteoid volume, *BV* bone volume, *TV* tissue volume, *Fb* fibrosis tissue volume, *BFR* bone formation rate

parathyroid cells accompanying a hyperglycemic state could inhibit PTH secretion [17]. However, currently, the molecular mechanism and physiological significance have yet to be clarified.

7.6 Bone Metabolic Markers

It is extremely important to grasp the histological type of ROD. However, bone biopsy, which is the current gold standard for diagnosing ROD, is highly invasive, and it is not practical to perform it in routine clinical practice. Therefore, bone metabolism marker measurement is recommended. The measurement of bone metabolism markers makes it possible to accurately and simply grasp the current state of bone metabolism. Bone metabolism markers are biological markers that reflect the state of bone resorption and formation at the time of measurement. As bone formation is stimulated by bone resorption, elevation of bone resorption and formation markers signifies the promotion of bone resorption-dominant bone metabolism.

For example, if PTH is extremely high and both formation and resorption markers greatly exceed the upper limit of the normal range, OF type is highly likely. Meanwhile, if PTH elevations are inhibited and bone formation markers have dropped to below the lower limit of the normal range, the case is likely low-turnover type – ABD. If bone metabolism markers are within the normal range but blood aluminum and/or iron levels are high, OM type should be taken into consideration and bone biopsy performed.

However, because there is the risk that in CKD patients, bone metabolic markers that accumulate in serum with decreased kidney function will exhibit false high values that are greater than the increased bone metabolism accompanying hyperparathyroidism onset, it is best to use bone-specific alkaline phosphatase (BAP) as a bone formation marker and tartrate-resistant acid phosphatase isoform 5b (TRACP 5b) as a bone resorption marker as these markers are not greatly influenced by decreased kidney function [18].

7.7 Bone Mass of DM HD Patients Is Maintained at a Higher Level Than Non-DM HD Patients

In general, secondary hyperparathyroidism starts to appear in CKD patients when GFR falls below 60 ml/min/1.73 m^2. Bone metabolism markers rise almost directly along with this (Fig. 7.1), causing marked high-turnover type decreased bone mass and OF type bone lesions. However, because PTH rises tend to be suppressed in DM patients, bone turnover is not as greatly increased as in non-DM patients. Accordingly, low-turnover, gradual bone mass decreases are seen in DM patients and ABD type bone lesions are exhibited.

We previously investigated the relationship between PTH and bone mass in 83 male HD patients (DM, 42 cases; non-DM, 41 cases). As expected, PTH levels were significantly low in DM HD patients and osteosono index (OSI) values were significantly higher in DM HD patients (Fig. 7.2). However, when discussing these results, one must remember that bone mass is not maintained in relation to poor glycemic control. In fact, the OSI values of the 42 male DM HD patients exhibited a significant negative correlation with GA (Fig. 7.3), suggesting that bone mass decreases more with poor glycemic control [19]. Thus, different mechanisms lead to bone metabolism abnormalities in DM and non-DM patients, and once secondary hyperparathyroidism begins to complicate the condition, non-DM patients exhibit greater acceleration of bone loss than DM patients. This leads to a bone loss reversal phenomenon with decreased kidney function.

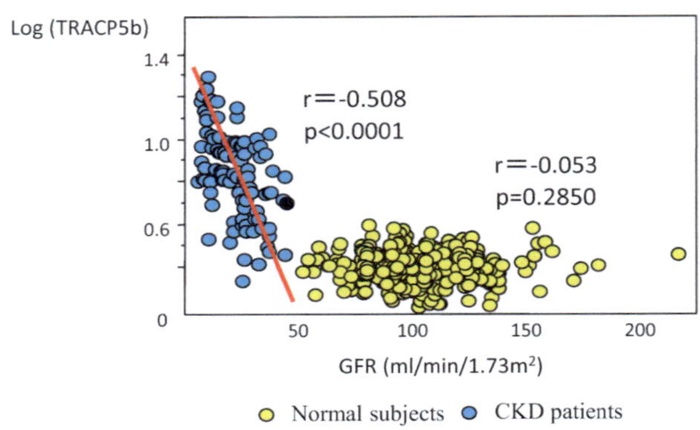

Fig. 7.1 Relationship between GFR and bone markers. Data from our past research. Generally, secondary hyperparathyroidism starts to develop when GFR drops below 60 ml/min/1.73 m^2. In accordance with this, bone markers rise in a relatively straight line, and OF bone lesions appear in CKD patients of stage 3 or greater

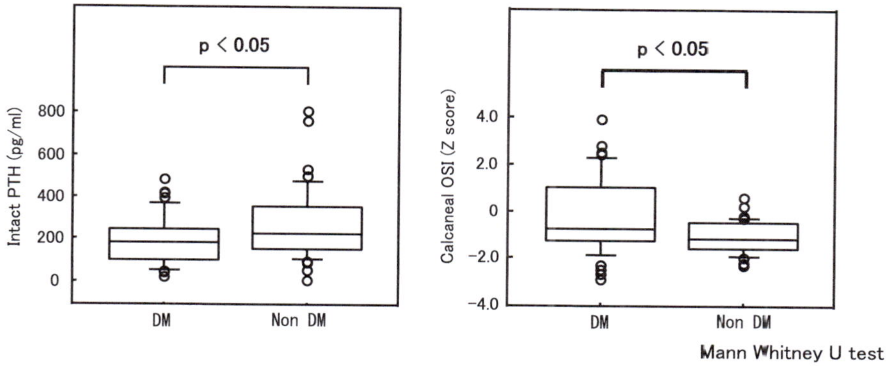

Fig. 7.2 Compared to non-DM HD patients, DM HD patients exhibited low intact PTH levels and high calcaneal OSI (Z score) levels (Cited from reference Yamada et al. [18]/partially revised). Because PTH elevation tends to be inhibited in DM HD patients, these patients exhibit more low-turnover, gradual bone loss than non-DM HD patients and bone mass tends to be maintained

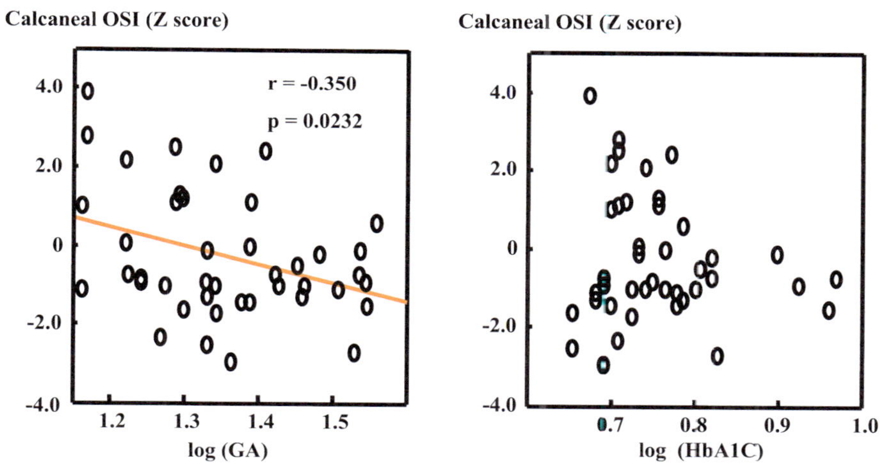

Fig. 7.3 Relationship between glycemic control and calcaneal OSI (Z score). Cited from reference Yamada et al. [18]/partially revised. Calcaneal OSI levels of DM HD patients exhibit a negative correlation with GA, rather than HbA1c. Thus, when glycemic control state is accurately evaluated with GA, one can see that poorer glycemic control indicates greater reduction in bone mass

7.8 Fracture Risk in DM Patients: Independent of Bone Mass

Although some reports have stated that the bone mineral density (BMD) of type 2 DM patients is greater than that of non-DM patients, other reports have stated that it is the same or even lower. Almost all reports, however, state that fracture risk is significantly high in the proximal femur [20], antebrachial [21], and vertebral [22]. Yamamoto et al. reported that in type 2 DM patients, there was no correlation between BMD and fracture risk in the proximal femur, radius, or vertebral and that fracture risk could not be predicted with BMD [21].

We also previously investigated the presence of a relationship between BMD and lumbar spine fractures in postmenopausal female HD patients aged 65 years or older (DM, 31 cases; non-DM, 83 cases) [22]. As a result, we found that the fracture rate was approximately 13 % (11/83 cases) in the non-DM group but approximately 32 % (10/31 cases) in the DM group, indicating significantly higher fracture risk in the DM group. As stated above, the DM group had maintained significantly high BMD in the lumbar, vertebral, and radius and no relationship was noted between fractures and BMD in the DM group despite cases of fractures in the non-DM group having significantly lower BMD (Table 7.3). Thus, it is difficult to determine fracture risk based on BMD in DM HD patients.

7.9 The Concept of Lifestyle-Related Osteoporosis

In recent years, the concept of bone quality being a more important factor than bone density in contributing to increased fractures in DM is becoming more widely accepted.

When a sustained hyperglycemic state causes increased oxidative stress, more advanced glycation end products (AGEs) are synthesized. Pentosidine, one of these AGEs, causes bones to lose their suppleness and become brittle by forming nonphysiological bridges between bone collagen fibers [23]. Oxidative stress is also said to suppress osteoblast function and encourage osteoclast function, leading to decreased bone mass. DM and CKD are representative types of "lifestyle-related osteoporosis" diseases as they cause increased oxidative stress. The deterioration of bone quality in DM CKD patients, who have these diseases, is likely to be quite pronounced.

Despite being such a crucial factor, there are currently no methods for objectively evaluating bone quality on a clinical level. Although various methods such as using blood pentosidine levels as a marker of bone quality or directly evaluating bone quality with ultrasound equipment have been tried, further research is required as none of these methods can currently be practically used in clinical practice.

7.10 Vascular Calcification Is Promoted by Osteoblast Deterioration

Okazaki et al. reported that type 2 DM patients with poor glycemic control exhibit high levels of BAP, which is secreted in the early stage of osteoblast differentiation, and low levels of osteocalcin (OC), which is secreted in the late stage of

Table 7.3 DM HD patients suffer fractures that are independent of BMD

	Non-DM HD patients			DM HD patients		
Fracture in lumbar spine	(−)	(+)	p	(−)	(+)	p
Numbers	72	11		21	10	
Age (years)	72.8 ± 5.7	79.0 ± 7.8	<0.005	72.1 ± 4.2	71.2 ± 5.3	n.s.
HD duration (years)	6.10 ± 6.31	3.13 ± 2.20	n.s.	4.24 ± 2.77	2.88 ± 3.46	n.s.
BMI (Kg/m2)	19.6 ± 3.4	20.2 ± 3.4	n.s.	20.9 ± 1.9	21.5 ± 2.7	n.s.
Hb_{A1C} (%)	N.D.	N.D.	–	6.33 ± 1.15	6.95 ± 1.75	n.s.
Serum PTH	146.2 ± 131.2	134.3 ± 179.8	n.s.	104.8 ± 62.4	109.6 ± 34.0	n.s.
Lumbar spine (L3) BMD (g/cm^2)	0.579 ± 0.121	0.490 ± 0.085	<0.05	0.597 ± 0.106	0.581 ± 0.086	n.s.
Distal radius 1/3 BMD (g/cm^2)	0.455 ± 0.090	0.392 ± 0.097	<0.05	0.480 ± 0.093	0.507 ± 0.091	n.s.

Cited from reference Yamamoto et al. [21]/partially revised

Although bone density was significantly decreased in cases in the non-DM HD patients group who suffered fractures, no relationship was observed between fractures and bone density in the DM HD patients group. Therefore, it is difficult to use bone density to determine the fracture risk of DM HD patients differentiation, but that these abnormalities could be improved with correct glycemic control [24]. However, in a previous study in which we evaluated serum OC levels before and after administering 1,25 dihydroxy vitamin D (1,25D) to DM patients, we found lower serum OC elevation rates after 1,25D administration and higher HbA1c levels [9]. These results suggest that poor glycemic control in DM patients impairs osteoblast differentiation and maturation, causing decreased osteoblast function. Conversely, OC-deficient mice were found to develop an insulin deficiency followed by onset of diabetes, suggesting that decreased OC is a factor in DM onset. Accordingly, osteoblast deterioration and decreased OC secretion, which occur in a hyperglycemic state, negatively affect glycometabolism and cause a malignant cycle to form between glycometabolism and bone metabolism. It has also been reported that a negative correlation exists between OC and arteriosclerosis, suggesting that OC may also affect the advance of arteriosclerosis in DM patients.

Jono et al. discovered that when vascular smooth muscle cells were cultured in high phosphate conditions, smooth muscle cells lost characteristics of smooth muscle and acquired osteoblastic characteristics instead [25]. Conventionally, it had been thought that ectopic calcification was simply a passive process caused by calcium deposits. However, after the release of this report, numerous types of transcription factors and extracellular matrix expression were confirmed to be involved in bone differentiation of regions of ectopic calcification in the blood vessels. Now, increased serum phosphate concentration is considered to be a powerful factor that induces bone differentiation of vascular smooth muscle cells.

Ishimura et al. reported that increased serum phosphate levels in non-DM HD patients were an independent risk factor for peripheral vascular calcification [26]. However, an investigation of whether peripheral artery calcification had occurred in the hands of 123 HD patients (DM, 49 cases; non-DM, 74 cases) found that the prevalence was approximately 27 % (20/74 cases) in the non-DM group but over 65 % (32/49 cases) in the DM group, indicating significantly high risk for vascular calcification in the DM group (Table 7.4). This indicated that the factor determining vascular calcification in DM patients was not serum phosphate level or HbA1c level, but GA elevation [27].

FGF-23, a phosphaturic hormone, is secreted from osteoblasts and osteocyte. Because osteoblast function decreases in a hyperglycemic state, secretion of FGF-23 may be decreased in DM patients with poor glycemic control in particular. Yoda et al. used an oral phosphate loading test on DM and non-DM patients to

Table 7.4 DM HD patients exhibit high vascular calcification rates

	Peripheral artery calcification in hands		
	Yes	No	Onset rate
DM patients	32 cases	17 cases	65.3 %
Non-DM patients	20 cases	54 cases	27.0 %

Cited from reference Yamada et al. [27]/partially revised
The vascular calcification rate of DM HD patients is much higher than that of non-DM HD patients

measure and comparatively investigate phosphate, PTH, and FGF-23 levels before loading and after 2 and 4 h of loading. Although no difference was noted between the groups for serum phosphate, PTH, and FGF-23 levels before loading, they found that both serum PTH and FGF-23 levels rose significantly after loading in the non-DM group and no significant changes were noted in the DM patients until 2 h after loading, when serum phosphate levels rose significantly in the DM patients only [28]. Thus, impairment of osteoblast and osteoclast function in DM patients lowers additional PTH and FGF-23 secretion ability, which may destroy the defense mechanism against postprandial hyperphosphatemia. This may cause not only impaired glucose tolerance but also promote vascular calcification by means of sustained exposure to hyperphosphatemia.

This suggests that although serum phosphate concentration is a direct risk factor for vascular calcification in non-DM dialysis patients [26], sustained hyperphosphatemia accompanying worsened glycemic control in diabetic patients on hemodialysis is the risk factor for such cases. Either way, because the appearance of vascular calcification has a markedly negative effect on prognosis [29], we believe that physicians should have a grasp of the above difference and implement not only phosphate control but also strict glycemic control for diabetic patients.

7.11 Treatment for ABD

Basically, from CKD stages 1–2 when GFR is 60 ml/min/1.73 m^2 or greater, the same treatment should be performed as for general osteoporosis patients. From CKD stages 3–5, patients should be treated in accordance with the CKD-mineral and bone disorder (CKD-MBD) concept, by appropriately managing levels of serum calcium, phosphate, and PTH. CKD-MBD is a clinical concept proposed by the international kidney treatment guideline creating body, Kidney Disease Improving Global Outcomes (KDIGO), which recommends that CKD be treated as a systemic disease including bones and blood vessels.

However, one must note that bone turnover is suppressed in patients in a hyperglycemic state, which negatively affects bones and blood vessels. Therefore, bone resorption inhibitors such as bisphosphonate are inappropriate for treating such patients. Although PTH preparations that promote bone formation may appear to be an appropriate selection, the physiological mechanism for PTH suppression in a sustained hyperglycemic state has yet to be clarified, and, in some cases, it may be lowered to correct some sort of nonphysiological state. Therefore, further research is needed to determine whether the use of PTH preparations is appropriate. With regard to the use of phosphorus adsorbents for hyperphosphatemia, if ABD is present, there is a risk that the administration of preparations containing calcium will cause the calcium to accumulate in blood vessels, promoting vascular calcification [30]. Therefore, types not containing calcium should be selected as much as possible. In a previous investigation, we switched 27 HD patients with PTH suppressing tendencies who were being treated with phosphorus adsorbents containing calcium to lanthanum carbonate which does not contain calcium, and observed their progress over 24 weeks. As a result, we found that serum calcium levels dropped, PTH rose, and bone formation and absorption markers indicated improvement from excessive suppression to within the normal range [31]. Furthermore, patients using sevelamer hydrochloride, an agent that does not contain calcium, have also been reported to have more inhibited coronary artery and aortic calcification than patients using phosphorus adsorbents containing calcium. In DM HD patients in whom ABD is suspected, it is important to eliminate excessive inhibition of PTH by removing calcium loading as much as possible to make bone turnover return to a normal level and maintain it at such a level.

7.12 Conclusions

When OF progresses, vertebral and femoral fractures and ectopic calcification of surrounding joints, soft tissue, heart valves, and blood vessels may occur. However, this has been reported as even more serious in DM complicated with ABD, as fractures occur frequently, patients are susceptible to vascular calcification, and there is a high likelihood of developing hypercalcemia if treated with calcium or vitamin D preparations. Prognosis has also been reported as poor in cases of decreased PTH secretion with suspected ABD. It appears that even once HD has been initiated, proactively implementing strict glycemic control is the best option as it not only prevents bone metabolism abnormalities but may also improve the prognosis of DM HD patients, who are in an extremely serious condition.

References

1. Plantinga LC, Crews DC, Coresh J et al (2010) Prevalence of chronic kidney disease in US adults with undiagnosed diabetes or prediabetes. Clin J Am Soc Nephrol 5:673–682
2. The Diabetes Control and Complications Trial Research Group (1993) The effect of intensive treatment of diabetes on the development and progression of long-term complications in insulin-dependent diabetes mellitus. The Diabetes Control and Complications Trial Research Group. N Engl J Med 30:977–986
3. Chujo K, Ichimiya C, Oohashi T et al (2002) Evaluation of reliable marker of the glycemic state in diabetic patients on hemodialysis. J Jpn Soc Dial Ther 35:1105–1110
4. Inaba M, Okuno S, Kumeda Y et al (2007) Glycated albumin is a better glycemic indicator than glycated hemoglobin values in hemodialysis patients with diabetes: effect of anemia and erythropoietin injection. J Am Soc Nephrol 18:896–903
5. Mehrotra R, Kalantar-Zadeh K, Adler S (2011) Assessment of glycemic control in dialysis patients with diabetes: glycosylated hemoglobin or glycated albumin? Clin J Am Soc Nephrol 6:1520–1522
6. Hui SL, Epstein S, Johnston CC (1985) A prospective study of bone mass in patients with type 1 diabetes. J Clin Endocrinol Metab 60:74–80
7. McNair P (1988) Bone mineral metabolism in human type 1 diabetes mellitus. Dan Med Bull 35:109–121

8. Tuominen JT, Impivaara O, Puukka P et al (1999) Bone mineral density in patients with type 1 and type 2 diabetes. Diabetes Care 22:1196–1200
9. Inaba M, Terada M, Koyama H et al (1995) Influence of high glucose on 1,25-dihydroxyvitamin D3-induced effect on human osteoblast-like MG-63 cells. J Bone Miner Res 10:1050–1056
10. Kobayashi K, Takahashi N, Jimi E et al (2000) Tumor necrosis factor α stimulates osteoclast differentiation by a mechanism independent of the ODF/RANKL-RANK interaction. J Exp Med 191:275–285
11. Okuno Y, Nishizawa Y, Sekiya K et al (1991) Total and regional bone mineral content in patients with non-insulin dependent diabetes mellitus. J Nutr Sci Vitaminol (Tokyo) 37:43–49
12. Imanishi Y, Inaba M, Nakatsuka K et al (2004) FGF-23 in patients with end-stage renal disease on hemodialysis. Kidney Int 65:1943–1946
13. Fukagawa M, Nakanishi S, Fujii H et al (2006) Regulation of parathyroid function in chronic kidney disease (CKD). Clin Exp Nephrol 10:175–179
14. Ishimura E, Nishizawa Y, Inaba M et al (1999) Serum levels of 1,25-dihydroxyvitamin D, 24,25-dihydroxyvitamin D, and 25-hydroxyvitamin D in nondialyzed patients with chronic renal failure. Kidney Int 55:1019–1027
15. Gonzalez EA, Ashutosh S, Martin KJ et al (2004) Vitamin D insufficiency and deficiency in chronic kidney disease. Am J Nephrol 24(5):503–510
16. Sherrard DJ, Hercz G, Pei Y et al (1993) The spectrum of bone disease in end-stage renal failure – an evolving disorder. Kidney Int 43:436–442
17. Sugimoto T, Ritter C, Morrissey J et al (1990) Effects of high concentrations of glucose on PTH secretion in parathyroid cells. Kidney Int 37:1522–1527
18. Yamada S, Inaba M, Kurajoh M et al (2008) Utility of serum tartrate-resistant acid phosphatase (TRACP5b) as a bone resorption marker in patients with chronic kidney disease: independence from renal dysfunction. Clin Endocrinol (Oxf) 69:189–196
19. Yamada S, Inaba M, Okada S et al (2010) Association of glycated albumin, but not glycated hemoglobin, with calcaneus quantitative ultrasound in male hemodialysis patients with type 2 diabetes mellitus. Metabolism 59:390–394
20. Vestergaard P, Rejnmark L, Mosekilde L (2005) Relative fracture risk in patients with diabetes mellitus, and the impact of insulin and oral antidiabetic medication on relative fracture risk. Diabetologia 48:1292–1299
21. Yamamoto M, Yamaguchi T, Yamauchi M et al (2007) Diabetic patients have an increased risk of vertebral fractures independent of BMD or diabetic complications. J Bone Miner Res 24:702–709
22. Inaba M, Okuno S, Kumeda Y et al (2005) Increased incidence of vertebral fracture in older female hemodialyzed patients with type 2 diabetes mellitus. Calcif Tissue Int 76:256–260
23. Saito M, Fujii K, Mori Y et al (2006) Role of collagen enzymatic and glycation induced cross-links as a determinant of bone quality in spontaneously diabetic WBN/Kob rats. Osteoporos Int 17:1514–1523
24. Okazaki R, Totsuka Y, Hamano K et al (1997) Metabolic improvement of poorly controlled noninsulin-dependent diabetes mellitus decreases bone turnover. J Clin Endocrinol Metab 82:2915–2920
25. Jono S, Shioi A, Ikari Y et al (2006) Vascular calcification in chronic kidney disease. J Bone Miner Metab 24:176–181
26. Ishimura E, Okuno S, Kitatani K et al (2002) Different risk factors for peripheral vascular calcification between diabetic and non-diabetic haemodialysis patients – importance of glycaemic control. Diabetologia 45:1446–1448
27. Yamada S, Inaba M, Shidara K et al (2008) Association of glycated albumin, but not glycated hemoglobin, with peripheral vascular calcification in hemodialysis patients with type 2 diabetes. Life Sci 83:516–519
28. Tanaka H, Hamano T, Fujii N et al (2009) The impact of diabetes mellitus on vitamin D metabolism in predialysis patients. Bone 45:949–955

29. Okuno S, Ishimura E, Kitatani K et al (2007) Presence of abdominal aortic calcification is significantly associated with all-cause and cardiovascular mortality in maintenance hemodialysis patients. Am J Kidney Dis 49:417–425
30. London GM, Marchais SJ, Guérin AP et al (2008) Association of bone activity, calcium load, aortic stiffness, and calcifications in ESRD. J Am Soc Nephrol 19:1827–1835
31. Inaba M, Okuno S, Nagayama H et al (2014) Restoration of parathyroid function after change of phosphate binder from calcium carbonate to lanthanum carbonate in hemodialysis patients with suppressed serum parathyroid hormone. J Ren Nutr 25:242–246

Chapter 8
Bone as an Endocrine Organ: Diabetic Bone Disease as a Cause of Endocrine Disorder via Osteocalcin, FGF23 Secreted from Osteocyte/Osteoblast

Koichiro Yoda

Abstract Endocrine effects occur when organs secrete humoral physiologically active substances into the blood or other bodily fluids, and these active substances exert their physiological activities in target tissues. Fibroblast growth factor (FGF) 23, which is secreted by osteocytes, acts on the renal tubule and is involved in phosphorus metabolism. Osteocalcin, which is secreted by osteoblasts, acts on pancreatic β-cells and adipocytes and plays a role in insulin secretion and glycometabolism, in addition to its conventional role as a bone matrix protein. Thus, FGF23 and osteocalcin secreted from bone tissues function as endocrine hormones. Osteocyte and osteoblast functions are decreased in diabetes. Consequently, the secretion of FGF23 and osteocalcin is hindered. The decreased function of FGF23 causes hyperphosphatemia and leads to the progression of arteriosclerosis. The decreased function of osteocalcin results in decreased insulin secretion and increased insulin resistance. In this article, we describe the role of bone as an endocrine organ and its association with diabetes.

Keywords Undercarboxylated osteocalcin (ucOC) • Fibroblast growth factor 23 (FGF23) • Diabetes • Atherosclerosis • Hyperphosphatemia

8.1 FGF23

8.1.1 Overview

FGF23 is a 251-amino acid endocrine hormone produced primarily in osteoblasts/osteocytes. This hormone is encoded by the FGF23 gene, which was identified as a causal gene in a linkage analysis of families with a history of autosomal dominant hypophosphatemic rickets or osteomalacia. FGF23 belongs to the FGF13

K. Yoda (✉)
Department of Metabolism, Endocrinology and Molecular Medicine, Osaka City University Graduate School of Medicine, 1-4-3, Asahi-machi, Abeno-ku, Osaka 545-8585, Japan
e-mail: y45162001@yahoo.co.jp

M. Inaba (ed.), *Musculoskeletal Disease Associated with Diabetes Mellitus*,
DOI 10.1007/978-4-431-55720-3_8

subfamily, which includes other structurally related homologues, FGF19 and FGF21. FGF23 is found in the serum of healthy people at a concentration of several tens of pg/mL. It regulates phosphorus metabolism, facilitates phosphorus excretion in the renal tubule, and further reduces phosphorus absorption from the digestive tract by suppressing the activity of vitamin D3 [1,25$(OH)_2D_3$]. As the functions of osteocytes and osteoblasts decrease in diabetes, FGF23 secretion resulting from phosphorus loading decreases, and serum phosphorus levels increase after meals. In chronic renal failure, in which the urinary secretion of phosphorus is decreased, the FGF23 level starts to increase when the glomerular filtration rate reaches approximately 60 mL/min. This is prior to PTH, which plays a similar role in the urinary secretion of phosphorus. Decreased FGF23 secretion facilitates the stimulation of bone metabolism turnover caused by the increase in PTH, resulting in the stimulation of Ca recruitment to blood from bone. This increased serum phosphorus or Ca level can be a risk factor for Monckeberg medial calcific sclerosis, a characteristic feature of patients with diabetes or chronic renal failure. In summary, decreased FGF23 function is associated with arteriosclerosis progression, cardiovascular events, and an increase in the mortality rate.

8.1.2 *Localization*

FGF23 is considered to be mainly located within bone tissues in vivo. The expression of FGF23 mRNA increases in a concentration-dependent manner in human osteoblast-like cells in response to increased levels of extracellular phosphate [1]. Furthermore, elevated FGF23 expression in osteocytes and osteoblasts has been confirmed in a murine model of X-linked dominant hypophosphatemic rickets, in which FGF23 is overexpressed due to an abnormality in the phosphate-regulating gene with homologies to endopeptidase on the X chromosome (PHEX) gene [2]. Functions of FGF23-producing osteocytes and osteoblasts decrease in diabetes (Fig. 8.1). Mesenchymal stem cells normally differentiate into osteocytes

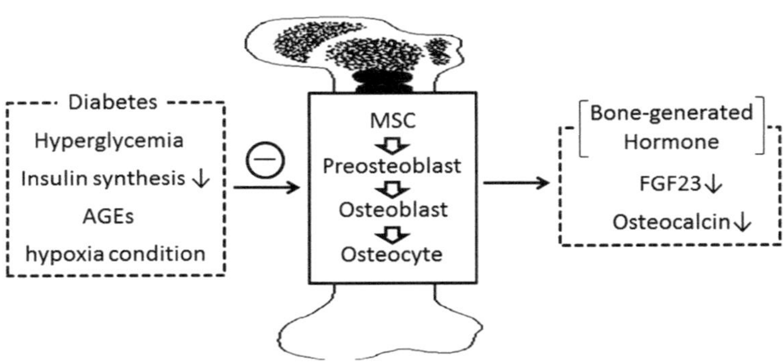

Fig. 8.1 Diabetes and bone-generated hormone interaction via osteoblast/osteocyte impairment. Several factors associated with diabetes impair osteoblast/osteocyte differentiation and function where FGF23 and osteocalcin were generated. *AGEs* advanced glycation end products, *MSC* mesenchymal stem cell

via preosteoblasts, immature osteoblasts, and mature osteoblasts. The differentiation of osteoblasts is inhibited by conditions commonly found in diabetes, such as hyperglycemia, impaired insulin function, and decreased blood flow to bones that accompanies microangiopathy. Hyperglycemia is directly toxic to osteoblasts themselves. Acute hyperglycemia and its associated hyperosmolality suppress the expression of genes involved in osteoblast maturation [3]. High blood glucose leads to the enhanced formation and accumulation of advanced glycation end products (AGEs) in bone. It has been shown that AGEs stimulate osteoblast apoptosis [4]. Hyperglycemia and oxidative stress may also affect mesenchymal stem cell differentiation. Culturing mesenchymal stem cells in high glucose media reduced the levels of osteoplastic markers such as osteocalcin and osteopontin [5]. Diabetes is also linked to generalized damage of blood vessel walls, which results in micro- and macrovascular complications. Oxygen tension within the marrow microenvironment is physiologically lower than that in other tissues, and the presence of diabetes may further alter cellular homeostasis. Indeed, it has been reported that differentiation of mesenchymal stem cells toward either the adipose or osteoblast phenotypes is reduced under hypoxic conditions [6].

8.1.3 Regulation of Phosphorus Metabolism

Serum phosphorus levels are mainly regulated by phosphorus absorption from the digestive tract and phosphorus reabsorption in the renal tubule (Fig. 8.2). Most of the phosphorus filtered in the glomerulus is reabsorbed in the proximal renal tubule. Type 2a and 2c sodium–phosphate cotransporters are responsible for the physiological reabsorption of phosphorus in the proximal renal tubule. FGF23 acts on the Klotho–FGF receptor (FGFR) complex in the renal tubule and suppresses phosphorus reabsorption by decreasing the expression of type 2a and 2c sodium–phosphate cotransporters [7]. In the kidney of streptozotocin-induced diabetic rats, decrease of Klotho and FGFR expression by high glucose has been documented [8]. FGF23 also decreases the level of activated vitamin D3 [1,25 $(OH)_2D_3$], which accelerates phosphorous absorption from the digestive tract, by decreasing the expression of Cyp27b1 (1α-hydroxylase), an enzyme producing 1,25 $(OH)_2D_3$, and by facilitating the expression of Cyp24 (24-hydroxylase), which transforms 1,25$(OH)_2D_3$ into a metabolite with lower activity [9]. As shown above, FGF23 decreases serum phosphorus levels by suppressing phosphorus reabsorption in the renal tubule as well as phosphorus absorption from the digestive tract by decreasing the serum 1,25$(OH)_2D_3$ level.

We previously reported a decrease in FGF23 responsiveness to phosphorus loading in patients with diabetes (Fig. 8.3) [10]. Phosphorus (1 g) was orally administered to patients with type 2 diabetes ($n = 10$) and nondiabetic patients ($n = 10$), and then, the short-term effect was examined. Patients in both groups

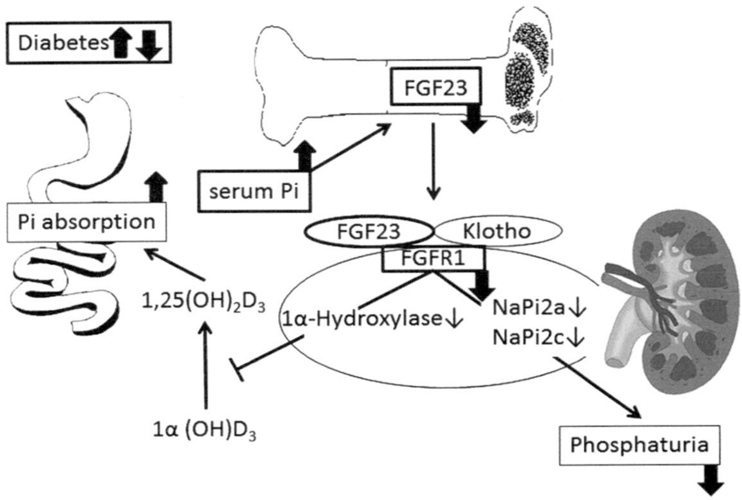

Fig. 8.2 Possible influence of diabetes on the regulation and action of FGF23. Increased serum Pi causes FGF23 to be released from skeletal osteoblasts/osteocytes. The major known effects of FGF23 are inhibition of Na–Pi cotransport in the kidney and the resultant phosphaturia and inhibition of 1α(OH)D3 hydroxylase, which reduces levels of activated vitamin D3 [1,25 $(OH)_2D_3$]. Reduced $1{,}25(OH)_2D_3$ levels decrease gastrointestinal Pi absorption. In diabetes, impaired production of FGF23 at osteoblasts/osteocytes and downregulation of FGF23-specific receptor that is composed of Klotho and FGF receptor 1 (FGFR1) may lead to decrement in phosphaturia and increment in Pi absorption

were confirmed to have no renal dysfunction. The serum FGF23 level was significantly increased in the nondiabetic group 2 and 4 h after the administration of phosphorus, whereas no increase was observed in the diabetic group. The serum iPTH level also increased significantly in the nondiabetic group 4 h after the load, whereas no increase was seen in the diabetic group. Serum phosphorus levels were significantly increased in both groups 2 h after phosphorus administration. Although the serum phosphorus level continued to increase in the diabetic group up to 4 h after the administration, it was suppressed in the nondiabetic group. Next, the long-term effect of phosphorus loading was examined by administering phosphorus (2 g per day) orally on two consecutive days. Significant increases in both serum FGF23 and iPTH levels were observed only in the nondiabetic group 3 days after the administration. When phosphorus was orally administered for 7 days to patients with chronic renal failure, the serum FGF23 level continued to increase from the basal value in the nondiabetic group during the investigation, whereas no such change was seen in the diabetic group [11].

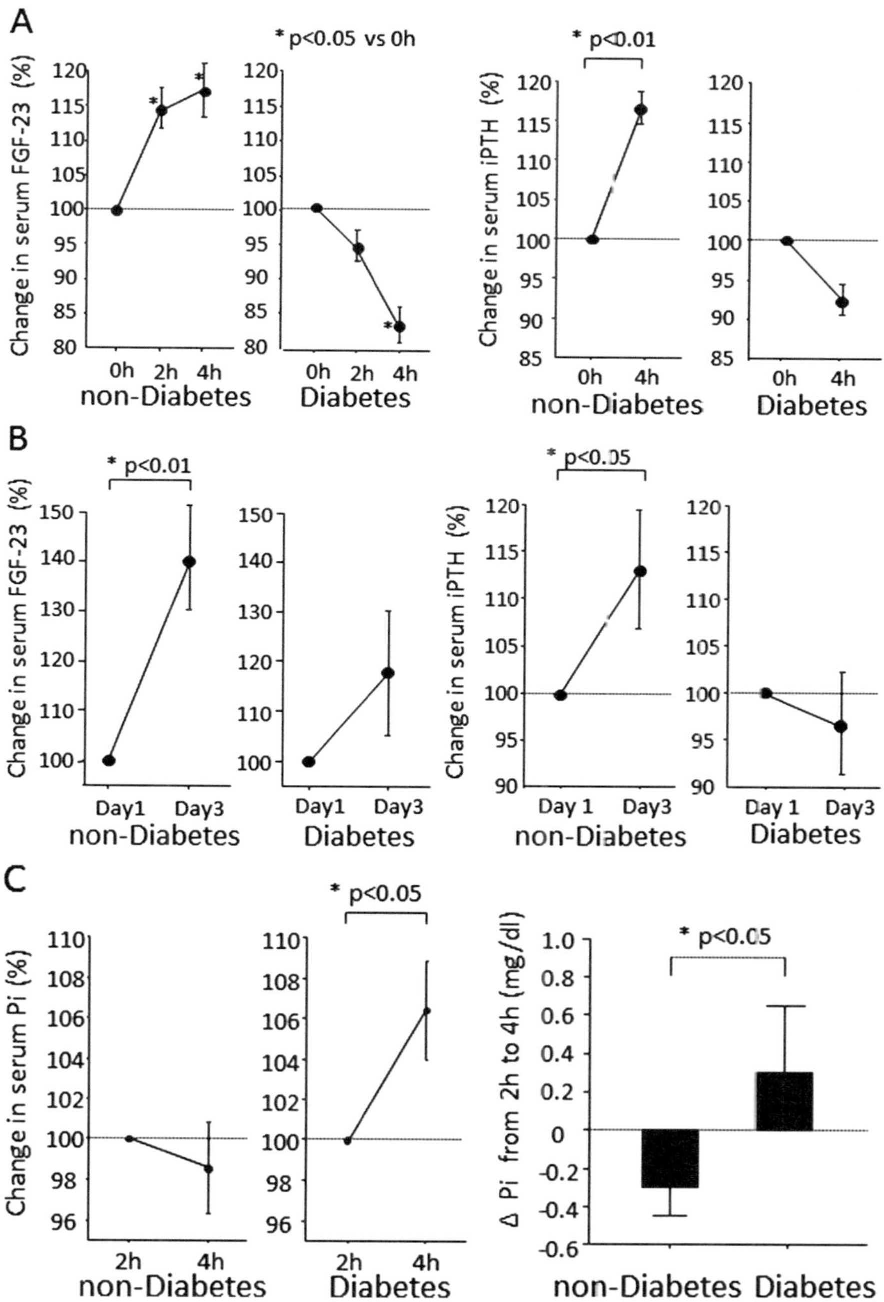

Fig. 8.3 Impaired responses of serum FGF23 and iPTH to oral Pi stimulation test. (**a**) Time courses of serum FGF23 and iPTH from 0 to 4 h after intake of Pi on day 1. In nondiabetic patients, serum FGF23 elevated significantly ($P = 0.046$ by ANOVA) and showed a significant increase at 2 h after Pi stimulation ($P < 0.05$ by Fisher test). In contrast, serum FGF23 was significantly reduced in diabetic patients ($P = 0.018$ by ANOVA) and showed a significant decrease at 4 h

8.1.4 Association with Arteriosclerosis

Because an increase in the serum phosphorus level is a risk factor for cardiovascular calcification and reduced life expectancy, the serum FGF23 level, which decreases the serum phosphorus level, helps predict the onset of cardiovascular calcification and reduced life expectancy. Chronic renal failure is one of the pathological conditions in which the serum phosphorus level is increased. When renal function decreases, this phosphaturic effect is hindered, and phosphorus accumulates in the body. In chronic renal failure, FGF23 increases when the estimated glomerular filtration rate reaches around 60 mL/min, which is before PTH [12], and this protects against an increase in the serum phosphorus level. For this reason, the FGF23 increase is a predictive factor for the progression of chronic renal failure, which is independent of the amount of albumin excreted into the urine [13]. When renal failure reaches the advanced stage, FGF23 levels are progressively increased to compensate for persistent phosphate retention, but this results in reduced renal production of activated vitamin D and decreased serum Ca and leads to secondary hyperparathyroidism (Fig. 8.4). As a result, Ca and phosphorus are recruited from bone to blood and increase the risk of cardiovascular calcification. Vessel calcification caused by this mechanism is called Monckeberg medial calcific sclerosis to distinguish it from the atherosclerotic plaques in the vascular intima. It is characterized by calcification within the vascular media. Increased areas of Monckeberg calcification are involved in the onset of cardiovascular events and the increase in the mortality rate [14]. The frequency of Monckeberg calcification in the peripheral artery (the artery in the hand) [15] and in the abdominal artery [16] reportedly increases in diabetic patients compared with nondiabetic patients. This suggests diabetes is a state where it is easy to accumulate phosphate and leads to secondary hyperparathyroidism. Based on this background, the increase in serum FGF23 can serve as a predictive factor for total death, in addition to cardiovascular events, in patients with chronic renal failure [17] or in patients on dialysis [18].

Some studies have suggested the direct involvement of FGF23 in the progression of vascular calcification, in addition to its indirect involvement via phosphorus metabolism. The FGF23 signal is transmitted through its binding to the Klotho–FGFR complex, which consists of membrane-bound Klotho and FGFR-1 and FGFR-3. Lim et al. reported that the Klotho–FGFR complex was expressed not

---

Fig. 8.3 (continued) ($P < 0.05$ by Fisher test). During oral Pi stimulation, serum iPTH significantly increased from 0 to 4 h in nondiabetic patients ($P = 0.007$) but not in diabetic patients ($P = 0.072$). (**b**) Comparison of serum FGF23 and iPTH levels on day 1 (0 h) and day 3 (0 h). An oral Pi load for 2 days significantly increased serum FGF23 and iPTH in nondiabetic patients ($P = 0.009$, $P = 0.048$) but not in diabetic patients ($P = 0.241$, $P = 0.507$). (**c**) Comparison of serum Pi changes in nondiabetic and diabetic patients. Serum Pi significantly increased between 2 and 4 h in diabetic patients ($P = 0.020$), whereas there was no significant change in nondiabetic patients ($P = 0.574$). The serum Pi changes from 2 to 4 h differed significantly between the two groups ($P = 0.027$)

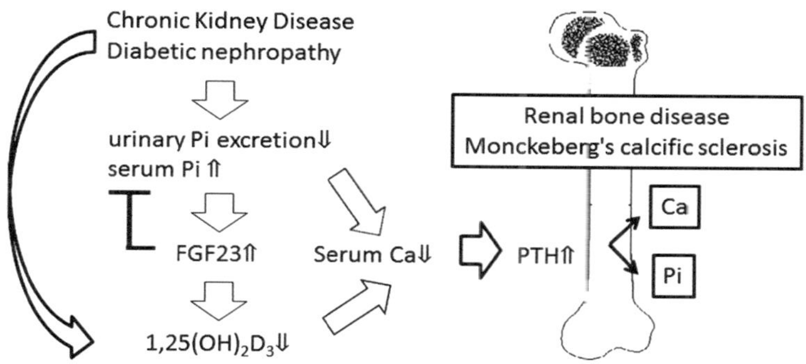

Fig. 8.4 The role of FGF23 in chronic kidney disease – mineral and bone disorder. In patients with chronic kidney disease, circulating FGF23 levels are progressively increased to compensate for persistent phosphate retention, but this results in reduced renal production of activated vitamin D3 [$1,25(OH)_2D_3$] and leads to secondary hyperparathyroidism. Ca and Pi are recruited from bone to blood and increase the risk of cardiovascular calcification known as Monckeberg calcific sclerosis

only in the renal tubule but also in the arteries of healthy people [19]. When examined in arterial smooth muscle cells, the sensitivity of the Klotho–FGFR complex toward FGF23 decreased, and the calcification of vascular media was accelerated under the condition of high glucose and/or uremia. Even in clinical trials, the decrease in FGF23 was reported to be a risk factor, independent of the increase in the Ca/phosphorus product, of the calcification of peripheral arteries [20] and the arch aorta [21], and these reports support the direct involvement of FGF23 in suppressing vascular calcification.

8.2 Osteocalcin

8.2.1 Overview

Osteocalcin was identified as a bone matrix protein mainly secreted by osteoblasts. Osteocalcin is carboxylated by γ-carboxylase, and most of it is embedded within the bone as part of the bone matrix. In blood, osteocalcin exists in the following two forms: one with all three glutamic acid residues carboxylated and the other with less carboxylation of the residues. Undercarboxylated osteocalcin (ucOC) facilitates the synthesis and secretion of insulin in the pancreas and increases the insulin sensitivity of peripheral tissues. In addition, insulin signaling in osteoblasts activates osteocalcin by regulating the interaction between osteoblasts and osteoclasts. In this manner, bone tissue creates a positive feedback mechanism that acts on pancreatic β-cells and adipose tissues via hormones such as ucOC and insulin. Some reports on clinical studies in humans have also suggested that ucOC facilitates insulin secretion and enhances insulin sensitivity.

8.2.2 Feedback Mechanism of Insulin and ucOC (Fig. 8.5)

In murine research, insulin directly acts on osteoblasts to facilitate osteocalcin synthesis [22]. Furthermore, it inhibits the synthesis of osteoprotegerin (OPG), which has a suppressive effect on osteoclast differentiation factor (RANKL) [23]. Osteocalcin synthesized in osteoblasts is further modified with the addition of a carbonate ion to a γ-glutamic acid residue by vitamin K-dependent carboxylase, which is then secreted as γ-carboxylated osteocalcin (cOC) [24]. cOC binds to hydroxyapatite within the bone matrix and accumulates in bone tissues. Meanwhile, because a decrease in OPG secretion enhances the function of RANKL, osteoclast formation is facilitated. As a result, bone resorption by osteoclasts is stimulated. Proton (H^+) and chloride ions (Cl^-) are secreted from the ruffled borders of osteoclasts into resorption cavities to form an acidic environment, which leads to the decalcification of bone minerals. In such an acidic environment, cOC bound to hydroxyapatite undergoes decarboxylation to yield ucOC, which is released into the

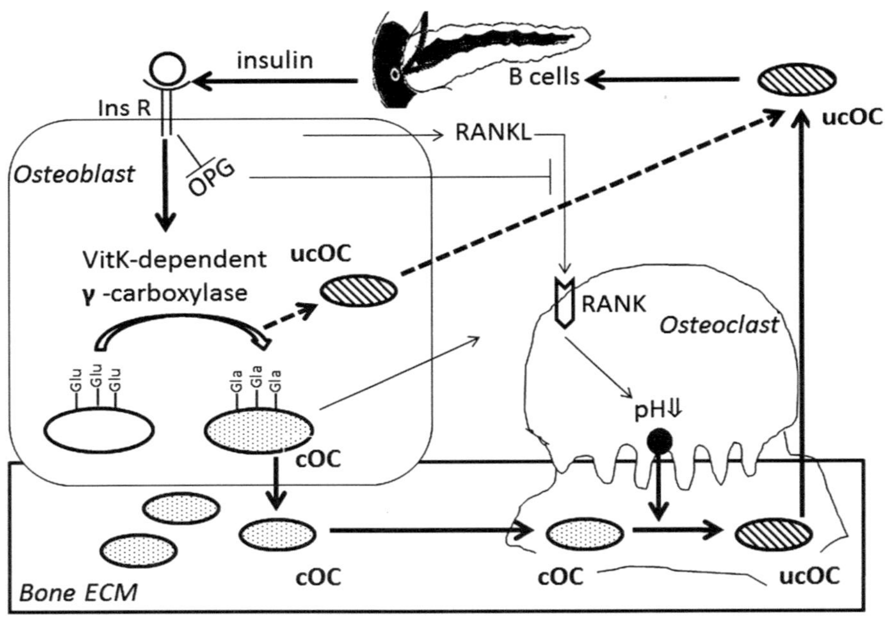

Fig. 8.5 A feedforward loop links insulin, bone resorption, and osteocalcin activity. Insulin signaling in osteoblasts acts on osteoblasts to facilitate osteocalcin synthesis via addition of a carbonate ion to a γ-glutamic acid residue by vitamin K-dependent **γ**-carboxylase, which is then secreted as γ-carboxylated osteocalcin (cOC). Secreted cOC is stored in the bone extracellular matrix (ECM). Furthermore, insulin signal inhibits the synthesis of osteoprotegerin (OPG). Because a decrease in OPG secretion enhances the function of osteoclast differentiation factor (RANKL), bone resorption by osteoclasts was activated. The acidic pH in resorption lacunae decarboxylates cOC stored in the bone EMC. Undercarboxylated osteocalcin (ucOC) then stimulates insulin secretion by the β-cells of the pancreatic islets. Ins R, insulin receptor

blood [23]. ucOC functions as an endocrine hormone for pancreatic β-cells and adipocytes. In pancreatic β-cells, ucOC facilitates insulin secretion, whereas it facilitates the secretion of adiponectin in adipocytes. For this reason, when ucOC is administered to mice, insulin sensitivity is increased, and blood glucose increases after glucose loading is suppressed [25]. Furthermore, ucOC administration causes a decrease in the amount of fat [25]. These results suggest that bone tissue creates a positive feedback mechanism that acts on pancreatic β-cells and adipose tissues via hormones such as ucOC and insulin, implying the presence of a close relationship between bone metabolism and glycometabolism.

8.2.3 Association of Osteocalcin with Diabetes

Clinical examinations have also been conducted to investigate the association of osteocalcin with glycometabolism and insulin sensitivity in humans. A cross-sectional study in patients with type 2 diabetes revealed that a decrease in ucOC was associated with fasting blood sugar levels and high HbA1c levels. In addition, its association with increases in body fat and the ratio of visceral fat to subcutaneous fat was revealed using a dual-energy X-ray absorptiometry method and CT, respectively [26]. In a large-scale cross-sectional study that involved 2,966 elderly males (70–89 years old), the levels of ucOC, total osteocalcin (TOC), and collagen type IC-terminal cross-linked telopeptide (CTX), which is a bone resorption marker, were all significantly reduced in patients with diabetes compared with those in nondiabetic patients, and these levels were associated with an increased risk of developing diabetes, independently of age, BMI, and renal function. In a multivariate model in which ucOC, TOC, and CTX were simultaneously incorporated, although both ucOC and CTX were risk factors for developing diabetes, TOC demonstrated no significant association, indicating that ucOC was involved in glycometabolism independently of bone metabolism turnover [27]. Even in hemodialysis patients with abnormalities of bone metabolism, increased levels of ucOC, which were associated with bone metabolism markers, were inversely associated with indices of glucose metabolism such as plasma glucose, hemoglobin A1c, and glycated albumin [28]. Concerning its association with insulin sensitivity, a longitudinal study in elderly males (55–80 years old) demonstrated that the rate of ucOC increase was related to the rate of HOMA-IR decrease [29], which is an index of insulin resistance. According to a study by Levinger et al., a significant increase in ucOC was observed together with increased insulin sensitivity after a 60-min exercise load, whereas no change was observed in TOC. In addition, an association was observed between the ucOC increase and the increase in insulin sensitivity before and after exercise [30]. These reports suggest that ucOC affects both insulin secretion and insulin sensitivity enhancement.

References

1. Mirams M, Robinson BG, Mason RS, Nelson AE (2004) Bone as a source of FGF23: regulation by phosphate? Bone 35(5):1192–1199. doi:10.1016/j.bone.2004.06.014
2. Liu S, Zhou J, Tang W, Jiang X, Rowe DW, Quarles LD (2006) Pathogenic role of Fgf23 in Hyp mice. Am J Physiol Endocrinol Metab 291(1):E38–E49. doi:10.1152/ajpendo.00008.2006
3. Terada M, Inaba M, Yano Y, Hasuma T, Nishizawa Y, Morii H, Otani S (1998) Growth-inhibitory effect of a high glucose concentration on osteoblast-like cells. Bone 22(1):17–23
4. Alikhani M, Alikhani Z, Boyd C, MacLellan CM, Raptis M, Liu R, Pischon N, Trackman PC, Gerstenfeld L, Graves DT (2007) Advanced glycation end products stimulate osteoblast apoptosis via the MAP kinase and cytosolic apoptotic pathways. Bone 40(2):345–353. doi:10.1016/j.bone.2006.09.011
5. Aguiari P, Leo S, Zavan B, Vindigni V, Rimessi A, Bianchi K, Franzin C, Cortivo R, Rossato M, Vettor R, Abatangelo G, Pozzan T, Pinton P, Rizzuto R (2008) High glucose induces adipogenic differentiation of muscle-derived stem cells. Proc Natl Acad Sci U S A 105 (4):1226–1231. doi:10.1073/pnas.0711402105
6. Malladi P, Xu Y, Chiou M, Giaccia AJ, Longaker MT (2006) Effect of reduced oxygen tension on chondrogenesis and osteogenesis in adipose-derived mesenchymal cells. Am J Physiol Cell Physiol 290(4):C1139–C1146. doi:10.1152/ajpcell.00415.2005
7. Urakawa I, Yamazaki Y, Shimada T, Iijima K, Hasegawa H, Okawa K, Fujita T, Fukumoto S, Yamashita T (2006) Klotho converts canonical FGF receptor into a specific receptor for FGF23. Nature 444(7120):770–774. doi:10.1038/nature05315
8. Cheng MF, Chen LJ, Wang MC, Hsu CT, Cheng JT (2014) Decrease of FGF receptor (FGFR) and interstitial fibrosis in the kidney of streptozotocin-induced diabetic rats. Horm Metab Res 46(1):1–7. doi:10.1055/s-0033-1349090
9. Quarles LD (2012) Role of FGF23 in vitamin D and phosphate metabolism: implications in chronic kidney disease. Exp Cell Res 318(9):1040–1048. doi:10.1016/j.yexcr.2012.02.027
10. Yoda K, Imanishi Y, Yoda M, Mishima T, Ichii M, Yamada S, Mori K, Emoto M, Inaba M (2012) Impaired response of FGF-23 to oral phosphate in patients with type 2 diabetes: a possible mechanism of atherosclerosis. J Clin Endocrinol Metab 97(11):E2036–E2043. doi:10.1210/jc.2012-2024
11. Muras K, Masajtis-Zagajewska A, Nowicki M (2013) Diabetes modifies effect of high-phosphate diet on fibroblast growth factor-23 in chronic kidney disease. J Clin Endocrinol Metab 98(12):E1901–E1908. doi:10.1210/jc.2013-2418
12. Isakova T, Wahl P, Vargas GS, Gutierrez OM, Scialla J, Xie H, Appleby D, Nessel L, Bellovich K, Chen J, Hamm L, Gadegbeku C, Horwitz E, Townsend RR, Anderson CA, Lash JP, Hsu CY, Leonard MB, Wolf M (2011) Fibroblast growth factor 23 is elevated before parathyroid hormone and phosphate in chronic kidney disease. Kidney Int 79(12):1370–1378. doi:10.1038/ki.2011.47
13. Agarwal R, Duffin KL, Laska DA, Voelker JR, Breyer MD, Mitchell PG (2014) A prospective study of multiple protein biomarkers to predict progression in diabetic chronic kidney disease. Nephrol Dial Transplant 29(12):2293–2302. doi:10.1093/ndt/gfu255
14. Hashimoto H, Iijima K, Hashimoto M, Son BK, Ota H, Ogawa S, Eto M, Akishita M, Ouchi Y (2009) Validity and usefulness of aortic arch calcification in chest X-ray. J Atheroscler Thromb 16(3):256–264
15. Ishimura E, Okuno S, Kitatani K, Kim M, Shoji T, Nakatani T, Inaba M, Nishizawa Y (2002) Different risk factors for peripheral vascular calcification between diabetic and non-diabetic haemodialysis patients – importance of glycaemic control. Diabetologia 45(10):1446–1448. doi:10.1007/s00125-002-0920-8
16. Chen NX, Moe SM (2003) Arterial calcification in diabetes. Curr Diabetes Rep 3(1):28–32

17. Kendrick J, Cheung AK, Kaufman JS, Greene T, Roberts WL, Smits G, Chonchol M, Investigators H (2011) FGF-23 associates with death, cardiovascular events, and initiation of chronic dialysis. J Am Soc Nephrol: JASN 22(10):1913–1922. doi:10.1681/ASN.2010121224
18. Gutierrez OM, Mannstadt M, Isakova T, Rauh-Hain JA, Tamez H, Shah A, Smith K, Lee H, Thadhani R, Juppner H, Wolf M (2008) Fibroblast growth factor 23 and mortality among patients undergoing hemodialysis. N Engl J Med 359(6):584–592. doi:10.1056/NEJMoa0706130
19. Lim K, Lu TS, Molostvov G, Lee C, Lam FT, Zehnder D, Hsiao LL (2012) Vascular Klotho deficiency potentiates the development of human artery calcification and mediates resistance to fibroblast growth factor 23. Circulation 125(18):2243–2255. doi:10.1161/CIRCULATIONAHA.111.053405
20. Inaba M, Okuno S, Imanishi Y, Yamada S, Shioi A, Yamakawa T, Ishimura E, Nishizawa Y (2006) Role of fibroblast growth factor-23 in peripheral vascular calcification in non-diabetic and diabetic hemodialysis patients. Osteoporos Int 17(10):1506–1513. doi:10.1007/s00198-006-0154-6
21. Tamei N, Ogawa T, Ishida H, Ando Y, Nitta K (2011) Serum fibroblast growth factor-23 levels and progression of aortic arch calcification in non-diabetic patients on chronic hemodialysis. J Atheroscler Thromb 18(3):217–223
22. Fulzele K, Riddle RC, DiGirolamo DJ, Cao X, Wan C, Chen D, Faugere MC, Aja S, Hussain MA, Bruning JC, Clemens TL (2010) Insulin receptor signaling in osteoblasts regulates postnatal bone acquisition and body composition. Cell 142(2):309–319. doi:10.1016/j.cell.2010.06.002
23. Ferron M, Wei J, Yoshizawa T, Del Fattore A, DePinho RA, Teti A, Ducy P, Karsenty G (2010) Insulin signaling in osteoblasts integrates bone remodeling and energy metabolism. Cell 142(2):296–308. doi:10.1016/j.cell.2010.06.003
24. Engelke JA, Hale JE, Suttie JW, Price PA (1991) Vitamin K-dependent carboxylase: utilization of decarboxylated bone Gla protein and matrix Gla protein as substrates. Biochim Biophys Acta 1078(1):31–34
25. Lee NK, Sowa H, Hinoi E, Ferron M, Ahn JD, Confavreux C, Dacquin R, Mee PJ, McKee MD, Jung DY, Zhang Z, Kim JK, Mauvais-Jarvis F, Ducy P, Karsenty G (2007) Endocrine regulation of energy metabolism by the skeleton. Cell 130(3):456–469. doi:10.1016/j.cell.2007.05.047
26. Kanazawa I, Yamaguchi T, Yamauchi M, Yamamoto M, Kurioka S, Yano S, Sugimoto T (2011) Serum undercarboxylated osteocalcin was inversely associated with plasma glucose level and fat mass in type 2 diabetes mellitus. Osteoporos Int 22(1):187–194. doi:10.1007/s00198-010-1184-7
27. Yeap BB, Alfonso H, Chubb SA, Gauci R, Byrnes E, Beilby JP, Ebeling PR, Handelsman DJ, Allan CA, Grossmann M, Norman PE, Flicker L (2015) Higher serum undercarboxylated osteocalcin and other bone turnover markers are associated with reduced diabetes risk and lower estradiol concentrations in older men. J Clin Endocrinol Metab 100(1):63–71. doi:10.1210/jc.2014-3019
28. Okuno S, Ishimura E, Tsuboniwa N, Norimine K, Yamakawa K, Yamakawa T, Shoji S, Mori K, Nishizawa Y, Inaba M (2013) Significant inverse relationship between serum undercarboxylated osteocalcin and glycemic control in maintenance hemodialysis patients. Osteoporos Int 24(2):605–612. doi:10.1007/s00198-012-2003-0
29. Bullo M, Moreno-Navarrete JM, Fernandez-Real JM, Salas-Salvado J (2012) Total and undercarboxylated osteocalcin predict changes in insulin sensitivity and beta cell function in elderly men at high cardiovascular risk. Am J Clin Nutr 95(1):249–255. doi:10.3945/ajcn.111.016642
30. Levinger I, Jerums G, Stepto NK, Parker L, Serpiello FR, McConell GK, Anderson M, Hare DL, Byrnes E, Ebeling PR, Seeman E (2014) The effect of acute exercise on undercarboxylated osteocalcin and insulin sensitivity in obese men. J Bone Mineral Res 29(12):2571–2576. doi:10.1002/jbmr.2285

Part II
Muscle Diseases

Chapter 9
Overview

Nobuharu L. Fujii

Abstract The skeletal muscle is the largest site for glucose metabolism in the human body. According to insulin-clamp measurements, the contribution by the skeletal muscle accounts for 70 % of the total glucose utilization rate, substantially exceeding the contribution by other organs such as the brain (~15 %) and adipose tissue (~5 %). Therefore, impaired glucose metabolism in the skeletal muscle greatly affects blood glucose control in the body. Glucose metabolism is an intracellular event. The extra- to intracellular passage of glucose is facilitated by glucose transporters (GLUTs). Glucose transporter 1 (GLUT1) and 4 (GLUT4) are expressed in the skeletal muscle. GLUT1 constitutively spans the cell membrane and takes up glucose into the skeletal cell in accordance with the glucose concentration gradient between the inside and outside of the cell. In contrast, GLUT4 is usually incorporated into small vesicles and localized in the cell and is translocated and incorporated into the cell membrane upon stimulation by insulin, which induces glucose uptake. Among multiple GLUTs, GLUT4 is the only isoform that is regulated by translocation, and its distribution is also limited to the skeletal muscle, heart, and adipose tissue. GLUT4 acts as a master regulator of glucose metabolism in response to changes in blood glucose. Several factors regulate GLUT4 expression and its translocation to, and retention in, the cell membrane. These factors include intracellular insulin signal transduction, insulin-independent glucose metabolism, and ectopic fat. A failure in any of these factors leads to the development of diabetic conditions in the body. Exercise and physical activity can coordinate these factors, acting favorably to turn the diabetic condition to a healthier state.

Keywords Skeletal muscle • Insulin • Contraction • Intracellular signal transduction • Glucose uptake

N.L. Fujii (✉)
Department of Health Promotion Sciences, Graduate School of Human Health Sciences, Tokyo Metropolitan University, Minami-Osawa, Hachioji, Tokyo 192-0397, Japan
e-mail: fujiin@tmu.ac.jp

M. Inaba (ed.), *Musculoskeletal Disease Associated with Diabetes Mellitus*,
DOI 10.1007/978-4-431-55720-3_9

9.1 Insulin Signal Transduction in the Skeletal Muscle

Insulin is an essential hormone for maintaining glucose homeostasis [1]. When the blood glucose level rises, insulin is released from pancreatic β-cells and then acts on various organs to bring the blood glucose back to the basal level. The skeletal muscle, in particular, is the largest target organ for insulin, where insulin facilitates the uptake of a large amount of glucose by muscle cells, to be used for ATP production or stored in cells as an energy source after conversion to glycogen [2]. Glycogen, a polymer synthesized through the dehydration of glucose, has a multibranched structure consisting of many glucose molecules. If glucose is stored without being converted to glycogen, its intracellular concentration increases to the order of millimolars, impacting the osmotic pressure of the cell. When glucose is stored in the form of glycogen, the impact on osmotic pressure can be eliminated. Before glycogen is used as an energy substrate in the skeletal muscle, it is first converted to glucose-6-phosphate. Because the liver has glucose-6-phosphatase that converts glucose-6-phosphate into glucose, it can release glucose into the circulating blood as an energy substrate for other organs. However, glucose-6-phosphatase is not expressed in the skeletal muscle, and therefore, glucose-6-phosphate enters the glycolytic pathway and subsequently is used in energy production for the skeletal muscle. Because the skeletal muscle is a large organ, accounting for 40–45 % of body weight, its potential for glucose consumption is very high. The initial rate-determining step for glucose utilization by the skeletal muscle constitutes glucose uptake into the skeletal muscle cells.

The extra- to intracellular passage of glucose is facilitated by glucose transporters (GLUTs) in the skeletal muscle [3, 4]. Thus far, at least 14 types of GLUTs have been identified [5], and glucose transporter 1 (GLUT1) and glucose transporter 4 (GLUT4) are the main isoforms expressed in the skeletal muscle. GLUT4 is responsive to insulin and promotes glucose uptake [3–5]. When blood glucose is at basal levels, a large amount of GLUT4 is localized intracellularly. Once the blood glucose level increases with food consumption, insulin is secreted from pancreatic β-cells and binds to the insulin receptor (IR) on the cell membrane of the skeletal muscle. The activated IR phosphorylates the tyrosine residue of insulin receptor substrate (IRS) [6]. IRS functions as a platform for insulin signal transduction [7]. Phosphoinositide 3-kinase (PI3-K) binds to the phosphorylated IRS to make it active. PI3-K promotes the production of phosphatidylinositol (3,4,5)-trisphosphate (PIP3) on the cell membrane [8], and then the downstream Akt is activated [9]. While there are several Akt isoforms, Akt2 is considered to play the most important role in regulating glucose metabolism and in anabolic events such as cell proliferation and hypertrophy [10]. The activated Akt suppresses GAP activity of molecules containing the Rab-GAP domain, namely, Akt substrate 160 (AS160) and TBC1 domain family member 1 (TBC1D1), resulting in Rab activation and GLUT4 translocation [11].

Besides this signal transduction pathway from IR to Akt, studies indicate that PKCλ/δ [12], a member of the atypical PKC family, and the CAP/c-Cbl/TC10 signaling pathway [13] are also involved in the process of glucose metabolism. However, very few studies have been conducted after publication of the original paper, and no significant developments have been reported.

9.2 Insulin Resistance

Lowered insulin sensitivity of cells, coupled with decreased insulin response, is known as insulin resistance where the insulin-dependent stimulation of glucose uptake is reduced in the skeletal muscle. Insulin resistance is closely associated with a number of diseases, including diabetes. The foremost role of insulin is to promote anabolic processes. Therefore, insulin facilitates absorption and storage of glucose, lipids, and amino acids and suppresses their catabolism. In obese people with an imbalance between food intake and the amount of energy exerted through physical activity, a sufficient amount of nutrients has already been stored in cells, with no need for additional supply, and a mechanism at the cellular level is likely triggered in the form of insulin resistance (Fig. 9.1).

The working mechanism of insulin resistance is complex, probably involving numerous factors, including defective tyrosine phosphorylation of IRS-1. IRS-1 is phosphorylated on a tyrosine residue for signal transduction to the downstream pathway. More than 50 phosphorylation sites exist on serine/threonine residues and hinder the phosphorylation of tyrosine residues. C-Jun N-terminal kinase (JNK) and nuclear factor-kB (IkB) are representative serine/threonine kinases for IRS-1 [14]. At first, JNK is activated by TNFα, and then JNK phosphorylates serine 307 of IRS-1, which suppresses phosphorylation of the major tyrosine residue of IRS-1 and subsequently attenuates insulin signaling [14]. Further, when S6kinase

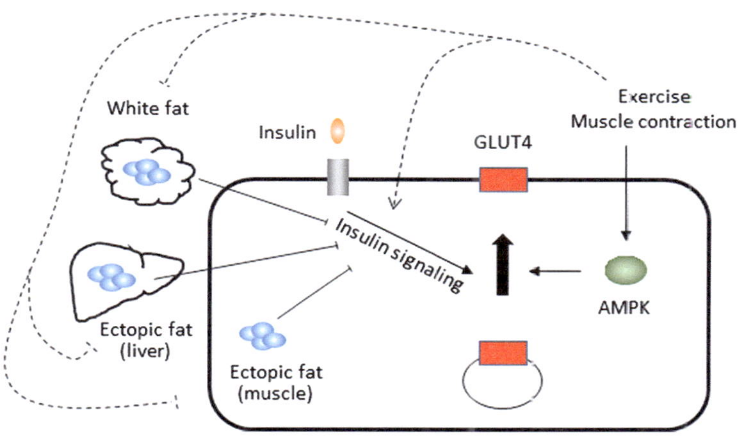

Fig. 9.1 The factors that affect to GLUT4 translocation and glucose utilization in the skeletal muscle

(S6K) is activated by insulin and amino acids, phosphorylation of serine 636/639 of IRS1 is accelerated, leading to attenuation of insulin signaling [15]. Phosphorylation of IRS-1 serine/threonine residues inhibits binding to PI3-K and accelerates proteasomal degradation of IRS-1 [16]. However, recent detailed analysis of the IRS phosphorylation sites suggests that serine/threonine phosphorylation does not necessarily lead to negative regulation of insulin signaling and that, in contrast, insulin signaling may be enhanced depending on the combinations of different phosphorylation sites. Under diverse physiological/pathological conditions, IRS-1 appears to modulate insulin signaling by transmitting the message for enhancing or suppressing insulin signals [17].

The findings available so far concerning how Class IA PI3-K is involved in insulin resistance are confusing [18]. PI3-K consists of a catalytic subunit with lipid kinase activity and a regulatory subunit that binds to the phosphorylated tyrosine residue of IRS. In mammals, the regulatory subunit is encoded by three genes, namely, pik3r1, pik3r2, and p55PIK [19]. While pik3r1 encodes three splice variants (p85α, AS53, and p50α), pik3r2 and p55PIK encode p85 and p55PIK, respectively [19]. Short isoforms, AS53, p50, and p55PIK, are expressed in limited cells or tissues while p85α and p85β are ubiquitously expressed, though expression of p85α is considered significant. In the skeletal muscle of patients with type 2 diabetes, the expression of these regulatory subunits increases [20]. Surprisingly, even in p85alpha [21] and p85beta [22] knockout mice, insulin sensitivity can be strengthened. It is difficult to fully explain these results. It is possible that p85 plays an essential role in insulin signaling by guiding P13-K toward IRS, though excess p85 suppresses insulin signaling. Phosphatase and tensin homolog (PTEN) deleted on chromosome ten is a phosphatase that antagonizes P13-K by dephosphorylating PIP3. It was difficult to induce insulin resistance in the skeletal muscle-specific PTEN knockout mice with a high-fat diet [23]. Therefore, insufficient regulation of the PIP3 production by PI3-K and PTEN may cause insulin resistance.

Protein-Tyrosine phosphatase 1B (PTP1B) is a phosphatase that dephosphorylates tyrosine residues of IR and IRS. Expression of PTP1B is increased in human insulin-resistant skeletal muscle [24]. Insulin sensitivity increases in skeletal muscle-specific PTP1B knockout mice and protects the body from high-fat diet-induced obesity and diabetes [25] and from TNFα-induced insulin resistance [26]. Based on these findings, PTP1B is being considered as a therapeutic target for treating insulin resistance.

9.3 Ectopic Fat

Males and postmenopausal women do not have sufficient estrogen, which functions to facilitate the accumulation of subcutaneous fat; therefore, visceral fat is easily accumulated. When this fat reaches a certain level, the energy that can no longer be stored as visceral fat must accumulate in the skeletal muscle and the liver, which do not primarily function as sites of fat storage. This accumulated fat can be consumed as a source of energy, but when the fat remains in these tissues for an extended period, insulin resistance intensifies. Asian populations, including the Japanese, have a low capacity for accumulating subcutaneous fat and instead have a tendency to accumulate ectopic fat; therefore, they are predisposed to diabetes. Accordingly, ectopic fat, along with visceral fat, should be strictly monitored.

We do not fully understand how the lipid in the skeletal muscle induces insulin resistance. However, new findings rule out the traditional explanation, and new hypotheses have been developed (see a review by Sulman for a detailed explanation [27]). According to the traditional theory, ectopic lipids accumulate in skeletal muscle and fatty acid oxidation increases. This causes the concentration of mitochondrial acetyl-coenzyme A to increase, which is followed by the following sequence of events: supression of pyruvate dehydrogenase (PDH), inhibition of glucose oxidation and intracelluar citrate concentration, suppression of phosphofructokinase (PFK), increase in intracellular glucose-6-phosphate concentration, suppression of hexokinase (HK) activity, increase in intracellular glucose concentration, and suppression of glucose transport (the so-called Randle's hypothesis [28]). However, according to recent reports, the concentrations of intracellular glucose-6-phosphate and glucose are in fact reduced by lipid accumulation. Based on this result, the following alternate hypothesis was proposed: the increase in intracellular diacylglycerol (DAG) concentration activates PKCθ, serine 1101 of IRS-1 is phosphorylated, and insulin signaling is suppressed.

The author's group performed three different lipidomics analyses in rats comparing the effects of a 10-week running exercise regime and a 16-week high-fat diet to determine the difference in the profiles of lipid species in the skeletal muscle [29]. The authors found that DAG content was not affected by either exercise or by high-fat diet, while insulin sensitivity of skeletal muscle was increased by exercise and suppressed by high-fat diet. These results indicate that DAG may not be the only causal agent in insulin resistance. Further, linoleic acid-containing phosphatidylcholine, sphingomyelin, and docosahexaenoic acid-containing phosphatidylcholine were found to be chronic exercise-induced lipids. In contrast, arachidonic acid-containing phosphatidylcholines, phosphatidylethanolamines, and phosphatidylinositol were found to be high-fat diet-induced lipids. In addition, minor sphingomyelin, which has long-chain fatty acids, was identified as a high-fat diet-specific lipid. There are numerous lipid species in the skeletal muscle, and their physiological activities vary. Therefore, a detailed analysis of the behaviors of these lipid species by mass spectrometry or by other methods would further delineate the mechanisms that lead to insulin resistance.

9.4 Effect of Exercise (Muscle Contraction) on Glucose Transport in the Skeletal Muscle

The importance of exercise in the control of blood glucose has been widely recognized. Dynamic contraction of large muscle groups, even for a relatively short time, promotes glucose uptake into the skeletal muscle. When the skeletal muscle from rodent hind limb was cultured in the presence of oxygen and electrically stimulated to induce contraction, glucose uptake occurred, as in the case of insulin stimulation [30]. Glucose uptake in response to muscle contraction has the same effect as glucose uptake in response to insulin, because GLUT4 translocation eventually occurs, though the signal transduction pathway to the final step is different. Even in insulin-resistant patients with type 2 diabetes, normal glucose uptake into the skeletal muscle can often be maintained by exercise, as long as their condition is not serious [31]. This is because of the activation of different signal transduction pathways by exercise and by insulin. This difference can be demonstrated by a classical experiment in which muscle contraction-induced glucose uptake is not suppressed by the PI3-K inhibitor [32–34]. Further, in the skeletal muscle of IR knockout mice, normal muscle contraction-induced glucose uptake is maintained [35]. In general, there are some factors that can evoke or intermediate exercise- and contraction-induced intracellular signaling (Fig. 9.2). Nevertheless, the identity of the specific intracellular molecules that are involved in this process remained unknown for a long time. A major breakthrough occurred when the role of AMP-activated protein kinase (AMPK) was discovered [30].

AMPK is the serine/threonine kinase that is activated when intracellular energy decreases [30]. AMPK is a heterotrimer consisting an α subunit, which contains the catalytic domain; a γ subunit, which mediates binding to ATP/ADP/AMP; and a β

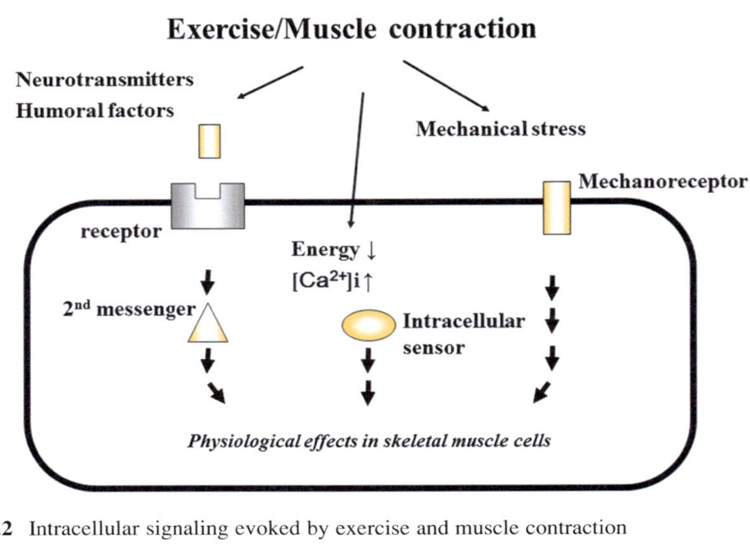

Fig. 9.2 Intracellular signaling evoked by exercise and muscle contraction

subunit, which links the other two subunits and contains a glycogen binding domain [36]. Kinase activity is enhanced or suppressed when AMP or ATP, respectively, binds to the γ subunit. When AMPK is activated, catabolic action is enhanced for energy production, while anabolic action for energy consumption is concurrently suppressed, so that the intracellular energy level increases. In summary, upon AMPK activation, glucose and fatty acid uptake, glycolysis, and oxidation are promoted, whereas the synthesis of lipids, glycogen, and protein is suppressed. A number of studies into the regulation of muscle contraction-associated glucose uptake were the starting point for understanding the multiple physiological activities of AMPK.

At the time of muscle contraction, the intracellular energy level goes down while the ratio of AMP to ATP increases. Subsequently, AMPK is activated, and an intracellular signaling cascade for GLUT4 translocation is initiated. AMPK phosphorylates downstream TBC1 domain family member 1 (TBC1D1) [37] and member 4 (AS160) [38] and suppresses the GTP hydrolytic enzymes of these proteins. These molecules become active when dephosphorylated. Usually activated in the state of abundant intracellular energy, these molecules suppress the downstream Ras homologous from brain (Rab) and prevent the translocation of GLUT4 to cell membrane. Rab8A, Rab13, Rab14, and other Rab proteins are known to be involved in GLUT4 regulation in the skeletal muscle [4], but additional molecules may be identified in the future. The GTP-bound and GDP-bound forms are the active and inactive forms of Rab, respectively. Therefore, when TBC1D1 and AS160 are phosphorylated and the GTPase activity is inactivated, the GTP-bound, active form of Rab increases and accelerates the translocation of GLUT4. Further, upon phosphorylation, TBC1D1 and AS160 bind to 14-3-3 and are prevented access to Rab [39].

A recent study suggests that sucrose nonfermenting AMPK-related kinase (SNARK) is an upstream factor involved in inactivation of TBC1D1 and AS160 [40]. SNARK, a member of the AMPK-related kinase family, is a serine/threonine kinase that, like AMPK, is phosphorylated by LKB-1. However, since LKB1 is constitutively activated, the status of the downstream target molecule likely determines whether the signal is transmitted. For instance, the site at which LKB-1 phosphorylates AMPK is exposed when AMPK is in the AMP-bound state (when the intracellular energy is low). Phosphorylation of threonine at this site works as a switch for the activation of AMPK. In contrast, in the case of SNARK, it is not known which signal, for example, a change in the cell environment or the presence of a second messenger, is a trigger for phosphorylation by LKB-1. In either case, AMPK and SNARK are the molecules that transmit the glucose uptake signal induced by muscle contraction. AMPK is stable as a heterotrimer of the α, β, and γ subunits. When the α-γ linking β subunit is missing, the trimer cannot be formed, leading to collapse of AMPK. In AMPK β1/β2 double knockout mice that lack the two β subunit isoforms (β1, β2), the muscle contraction-induced glucose uptake is reduced to approximately half [41]. A similar reduction is found in the LKB-1 knockout mouse [40]. Based on these findings, there may be other signaling molecules besides AMPK and SNARK that are associated with muscle contraction-induced glucose uptake.

9.5 Effect of Exercise (Muscle Contraction) on Insulin Sensitivity in the Skeletal Muscle

It has been widely recognized that continuous, daily exercise can enhance insulin sensitivity in the skeletal muscle and improve insulin resistance. Nevertheless, the underlying mechanism for this phenomenon is mostly unknown. In a recent study, a test subject rode a bicycle with one foot for 1 h (no movement of the other resting foot), and an insulin clamp test was conducted 6 h afterwards. In the foot that was actively cycling, insulin sensitivity increased when compared to the sensitivity in the foot that was at rest [42]. Such improvement in insulin sensitivity probably continued to gradually increase after each repetitive exercise.

To enhance insulin sensitivity by muscle contraction, cross talk between muscle contraction-induced intracellular signal and the insulin-signaling pathway should exist. Both TBC1D1 and AS160 are multiply phosphorylated, and the phosphorylation sites are specific to the insulin pathway or the muscle contraction pathway, though some of phosphorylated amino acid residues are overlapping. Akt phosphorylates the molecules in the insulin pathway, while AMPK phosphorylates the molecules in the muscle contraction pathway. Therefore, the amino acid residues that are phosphorylated by AMPK likely enhance the efficiency of insulin signaling and GLUT4 translocation via a unique mechanism.

Alternative explanations for enhancement of insulin sensitivity by continuous exercise include the increase in GLUT4 expression level [43] and an increase in the number of mitochondria [44]. When lipids accumulate in the skeletal muscle, insulin resistance occurs, as is widely known. Continuous exercise generally reduces the accumulated lipid and is thus expected to alleviate insulin resistance. However, despite a high level of insulin sensitivity, the intracellular lipid content of highly trained athletes that are middle-distance and long-distance runners is large. This phenomenon is called the athlete's paradox [45] and indicates that not all lipids in the skeletal muscle work to induce insulin resistance. In fact, in studies with rat, lipid molecular species that specifically increased with running exercise and those that specifically increased with high fatty food were identified, and therefore, differences in lipid composition may be an important matter for consideration (Fig. 9.3) [29].

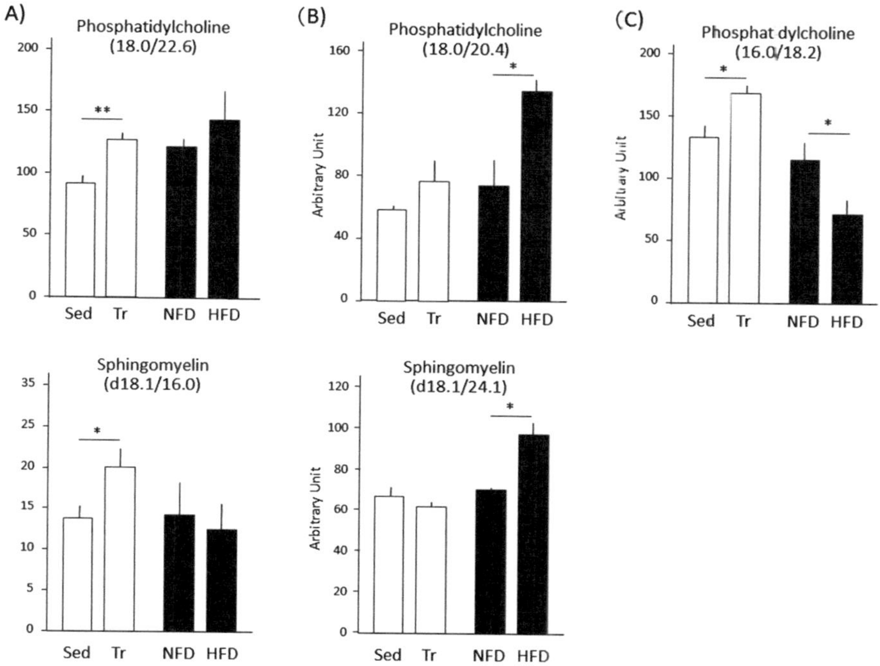

Fig. 9.3 Changes in lipid species content in the skeletal muscle by exercise training and high-fat diet. (**a**) Exercise training-specific increase in lipid contents. (**b**) High-fat-specific increase in lipid content. (**c**) A lipid that is increased by exercise training but decreased by high-fat diet. *Sed* Sedentary, *Tr* Training, *NFD* Normal-fat diet, *HFD* High-fat diet. *$p < 0.05$, **$p < 0.01$ [29]

References

1. Schwartz MW, Seeley RJ, Tschöp MH, Woods SC, Morton GJ, Myers MG, D'Alessio D (2013) Cooperation between brain and islet in glucose homeostasis and diabetes. Nature 503 (7474):59–66
2. Ørtenblad N, Westerblad H, Nielsen J (2013) Muscle glycogen stores and fatigue. J Physiol 591(Pt 18):4405–4413
3. Richter EA, Hargreaves M (2013) Exercise, GLUT4, and skeletal muscle glucose uptake. Physiol Rev 93(3):993–1017
4. Klip A, Sun Y, Chiu TT, Foley KP (2014) Signal transduction meets vesicle traffic: the software and hardware of GLUT4 translocation. Am J Physiol Cell Physiol 306(10):C879–C886
5. Augustin R (2010) The protein family of glucose transport facilitators: it's not only about glucose after all. IUBMB Life 62(5):315–333
6. Taniguchi CM, Emanuelli B, Kahn CR (2006) Critical nodes in signalling pathways: insights into insulin action. Nat Rev Mol Cell Biol 7(2):85–96
7. Copps KD, White MF (2012) Regulation of insulin sensitivity by serine/threonine phosphorylation of insulin receptor substrate proteins IRS1 and IRS2. Diabetologia 55(10):2565–2582

8. Shepherd PR (2005) Mechanisms regulating phosphoinositide 3-kinase signalling in insulin-sensitive tissues. Acta Physiol Scand 183(1):3–12
9. Wu M, Falasca M, Blough ER (2011) Akt/protein kinase B in skeletal muscle physiology and pathology. J Cell Physiol 226(1):29–36
10. Cho H, Mu J, Kim JK, Thorvaldsen JL, Chu Q, Crenshaw EB 3rd, Kaestner KH, Bartolomei MS, Shulman GI, Birnbaum MJ (2001) Insulin resistance and a diabetes mellitus-like syndrome in mice lacking the protein kinase Akt2 (PKB beta). Science 292(5522):1728–1731
11. Bogan JS (2012) Regulation of glucose transporter translocation in health and diabetes. Annu Rev Biochem 81:507–532
12. Farese RV, Sajan MP, Standaert ML (2005) Atypical protein kinase C in insulin action and insulin resistance. Biochem Soc Trans 33(Pt 2):350–353
13. Baumann CA, Ribon V, Kanzaki M, Thurmond DC, Mora S, Shigematsu S, Bickel PE, Pessin JE, Saltiel AR (2000) CAP defines a second signaling pathway required for insulin-stimulated glucose transport. Nature 407(6801):202–207
14. Aguirre V, Uchida T, Yenush L, Davis R, White MF (2000) The c-Jun NH(2)-terminal kinase promotes insulin resistance during association with insulin receptor substrate-1 and phosphorylation of Ser(307). J Biol Chem 275(12):9047–9054
15. Um SH, Frigerio F, Watanabe M, Picard F, Joaquin M, Sticker M, Fumagalli S, Allegrini PR, Kozma SC, Auwerx J, Thomas G (2004) Absence of S6K1 protects against age- and diet-induced obesity while enhancing insulin sensitivity. Nature 431(7005):200–205
16. Pederson TM, Kramer DL, Rondinone CM (2001) Serine/threonine phosphorylation of IRS-1 triggers its degradation: possible regulation by tyrosine phosphorylation. Diabetes 50 (1):24–31
17. Roberts CK, Hevener AL, Barnard RJ (2013) Metabolic syndrome and insulin resistance: underlying causes and modification by exercise training. Compr Physiol 3(1):1–58
18. Ueki K, Fruman DA, Yballe CM, Fasshauer M, Klein J, Asano T, Cantley LC, Kahn CR (2003) Positive and negative roles of p85 alpha and p85 beta regulatory subunits of phosphoinositide 3-kinase in insulin signaling. J Biol Chem 278(48):48453–48466
19. Shepherd PR, Withers DJ, Siddle K (1998) Phosphoinositide 3-kinase: the key switch mechanism in insulin signalling. Biochem J 333:471–490
20. Bandyopadhyay GK, Yu JG, Ofrecio J, Olefsky JM (2005) Increased p85/55/50 expression and decreased phosphatidylinositol 3-kinase activity in insulin-resistant human skeletal muscle. Diabetes 54(8):2351–2359
21. Mauvais-Jarvis F, Ueki K, Fruman DA, Hirshman MF, Sakamoto K, Goodyear LJ, Iannacone M, Accili D, Cantley LC, Kahn CR (2002) Reduced expression of the murine p85alpha subunit of phosphoinositide 3-kinase improves insulin signaling and ameliorates diabetes. J Clin Invest 109(1):141–149
22. Ueki K, Yballe CM, Brachmann SM, Vicent D, Watt JM, Kahn CR, Cantley LC (2002) Increased insulin sensitivity in mice lacking p85beta subunit of phosphoinositide 3-kinase. Proc Natl Acad Sci U S A 99(1):419–424
23. Wijesekara N, Konrad D, Eweida M, Jefferies C, Liadis N, Giacca A, Crackower M, Suzuki A, Mak TW, Kahn CR, Klip A, Woo M (2005) Muscle-specific Pten deletion protects against insulin resistance and diabetes. Mol Cell Biol 25(3):1135–1145
24. Ahmad F, Azevedo JL, Cortright R, Dohm GL, Goldstein BJ (1997) Alterations in skeletal muscle protein-tyrosine phosphatase activity and expression in insulin-resistant human obesity and diabetes. J Clin Invest 100(2):449–458
25. Delibegovic M, Bence KK, Mody N, Hong EG, Ko HJ, Kim JK, Kahn BB, Neel BG (2007) Improved glucose homeostasis in mice with muscle-specific deletion of protein-tyrosine phosphatase 1B. Mol Cell Biol 27(21):7727–7734
26. Nieto-Vazquez I, Fernández-Veledo S, de Alvaro C, Rondinone CM, Valverde AM, Lorenzo M (2007) Protein-tyrosine phosphatase 1B-deficient myocytes show increased insulin sensitivity and protection against tumor necrosis factor-alpha-induced insulin resistance. Diabetes 56(2):404–413
27. Shulman GI (2014) Ectopic fat in insulin resistance, dyslipidemia, and cardiometabolic disease. N Engl J Med 371(12):1131–1141

28. Randle PJ, Garland PB, Hales CN, Newsholme EA (1962) The glucose fatty-acid cycle. Its role in insulin sensitivity and the metabolic disturbances of diabetes mellitus. Lancet 1 (7285):785–789
29. Goto-Inoue N, Yamada K, Inagaki A, Furuichi Y, Ogino S, Manabe Y, Setou M, Fujii NL (2013) Lipidomics analysis revealed the phospholipid compositional changes in muscle by chronic exercise and high-fat diet. Sci Rep 3:3267
30. Fujii N, Jessen N, Goodyear LJ (2006) AMP-activated protein kinase and the regulation of glucose transport. Am J Physiol Endocrinol Metab 291(5):E867–E877
31. Martin IVAK, Katz A, Wahren J, Iva K (1995) Splanchnic and muscle metabolism during exercise in NIDDM patients. Am J Physiol Endocrinol Metab 269:583–590
32. Lund S, Holman GD, Schmitz O, Pedersen O (1995) Contraction stimulates translocation of glucose transporter GLUT4 in skeletal muscle through a mechanism distinct from that of insulin. Proc Natl Acad Sci U S A 92(13):5817–5821
33. Lee AD, Hansen PA, Holloszy JO (1995) Wortmannin inhibits insulin-stimulated but not contraction-stimulated glucose transport activity in skeletal muscle. FEBS Lett 361(1):51–54
34. Yeh JI, Gulve EA, Rameh L, Birnbaum MJ (1995) The effects of wortmannin on rat skeletal muscle. Dissociation of signaling pathways for insulin- and contraction-activated hexose transport. J Biol Chem 270(5):2107–2111
35. Wojtaszewski JF, Higaki Y, Hirshman MF, Michael MD, Dufresne SD, Kahn CR, Goodyear LJ (1999) Exercise modulates postreceptor insulin signaling and glucose transport in muscle-specific insulin receptor knockout mice. J Clin Invest 104(9):1257–1264
36. Hardie DG (2013) AMPK: a target for drugs and natural products with effects on both diabetes and cancer. Diabetes 62(7):2164–2172
37. Taylor EB, An D, Kramer HF, Yu H, Fujii NL, Roeckl KS, Bowles N, Hirshman MF, Xie J, Feener EP, Goodyear LJ (2008) Discovery of TBC1D1 as an insulin-, AICAR-, and contraction-stimulated signaling nexus in mouse skeletal muscle. J Biol Chem 283 (15):9787–9796
38. Kramer HF, Witczak CA, Fujii N, Jessen N, Taylor EB, Arnolds DE, Sakamoto K, Hirshman MF, Goodyear LJ (2006) Distinct signals regulate AS160 phosphorylation in response to insulin, AICAR, and contraction in mouse skeletal muscle. Diabetes 55(7):2067–2076
39. Geraghty KM, Chen S, Harthill JE, Ibrahim AF, Toth R, Morrice NA, Vandermoere F, Moorhead GB, Hardie DG, MacKintosh C (2007) Regulation of multisite phosphorylation and 14-3-3 binding of AS160 in response to IGF-1, EGF, PMA and AICAR. Biochem J 407 (2):231–241
40. Koh HJ, Toyoda T, Fujii N, Jung MM, Rathod A, Middelbeek RJ, Lessard SJ, Treebak JT, Tsuchihara K, Esumi H, Richter EA, Wojtaszewski JF, Hirshman MF, Goodyear LJ (2010) Sucrose nonfermenting AMPK-related kinase (SNARK) mediates contraction-stimulated glucose transport in mouse skeletal muscle. Proc Natl Acad Sci U S A 107(35):15541–15546
41. O'Neill HM, Maarbjerg SJ, Crane JD, Jeppesen J, Jørgensen SB, Schertzer JD, Shyroka O, Kiens B, van Denderen BJ, Tarnopolsky MA, Kemp BE, Richter EA, Steinberg GR (2011) AMP-activated protein kinase (AMPK) beta1beta2 muscle null mice reveal an essential role for AMPK in maintaining mitochondrial content and glucose uptake during exercise. Proc Natl Acad Sci U S A 108(38):16092–16097
42. Richter EA, Mikines KJ, Galbo H, Kiens B (1985) Effect of exercise on insulin action in human skeletal muscle. J Appl Physiol 66(2):876–885
43. Daugaard JR, Nielsen JN, Kristiansen S, Andersen JL, Hargreaves M, Richter EA (2000) Fiber type-specific expression of GLUT4 in human skeletal muscle: influence of exercise training. Diabetes 49(7):1092–1095
44. Yan Z, Lira VA, Greene NP (2012) Exercise training-induced regulation of mitochondrial quality. Exerc Sport Sci Rev 40(3):159–164
45. Dubé JJ, Amati F, Stefanovic-Racic M, Toledo FG, Sauers SE, Goodpaster BH (2008) Exercise-induced alterations in intramyocellular lipids and insulin resistance: the athlete's paradox revisited. Am J Physiol Endocrinol Metab 294(5):E882–E888

Chapter 10
Mechanism of Skeletal Muscle Contraction: Intracellular Signaling in Skeletal Muscle Contraction

Yasuko Manabe

Abstract Regular exercise contributes to maintaining the skeletal muscle mass and quality, which may prevent type II diabetes, hypertension, coronary heart disease, and/or sarcopenia. Exercise/muscle contraction induces activation or inactivation of the intracellular molecules for a short period, which results in an increased glucose uptake, fatty acid oxidation, and protein synthesis. Exercise also affects transcription factors and coactivators, which change the target gene expression and are related to muscle adaptations such as increasing glucose transport-related protein, mitochondrial biogenesis, and the muscle fiber type transition over a long period. Alterations of these molecules are mediated by changes in the intracellular Ca^{2+} level, energy status level, and/or the activated mitogen-activated protein kinase (MAPK) signaling pathway. In this section, the intracellular signaling pathway induced by skeletal muscle contraction is discussed.

Keywords AMPK • Calcium signaling • MAPK

10.1 Introduction

Skeletal muscle contraction induces dynamic metabolic changes including glucose metabolism, fatty acid metabolism, and protein synthesis. These metabolic changes are caused by biochemical modulations of the intracellular molecules for a short period and alterations of gene expression for a long period.

Exercise/muscle contraction increases intracellular Ca^{2+} levels from the sarcoplasmic reticulum. Increased levels of Ca^{2+} activate different kinds of signaling molecules such as Ca^{2+}/calmodulin-dependent protein kinase (CaMK), calcineurin (Ca^{2+}/calmodulin-dependent phosphatase), and protein kinase C (PKC), which results in an increase in glucose uptake, mitochondrial biogenesis, and/or fiber type transition (Fig. 10.1).

Y. Manabe (✉)
Department of Health Promotion Sciences, Graduate School of Human Health Sciences, Tokyo Metropolitan University, 1-1 Minami-Osawa, Hachioji 192-0397, Japan
e-mail: ymanabe@tmu.ac.jp

M. Inaba (ed.), *Musculoskeletal Disease Associated with Diabetes Mellitus*,
DOI 10.1007/978-4-431-55720-3_10

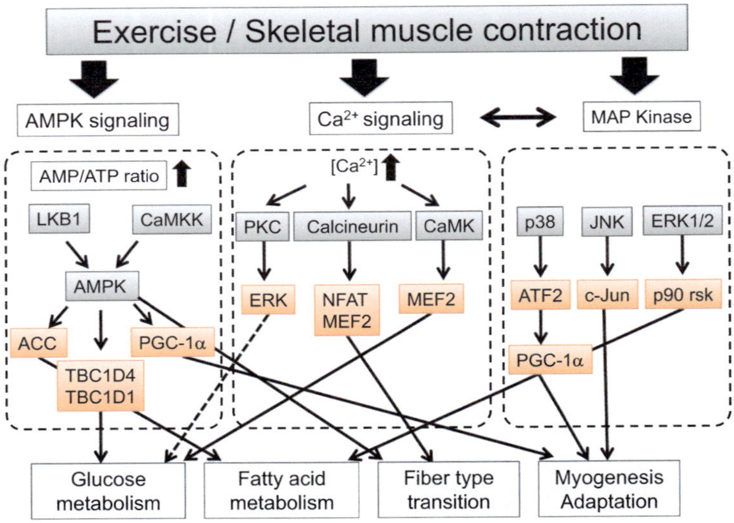

Fig. 10.1 Proposed model of exercise-induced signaling pathway in the skeletal muscle. Classified into three signaling pathways: AMP-activated protein kinase (*AMPK*), Ca^{2+}, and mitogen-activated protein kinase (*MAPK*). AMPK is activated by detection of an increased intracellular AMP/ATP ratio. LKB1 and Ca^{2+}/calmodulin kinase kinase (*CAMKK*) are also known as upstream kinases of AMPK. AMPK serves as a metabolic regulator, which activates and/or inactivates the downstream molecules related to metabolic regulation. Ca^{2+} activates Ca^{2+}/calmodulin-dependent protein kinase (*CaMK*), calcineurin, and protein kinase C (*PKC*). These signaling pathways regulate transcriptional factors and regulate glucose metabolism and fiber type transition. The MAPK signaling pathway including p38, c-jun NH2-terminal kinases (*JNK*), and extracellular signal-regulated kinase (*ERK*) is also activated by muscle contraction. MAPK mainly regulates downstream transcription factors and coactivators, which results in myogenesis and muscle adaptation

When skeletal muscles start contraction, intracellular energy levels are dynamically changed. Muscle contraction accelerates ATP consumption and increases AMP. Namely, the intracellular AMP/ATP ratio is increased, which results in the activation of AMP-activated protein kinase (AMPK). AMPK serves as a metabolic regulator, which activates and/or inactivates the different kinds of signaling proteins related to glucose, fatty acid, and protein metabolism (Fig. 10.1).

The mitogen-activated protein kinase (MAPK) signaling pathway, including p38, c-jun NH2-terminal kinases (JNK), and extracellular signal-regulated kinase (ERK), is known to transmit environmental changes into intracellular responses. MAPK is ubiquitously expressed and regulates gene transcriptions and metabolisms. Exercise/contraction also activates the MAPK signaling pathway, which regulates gene expressions and metabolism (Fig. 10.1). Understanding these signaling pathways and resultant metabolic regulations may contribute toward explaining the beneficial effects of exercise.

10.2 Ca^{2+} Signaling Pathway Induced by Muscle Contraction

Ca^{2+} is the first trigger to induce muscle contraction. The action potential traverses the T-system [1] and reaches the sarcoplasmic reticulum to release Ca^{2+}. An increase in sarcoplasmic Ca^{2+} plays a pivotal role to induce not only excitation–contraction coupling but also serves as the regulator for many cellular events via several pathways including the activation of CaMK, calcineurin, and PKC [2].

CaMK is a serine/threonine protein kinase which is classified into the following two categories: kinases with a single substrate such as phosphorylase kinase, CaMKIII, and myosin light chain kinase, and multifunctional kinases with several substrates such as CaMKI, CaMKII, and CaMKIV [3]. Of those, CaMKII is of particular interest in the skeletal muscle. CaMKII has four isoforms (α, β, γ, and δ) and each isoform is encoded by separate genes [3]. CaMKII consists of 8–12 similar homologous subunits held together by interactions between a C-terminal association domain and forms a pinwheel-like structure [3]. When one subunit is activated by binding a Ca^{2+}–calmodulin complex, it phosphorylates the other subunits in the same enzyme (inter-subunit autophosphorylation). This complex system results in the delayed regulation of CaMKII activity in response to elevated Ca^{2+}. Therefore, CaMKII is considered to act as the stimulation–frequency decoder in the skeletal muscle, which decodes the frequency of Ca^{2+} spikes into graded amounts of kinase activity [4].

CaMKII activation induced by acute exercise enhances glucose transport. In mice, overexpression of the specific inhibitor of CaMKII in the skeletal muscle decreased glucose transport induced by muscle contraction without affecting AMPK phosphorylation. This suggests that CaMKII has a critical role in the regulation of glucose uptake independent of the AMPK pathway [5]. CaMK also affects gene expression levels related to glucose transport and mitochondrial biogenesis. Myocyte enhancer factor-2 (MEF2), a transcription factor, and class II histone deacetylases (HDACs) are the key factors for regulating gene expressions related to glucose transport [6–8]. In the basal state, a complex of HDACs and MEF2 bind to the MEF2 target genes and deacetylates histones surrounding the MEF2 binding domain and represses the transcription of target genes [9]. When activated, CaMKII phosphorylates HDACs. Then, MEF2 is released from the phosphorylated HDACs and exported to the cytoplasm. The released MEF2 is able to associate with coactivators such as p300 and PGC-1α, which induce transcription [10, 11]. In rats, swimming exercises increased MEF2 binding to the glucose transport type 4 (Glut4) promoter, a critical glucose transporter in the skeletal muscle, and in the acetylation of histone H3 on the Glut4 gene [12]. Rats injected with KN-93, an inhibitor of CaMK, attenuated the MEF2 binding, histone acetylation, and Glut4 expression [12]. This suggests that CaMKII activation is important to increase Glut4 expression.

Calcineurin is a Ca^{2+}-dependent serine/threonine phosphatase which is the heterodimer of a catalytic unit, calcineurin A (α, β, or γ), and a regulatory subunit, calcineurin B (1 or 2). In the skeletal muscle, calcineurin A-α, calcineurin A-β, and calcineurin B1 are expressed [13]. Calcineurin is activated by calmodulin [14], which is related to muscle hypertrophy [15, 16] and muscle fiber transition [17, 18]. Calcineurin-deficient mice showed reduced type I fibers [19]. Mice overexpressing muscle-specific calcineurin showed an increase in type I fibers and mitochondrial oxidative function [17, 18], suggesting that calcineurin regulates type I fiber transition. In addition, calcineurin activated the myosin heavy chain (MHC) IIa promoter rather than the MHCIIb promoter [20, 21], suggesting that calcineurin also serves as the fiber type transition within the type II fiber. Two transcription factors, nuclear factor of activated T-cells (NFAT) and MEF2, are the downstream targets of calcineurin in muscle fiber type regulation. Calcineurin directly binds to dephosphorylate NFAT. Then NFAT is translocated to the nucleus and regulates gene expression including myf5, myoglobin, MHC, and troponin [22]. Calcineurin also stimulated the transcriptional activation function of MEF2 in the skeletal muscle using transgenic mice and cultured myocytes [6], and cyclosporin A, a calcineurin inhibitor, blocked this effect [23]. These studies suggest MEF2 and NFAT serve as important transcriptional factors in the fiber type transition. On the other hand, whether calcineurin is related to muscle hypertrophy is still controversial. With reference to many genetically modified mice models, some have reported that calcineurin is not related to muscle size [17, 19, 24], while others showed calcineurin was related to muscle size [15, 16]. There is a relationship between fiber type transition and muscle size as the type I fiber is resistant to muscle atrophy in comparison to the type II fiber [25]. Therefore, to determine whether calcineurin contributes to hypertrophy, a comprehensive understanding of the mechanism, including fiber type transition and atrophy, is needed.

PKC is classified into three groups. The conventional PKC (cPKCs, α, β1, β2, and γ isoforms) is directly activated by Ca^{2+}[26], the novel PKCs (nPKCs, δ, ε, θ, and η isoforms) are dependent on only diacylglycerol for activation, and the atypical PKCs (aPKCs, ζ, and λ isoforms) are activated independent of Ca^{2+} and diacylglycerol. cPKC activation is regulated by the frequency of Ca^{2+} spikes and the temporal coordination between Ca^{2+} spikes and diacylglycerol signals in rat basophilic leukemia 2H3 cells [27], although how this applies to the skeletal muscle still remains unclear. In early reports, total PKC was activated by muscle contraction in the rat skeletal muscle [28, 29]. However, recent studies suggested that isoform-specific analyses of cPKC and nPKC were not affected by exercise in humans [30, 31]. In contrast, aPKCs are reported to be activated by exercise in rats and humans [30–33]. In rat muscle and L6 myotubes, aPKCs were also activated by 5-aminoimidazole-4-carboxamide-1-β-D-riboside (AICAR), an activator of AMPK, and specific aPKC inhibitors blocked glucose uptake stimulated by AICAR. This suggests that glucose uptake via the AMPK pathway is mediated via aPKCs. Although some studies suggest that the effect of aPKC on glucose uptake was mediated by ERK signaling [32, 33], exercise-stimulated glucose uptake was not related to ERK signaling ([34] as described below). Therefore further studies to elucidate the effect of aPKC on glucose uptake will be required.

10.3 AMPK Signaling Pathway Induced by Muscle Contraction

Exercise/muscle contraction alters the energy status in the skeletal muscle. During exercise, AMPK senses an increased AMP level and decreased ATP level (an increase in the intracellular AMP/ATP ratio), and then AMPK is phosphorylated at the Thr172 site and regulates downstream molecules resulting in an increase in glucose uptake and fatty acid oxidation. Therefore, AMPK is considered as a fuel gauge regulating energy metabolism in the cells [35].

AMPK is a serine/threonine kinase that consists of a catalytic subunit (α-subunit) and regulatory subunit (β-subunit and γ-subunit). Each subunit has some isoforms: α-subunit (α1 and α2), β-subunit (β1 and β2), and γ-subunit (γ1, γ2, and γ3). Although the skeletal muscle expresses all isoforms, the major isoform is the heterodimer complex of α2β2γ1, α1β2 γ1, and α2 β2 γ3 in the human vastus lateralis muscle [36, 37]. The γ-subunit of AMPK has four cystathionine beta synthase (CBS) domains, which bind either AMP or ATP. When cellular energy status is low, such as from prolonged fasting or exercise, AMP binds to the CBS domain of γ-subunit. This results in a conformational change, activating AMPK, which turns on the ATP regenerative pathway and inhibits the ATP-consuming pathway.

In addition to detecting the energy status change, upstream molecules of the tumor suppressor protein kinase LKB1 [38] and Ca^{2+}/calmodulin kinase kinase (CaMKK) [39] also phosphorylate Thr172 in AMPK and regulate AMPK activity. Muscle-specific LKB1 knockout mice showed a significant decrease in AMPKα2 activity under basal and contractive stimulation [40, 41]. LKB1 is a constitutively active protein and is not rate limiting for activation of AMPK [42]. When AMPK undergoes a conformational change induced by AMP binding to a CBS domain, LKB1 can easily access AMPK and serves to accelerate AMPK phosphorylation. Unlike AMPKα2, AMPKα1 activity is not affected by LKB1 knockout mice, suggesting that LKB1 is the predominantly upstream kinase of AMPKα2.

Another upstream kinase is CaMKK. CaMKKII is considered to be a dominant upstream of AMPK [39, 43]. In endothelial cells, activated AMPK via CaMKKII was dependent on thrombin but independent of LKB1 [44]. In T lymphocytes, T-cell antigen receptor stimulus activates AMPK via the CaMKK-dependent pathway without change of energy status [45]. In the skeletal muscle, CaMKK inhibitors of KN-93 and STO-609 reduced AMPK phosphorylation and activity, while the inhibitors did not affect the AICAR-stimulated glucose uptake or LKB1 activity [46]. This suggests that CaMKK regulates AMPK phosphorylation and glucose uptake independent of energy status and LKB1 pathway.

AMPK has been of considerable interest with respect to exercise-induced glucose uptake. Exercise/contraction induced activation of AMPK in humans [47, 48] and rodents [49, 50] and increased glucose uptake independent of the insulin pathway. Interestingly, genetically modified mice with an ablation of AMPK activity showed a normal contraction-induced glucose uptake [51, 52]. On the other hand, contraction-induced glucose uptake was inhibited in LKB1 knockout mice [40, 41], suggesting that other downstream molecules of LKB1 besides AMPK are related to contraction-induced glucose uptake. A recent study suggests that sucrose nonfermenting AMPK-related kinase (SNARK) is another substrate of LKB1 for regulating glucose transport [53]. As downstream molecules of AMPK, GTPase-activating proteins of the TBC1 domain family, members 4 and 1 [TBC1D4 (AS160) and TBC1D1] have been reported (see the review [54]). Activated AMPK by muscle contraction phosphorylates TBC1D4/TBC1D, which enhances Glut4 translocation and an increase in glucose uptake.

Activation of AMPK also promotes fatty acid metabolism. Carnitine acyltransferase 1 (CPT1) is a mitochondrial fatty acid transporter, which is allosterically inhibited by the malonyl-CoA. Malonyl-CoA is synthesized from acetyl-CoA catalyzed by acetyl-CoA carboxylase (ACC). AMPK activation inhibits ACC activity via an increase in ACC phosphorylation, which therefore decreases malonyl-CoA synthesis, resulting in CPT1 activation and promotes fatty acid uptake into mitochondria and an increase in fatty acid oxidation. Although AMPK plays a role in ACC phosphorylation, the necessity of AMPK in fatty acid oxidation in the skeletal muscle remains unclear. Mice with skeletal muscle-specific AMPKα2-deficient and AMPKα1-dominant-negative transgenes showed increased fatty acid oxidation when stimulated by in vivo exercise and isolated muscle contraction [55]. It was also reported that ACC is not the only regulator of fatty acid oxidation [55]. Therefore, fatty acid activation stimulated by exercise is not fully explained with an inactivation of ACC by AMPK activation. Some redundant pathway may exist for fatty acid oxidation induced by contraction.

Activated AMPK regulates not only downstream phosphoproteins related to metabolism but also gene expressions via transcription factors and a transcriptional coactivator [56]. PGC-1α is one of the transcriptional coactivators that interacts with the transcription factors and regulates many genes of energy homeostasis related to fat oxidation and mitochondrial biogenesis [57]. Activated AMPK directly phosphorylates PGC-1α at thr177 and ser538 [57]. Phosphorylation of PGC-1α regulates the gene expression of glut4, mitochondrial genes such as cytochrome C, ucp1/2, and even pgc-1 itself. AMPK also affects the transcription factors. Activated AMPK enhances the nuclear respiratory factor-1 (NRF-1) binding activity to its promoter, which enhances mitochondrial biogenesis [58]. AMPK directly phosphorylates and activates glut4 enhancer factor, which recruits the MEF2 and enhances glut4 transcription [59]. These data suggest that AMPK indirectly regulates gene expression via enhancement of coactivator activity and transcriptional factors. It is also reported that AMPK is related to fiber type transition. Continuous dosing of AICAR in rats showed a decreased ratio of type IIb fibers and an increased ratio of type IIx fibers in the extensor digitorum longus muscle [60]. AMPKγ1 transgenic mice with a chronic activation of AMPK showed an increase in type IIa/x fiber [61]. As a downstream molecule related to fiber type transition, PGC-1α is known to regulate fast-to-slow fiber type transformation [62]. However, AMPKα2 knockout mice [63] and dominant-negative mice [61] showed an increase in exercise-induced PGC-1α gene expression in the skeletal muscle with only a little impairment in the exercise-induced fiber transition. Therefore, it is not well understood how AMPK regulates fiber type transition.

10.4 The Mitogen-Activated Protein Kinase Signaling Pathway Induced by Muscle Contraction

MAPK signaling cascades play important roles in various kinds of cells, which are stimulated by environmental stressors, cytokines, and growth factors. Activation of the MAPK signaling pathway phosphorylates downstream substrates and finally transmits the transcription factors and coactivators. This results in the regulation of physiological processes such as cell proliferation, cell differentiation, apoptosis, inflammation, hypertrophy, energy metabolism, and gene transcription [64]. In the skeletal muscle, the MAPK signaling pathway such as the ERK1/ERK2, p38, and JNK is rapidly induced by muscle contraction [65].

10.4.1 p38 MAPK

Four isoforms of p38 (p38α, p38β, p38γ, and p38δ) were reported. p38α and p38β were ubiquitously expressed, while p38γ is expressed mainly in the skeletal muscle and p38δ is expressed mainly in the lung and kidney [66]. Muscle contraction increases p38 phosphorylation in rodents [67, 68] and humans [69, 70]. In an early study, activation of p38 MAPK by muscle contraction was thought to regulate glucose metabolism, since SB203580, a p38α/β antagonist, inhibited glucose uptake stimulated by AICAR [71]. However, later studies suggested that overexpression of p38γ in the skeletal muscle negatively regulates Glut4 expression and contraction-mediated glucose uptake [72]. In another report, overexpression of dominant-negative p38α/β did not affect insulin-stimulated glucose uptake [73]. Therefore, inhibition of SB203580 in the early study is considered to come from the direct inhibition of the glucose transporter [74]. It seems that activation of p38 induced by muscle contraction is not directly related to glucose transport in the skeletal muscle.

Activation of p38 by muscle contraction induced PGC-1α expression via the activation of transcription factor 2 (ATF2), a transcription factor of PGC-1α in C2C12 cells [75], and is related to the muscle adaptation. Skeletal muscle-specific expression of MKK6E, a constitutively active activator of p38, increased PGC-1α and cytochrome c oxidase IV (COX IV) protein expression in fast type skeletal muscles [75]. Muscle-specific ablation of p38γ, but not p38α and p38β, reduced endurance exercise-induced pgc-1α mRNA expression and mitochondrial proteins such as COX IV and cytochrome c [76]. p38 activation is also involved in myogenic differentiation. Using the primary myoblasts from the skeletal muscle of neonatal mice deficient in p38α, p38β, p38γ, or p38δ, p38α plays a critical role in myogenesis and p38γ plays a role in cellular fusion [77]. Although the relative contribution of the p38 subtypes in response to physiological conditions such as contraction and proliferation still remains unclear, at least p38 seems to contribute to myogenesis.

10.4.2 c-jun NH2-Terminal Kinases

JNK, members of the stress-activated protein kinase family, are encoded by three genes, juk1, juk2, and juk3 and produce ten isoforms via alternative splicing [78]. Transcripts derived from three juk genes produce 46 kDa (JNK1) and 55 kDa (JNK2) isoforms [78], although the functional difference of two splice variants remains unclear. JNK activity is related to insulin resistance [79, 80]. JNK1 knockout mice were protected from obesity-induced insulin resistance [81]. These JNK KO mice that were fed a high-fat diet had a significantly lower blood glucose level and decreased adipose size than the control mice [81]. In the muscle-specific JNK KO mice study [82], the mice showed improved high fat-induced insulin resistance. However, these mice did not influence diet-induced obesity. In particular, adipose tissue-specific JNK1 KO also showed improved insulin sensitivity with the diet-induced obesity phenotype [83], while liver-specific JNK KO mice did not [84]. In the skeletal muscle, muscle contraction and physical exercise increase JNK activity in the rat and human skeletal muscle [65, 70, 85–87]. Considering that the JNK KO mice showed improved insulin resistance, the activation of JNK by muscle contraction is confusing. One interpretation is that JNK in the skeletal muscle is not directly related to glucose metabolism but regulates other events via regulation of gene expression. The glycogen content and glycogen synthase activity stimulated by contraction was not different between control and skeletal muscle-specific JNK overexpressed muscles [88]. In addition, glucose uptake stimulated by the insulin or muscle contraction was not significantly different between control and JNK KO muscles [88], suggesting that JNK activity is not related to glucose metabolism in the skeletal muscle. JNK activation induced by muscle contraction is associated with an increased mRNA level of c-Jun, a downstream molecule of JNK in humans and rats [87, 89]. c-Jun is known as the transcription factor which regulates various cell events including cellular proliferation, apoptosis, DNA repair, and inflammation [90–92]. Therefore, JNK activation stimulated by muscle contraction may contribute to these events via c-jun.

10.4.3 Extracellular Signal-Regulated Kinase 1/2

ERK, a major MAP kinase family, is also activated by exercise such as treadmill running in rodents [65, 67], in vitro contraction in rats [93, 94], cycle ergometer exercise and running in humans [95, 70], and a knee extensor resistance exercise

[96]. Phosphorylation of ERK is dependent on the intensity of exercise [97]. When one leg was exercised using a cycle ergometer and the other leg was rested, ERK activation was detected only in the exercised muscle [86, 70]. This suggested that ERK is activated as a local response to muscle contraction rather than as a systemic response. Insulin is also known as an activator of the ERK signaling pathway [65, 98, 99].

In response to exercise, the upstream kinase of ERK1/ERK2 phosphorylation, Raf-1, and the upstream kinase MAP/ERK kinase (MEK1/MEK2) are reported [86, 100]. Insulin also activates ERK phosphorylation via MEK activation, which is activated by the upstream molecules of Ras and Raf via classical receptor tyrosine kinase pathways [101, 102]. Although ERK phosphorylation induced by insulin stimulation was diminished by the pre-treatment of phosphatidylinositol (PI) 3-kinase inhibitors, wortmannin, and LY-294002, ERK phosphorylation induced by muscle contraction was not. This suggests that the ERK phosphorylation stimulated by contraction uses a different mechanism from that by insulin [34]. The ERK activation mechanism stimulated by contraction still remains unclear.

P90 ribosomal S6 kinase (p90rsk) is the downstream target of ERK1/ERK2 [93, 103]. In an isolated rat muscle, contraction-induced activation of p90rsk was concomitant with ERK1/ERK2 phosphorylation [93]. Inhibition of MEK-ERK inhibitor, PD98059, completely abolished the p90rsk activation induced by contraction, suggesting that the p90rsk is ERK dependent [93]. Mitogen- and stress-activated kinase 1/2 (MSK1/MSK2) is also reported as a downstream target of ERK1/ERK2. MSK1/MSK2 is activated in response to muscle contraction in the human skeletal muscle [69, 103]. The activation pattern of MSK1/MSK2 by exercise is related to the ERK phosphorylation pattern; therefore, MSK1/MSK2 is also considered to be regulated by ERK phosphorylation [104].

ERK activation is not related to glucose uptake induced by muscle contraction. Glucose uptake stimulated by contraction was not inhibited by PD-98059, a MEK inhibitor, in rat muscle [34]. On the other hand, some studies suggested that ERK activity is related to the fatty acid uptake in the skeletal muscle. Fatty acid uptake was significantly correlated with ERK1/ERK2 phosphorylation from low- to moderate-intensity muscle contraction in rat muscles [105]. To support this data, contraction-induced palmitate uptake was abolished by the PD-98059, suggesting that ERK phosphorylation is related to fatty acid uptake. Although muscle contraction has been shown to activate ERK1/ERK2, more studies will be required on how ERK activation induced by exercise contributes to metabolic regulations.

References

1. Lieber RL (2009) Skeletal muscle structure, function, and plasticity. Lippincott Williams & Wilkins, Philadelphia
2. Hawley JA, Hargreaves M, Zierath JR (2006) Signalling mechanisms in skeletal muscle: role in substrate selection and muscle adaptation. Essays Biochem 42:1–12. doi:10.1042/bse0420001

3. Hook SS, Means AR (2001) Ca(2+)/CaM-dependent kinases: from activation to function. Annu Rev Pharmacol Toxicol 41:471–505. doi:10.1146/annurev.pharmtox.41.1.471
4. Chin ER (2005) Role of Ca2+/calmodulin-dependent kinases in skeletal muscle plasticity. J Appl Physiol (1985) 99(2):414–423. doi:10.1152/japplphysiol.00015.2005
5. Witczak CA, Jessen N, Warro DM, Toyoda T, Fujii N, Anderson ME et al (2010) CaMKII regulates contraction- but not insulin-induced glucose uptake in mouse skeletal muscle. Am J Physiol Endocrinol Metab 298(6):E1150–E1160. doi:10.1152/ajpendo.00659.2009
6. Wu H, Naya FJ, McKinsey TA, Mercer B, Shelton JM, Chin ER et al (2000) MEF2 responds to multiple calcium-regulated signals in the control of skeletal muscle fiber type. EMBO J 19 (9):1963–1973. doi:10.1093/emboj/19.9.1963
7. Blaeser F, Ho N, Prywes R, Chatila TA (2000) Ca(2+)-dependent gene expression mediated by MEF2 transcription factors. J Biol Chem 275(1):197–209
8. Passier R, Zeng H, Frey N, Naya FJ, Nicol RL, McKinsey TA et al (2000) CaM kinase signaling induces cardiac hypertrophy and activates the MEF2 transcription factor in vivo. J Clin Invest 105(10):1395–1406. doi:10.1172/JCI8551
9. Lu J, McKinsey TA, Zhang CL, Olson EN (2000) Regulation of skeletal myogenesis by association of the MEF2 transcription factor with class II histone deacetylases. Mol Cell 6 (2):233–244
10. Ojuka EO, Goyaram V, Smith JA (2012) The role of CaMKII in regulating GLUT4 expression in skeletal muscle. Am J Physiol Endocrinol Metab 303(3):E322–E331. doi:10.1152/ajpendo.00091.2012
11. McKinsey TA, Zhang CL, Olson EN (2002) MEF2: a calcium-dependent regulator of cell division, differentiation and death. Trends Biochem Sci 27(1):40–47
12. Smith JA, Kohn TA, Chetty AK, Ojuka EO (2008) CaMK activation during exercise is required for histone hyperacetylation and MEF2A binding at the MEF2 site on the Glut4 gene. Am J Physiol Endocrinol Metab 295(3):E698–E704. doi:10.1152/ajpendo.00747.2007
13. Manalan AS, Krinks MH, Klee CB (1984) Calcineurin: a member of a family of calmodulin-stimulated protein phosphatases. Proc Soc Exp Biol Med 177(1):12–16
14. Klee CB, Crouch TH, Krinks MH (1979) Calcineurin: a calcium- and calmodulin-binding protein of the nervous system. Proc Natl Acad Sci U S A 76(12):6270–6273
15. Talmadge RJ, Otis JS, Rittler MR, Garcia ND, Spencer SR, Lees SJ et al (2004) Calcineurin activation influences muscle phenotype in a muscle-specific fashion. BMC Cell Biol 5:28. doi:10.1186/1471-2121-5-28
16. Kegley KM, Gephart J, Warren GL, Pavlath GK (2001) Altered primary myogenesis in NFATC3 (-/-) mice leads to decreased muscle size in the adult. Dev Biol 232(1):115–126. doi:10.1006/dbio.2001.0179
17. Naya FJ, Mercer B, Shelton J, Richardson JA, Williams RS, Olson EN (2000) Stimulation of slow skeletal muscle fiber gene expression by calcineurin in vivo. J Biol Chem 275(7):4545–4548
18. Jiang LQ, Garcia-Roves PM, de Castro BT, Zierath JR (2010) Constitutively active calcineurin in skeletal muscle increases endurance performance and mitochondrial respiratory capacity. Am J Physiol Endocrinol Metab 298(1):E8–E16. doi:10.1152/ajpendo.00403.2009
19. Parsons SA, Millay DP, Wilkins BJ, Bueno OF, Tsika GL, Neilson JR et al (2004) Genetic loss of calcineurin blocks mechanical overload-induced skeletal muscle fiber type switching but not hypertrophy. J Biol Chem 279(25):26192–26200. doi:10.1074/jbc.M313800200
20. Allen DL, Leinwand LA (2002) Intracellular calcium and myosin isoform transitions. Calcineurin and calcium-calmodulin kinase pathways regulate preferential activation of the IIa myosin heavy chain promoter. J Biol Chem 277(47):45323–45330. doi:10.1074/jbc.M208302200
21. Allen DL, Sartorius CA, Sycuro LK, Leinwand LA (2001) Different pathways regulate expression of the skeletal myosin heavy chain genes. J Biol Chem 276(47):43524–43533. doi:10.1074/jbc.M108017200

22. Rao A, Luo C, Hogan PG (1997) Transcription factors of the NFAT family: regulation and function. Annu Rev Immunol 15:707–747. doi:10.1146/annurev.immunol.15.1.707
23. Wu H, Rothermel B, Kanatous S, Rosenberg P, Naya FJ, Shelton JM et al (2001) Activation of MEF2 by muscle activity is mediated through a calcineurin-dependent pathway. EMBO J 20(22):6414–6423. doi:10.1093/emboj/20.22.6414
24. Parsons SA, Wilkins BJ, Bueno OF, Molkentin JD (2003) Altered skeletal muscle phenotypes in calcineurin Aalpha and Abeta gene-targeted mice. Mol Cell Biol 23(12):4331–4343
25. Sandri M (2008) Signaling in muscle atrophy and hypertrophy. Physiology (Bethesda) 23:160–170. doi:10.1152/physiol.00041.2007
26. Gundersen K (2011) Excitation-transcription coupling in skeletal muscle: the molecular pathways of exercise. Biol Rev Camb Philos Soc 86(3):564–600. doi:10.1111/j.1469-185X.2010.00161.x
27. Oancea E, Meyer T (1998) Protein kinase C as a molecular machine for decoding calcium and diacylglycerol signals. Cell 95(3):307–318
28. Cleland PJ, Appleby GJ, Rattigan S, Clark MG (1989) Exercise-induced translocation of protein kinase C and production of diacylglycerol and phosphatidic acid in rat skeletal muscle in vivo. Relationship to changes in glucose transport. J Biol Chem 264(30):17704–17711
29. Richter EA, Cleland PJ, Rattigan S, Clark MG (1987) Contraction-associated translocation of protein kinase C in rat skeletal muscle. FEBS Lett 217(2):232–236
30. Rose AJ, Michell BJ, Kemp BE, Hargreaves M (2004) Effect of exercise on protein kinase C activity and localization in human skeletal muscle. J Physiol 561(Pt 3):861–870. doi:10.1113/jphysiol.2004.075549
31. Perrini S, Henriksson J, Zierath JR, Widegren U (2004) Exercise-induced protein kinase C isoform-specific activation in human skeletal muscle. Diabetes 53(1):21–24
32. Nielsen JN, Frosig C, Sajan MP, Miura A, Standaert ML, Graham DA et al (2003) Increased atypical PKC activity in endurance-trained human skeletal muscle. Biochem Biophys Res Commun 312(4):1147–1153
33. Chen HC, Bandyopadhyay G, Sajan MP, Kanoh Y, Standaert M, Farese RV Jr et al (2002) Activation of the ERK pathway and atypical protein kinase C isoforms in exercise- and aminoimidazole-4-carboxamide-1-beta-D-riboside (AICAR)-stimulated glucose transport. J Biol Chem 277(26):23554–23562. doi:10.1074/jbc.M201152200
34. Wojtaszewski JF, Lynge J, Jakobsen AB, Goodyear LJ, Richter EA (1999) Differential regulation of MAP kinase by contraction and insulin in skeletal muscle: metabolic implications. Am J Physiol 277(4 Pt 1):E724–E732
35. Hardie DG, Carling D (1997) The AMP-activated protein kinase–fuel gauge of the mammalian cell? Eur J Biochem/FEBS 246(2):259–273
36. Birk JB, Wojtaszewski JF (2006) Predominant alpha2/beta2/gamma3 AMPK activation during exercise in human skeletal muscle. J Physiol 577(Pt 3):1021–1032. doi:10.1113/jphysiol.2006.120972
37. Wojtaszewski JF, Birk JB, Frosig C, Holten M, Pilegaard H, Dela F (2005) 5'AMP activated protein kinase expression in human skeletal muscle: effects of strength training and type 2 diabetes. J Physiol 564(Pt 2):563–573. doi:10.1113/jphysiol.2005.082669
38. Shaw RJ, Kosmatka M, Bardeesy N, Hurley RL, Witters LA, DePinho RA et al (2004) The tumor suppressor LKB1 kinase directly activates AMP-activated kinase and regulates apoptosis in response to energy stress. Proc Natl Acad Sci U S A 101(10):3329–3335. doi:10.1073/pnas.0308061100
39. Hurley RL, Anderson KA, Franzone JM, Kemp BE, Means AR, Witters LA (2005) The Ca2+/calmodulin-dependent protein kinase kinases are AMP-activated protein kinase kinases. J Biol Chem 280(32):29060–29066. doi:10.1074/jbc.M503824200
40. Koh HJ, Arnolds DE, Fujii N, Tran TT, Rogers MJ, Jessen N et al (2006) Skeletal muscle-selective knockout of LKB1 increases insulin sensitivity, improves glucose homeostasis, and decreases TRB3. Mol Cell Biol 26(22):8217–8227. doi:10.1128/MCB.00979-06

41. Sakamoto K, McCarthy A, Smith D, Green KA, Grahame Hardie D, Ashworth A et al (2005) Deficiency of LKB1 in skeletal muscle prevents AMPK activation and glucose uptake during contraction. EMBO J 24(10):1810–1820. doi:10.1038/sj.emboj.7600667
42. Woods A, Vertommen D, Neumann D, Turk R, Bayliss J, Schlattner U et al (2003) Identification of phosphorylation sites in AMP-activated protein kinase (AMPK) for upstream AMPK kinases and study of their roles by site-directed mutagenesis. J Biol Chem 278(31):28434–28442. doi:10.1074/jbc.M303946200
43. Woods A, Dickerson K, Heath R, Hong SP, Momcilovic M, Johnstone SR et al (2005) Ca2+/calmodulin-dependent protein kinase kinase-beta acts upstream of AMP-activated protein kinase in mammalian cells. Cell Metab 2(1):21–33. doi:10.1016/j.cmet.2005.06.005
44. Stahmann N, Woods A, Carling D, Heller R (2006) Thrombin activates AMP-activated protein kinase in endothelial cells via a pathway involving Ca2+/calmodulin-dependent protein kinase kinase beta. Mol Cell Biol 26(16):5933–5945. doi:10.1128/MCB.00383-06
45. Tamas P, Hawley SA, Clarke RG, Mustard KJ, Green K, Hardie DG et al (2006) Regulation of the energy sensor AMP-activated protein kinase by antigen receptor and Ca2+ in T lymphocytes. J Exp Med 203(7):1665–1670. doi:10.1084/jem.20052469
46. Jensen TE, Rose AJ, Jorgensen SB, Brandt N, Schjerling P, Wojtaszewski JF et al (2007) Possible CaMKK-dependent regulation of AMPK phosphorylation and glucose uptake at the onset of mild tetanic skeletal muscle contraction. Am J Physiol Endocrinol Metab 292(5): E1308–E1317. doi:10.1152/ajpendo.00456.2006
47. Wojtaszewski JF, Nielsen P, Hansen BF, Richter EA, Kiens B (2000) Isoform-specific and exercise intensity-dependent activation of 5'-AMP-activated protein kinase in human skeletal muscle. J Physiol 528(Pt 1):221–226
48. Fujii N, Hayashi T, Hirshman MF, Smith JT, Habinowski SA, Kaijser L et al (2000) Exercise induces isoform-specific increase in 5'AMP-activated protein kinase activity in human skeletal muscle. Biochem Biophys Res Commun 273(3):1150–1155. doi:10.1006/bbrc.2000.3073
49. Hayashi T, Hirshman MF, Fujii N, Habinowski SA, Witters LA, Goodyear LJ (2000) Metabolic stress and altered glucose transport: activation of AMP-activated protein kinase as a unifying coupling mechanism. Diabetes 49(4):527–531
50. Hayashi T, Hirshman MF, Kurth EJ, Winder WW, Goodyear LJ (1998) Evidence for 5' AMP-activated protein kinase mediation of the effect of muscle contraction on glucose transport. Diabetes 47(8):1369–1373
51. Jorgensen SB, Viollet B, Andreelli F, Frosig C, Birk JB, Schjerling P et al (2004) Knockout of the alpha2 but not alpha1 5'-AMP-activated protein kinase isoform abolishes 5-aminoimidazole-4-carboxamide-1-beta-4-ribofuranoside but not contraction-induced glucose uptake in skeletal muscle. J Biol Chem 279(2):1070–1079. doi:10.1074/jbc.M306205200
52. Fujii N, Hirshman MF, Kane EM, Ho RC, Peter LE, Seifert MM et al (2005) AMP-activated protein kinase alpha2 activity is not essential for contraction- and hyperosmolarity-induced glucose transport in skeletal muscle. J Biol Chem 280(47):39033–39041. doi:10.1074/jbc.M504208200
53. Koh HJ, Toyoda T, Fujii N, Jung MM, Rathod A, Middelbeek RJ et al (2010) Sucrose nonfermenting AMPK-related kinase (SNARK) mediates contraction-stimulated glucose transport in mouse skeletal muscle. Proc Natl Acad Sci U S A 107(35):15541–15546. doi:10.1073/pnas.1008131107
54. Friedrichsen M, Mortensen B, Pehmoller C, Birk JB, Wojtaszewski JF (2013) Exercise-induced AMPK activity in skeletal muscle: role in glucose uptake and insulin sensitivity. Mol Cell Endocrinol 366(2):204–214. doi:10.1016/j.mce.2012.06.013
55. Olson DP, Pulinilkunnil T, Cline GW, Shulman GI, Lowell BB (2010) Gene knockout of Acc2 has little effect on body weight, fat mass, or food intake. Proc Natl Acad Sci U S A 107 (16):7598–7603. doi:10.1073/pnas.0913492107

56. Hardie DG (2004) The AMP-activated protein kinase pathway–new players upstream and downstream. J Cell Sci 117(Pt 23):5479–5487. doi:10.1242/jcs.01540
57. Jager S, Handschin C, St-Pierre J, Spiegelman BM (2007) AMP-activated protein kinase (AMPK) action in skeletal muscle via direct phosphorylation of PGC-1alpha. Proc Natl Acad Sci U S A 104(29):12017–12022. doi:10.1073/pnas.0705070104
58. Bergeron R, Ren JM, Cadman KS, Moore IK, Perret P, Pypaert M et al (2001) Chronic activation of AMP kinase results in NRF-1 activation and mitochondrial biogenesis. Am J Physiol Endocrinol Metab 281(6):E1340–E1346
59. Holmes BF, Sparling DP, Olson AL, Winder WW, Dohm GL (2005) Regulation of muscle GLUT4 enhancer factor and myocyte enhancer factor 2 by AMP-activated protein kinase. Am J Physiol Endocrinol Metab 289(6):E1071–E1076. doi:10.1152/ajpendo.00606.2004
60. Suwa M, Nakano H, Kumagai S (2003) Effects of chronic AICAR treatment on fiber composition, enzyme activity, UCP3, and PGC-1 in rat muscles. J Appl Physiol (1985) 95 (3):960–968. doi:10.1152/japplphysiol.00349.2003
61. Rockl KS, Hirshman MF, Brandauer J, Fujii N, Witters LA, Goodyear LJ (2007) Skeletal muscle adaptation to exercise training: AMP-activated protein kinase mediates muscle fiber type shift. Diabetes 56(8):2062–2069. doi:10.2337/db07-0255
62. Lin J, Wu H, Tarr PT, Zhang CY, Wu Z, Boss O et al (2002) Transcriptional co-activator PGC-1 alpha drives the formation of slow-twitch muscle fibres. Nature 418(6899):797–801. doi:10.1038/nature00904
63. Jorgensen SB, Wojtaszewski JF, Viollet B, Andreelli F, Birk JB, Hellsten Y et al (2005) Effects of alpha-AMPK knockout on exercise-induced gene activation in mouse skeletal muscle. FASEB J 19(9):1146–1148. doi:10.1096/fj.04-3144fje
64. Sakamoto K, Goodyear LJ (2002) Invited review: intracellular signaling in contracting skeletal muscle. J Appl Physiol (1985) 93(1):369–383. doi:10.1152/japplphysiol.00167.2002
65. Goodyear LJ, Chang PY, Sherwood DJ, Dufresne SD, Moller DE (1996) Effects of exercise and insulin on mitogen-activated protein kinase signaling pathways in rat skeletal muscle. Am J Physiol 271(2 Pt 1):E403–E408
66. Jiang Y, Gram H, Zhao M, New L, Gu J, Feng L et al (1997) Characterization of the structure and function of the fourth member of p38 group mitogen-activated protein kinases, p38delta. J Biol Chem 272(48):30122–30128
67. Nader GA, Esser KA (2001) Intracellular signaling specificity in skeletal muscle in response to different modes of exercise. J Appl Physiol (1985) 90(5):1936–1942
68. Boppart MD, Hirshman MF, Sakamoto K, Fielding RA, Goodyear LJ (2001) Static stretch increases c-Jun NH2-terminal kinase activity and p38 phosphorylation in rat skeletal muscle. Am J Physiol Cell Physiol 280(2):C352–C358
69. Yu M, Blomstrand E, Chibalin AV, Krook A, Zierath JR (2001) Marathon running increases ERK1/2 and p38 MAP kinase signalling to downstream targets in human skeletal muscle. J Physiol 536(Pt 1):273–282
70. Widegren U, Jiang XJ, Krook A, Chibalin AV, Bjornholm M, Tally M et al (1998) Divergent effects of exercise on metabolic and mitogenic signaling pathways in human skeletal muscle. FASEB J 12(13):1379–1389
71. Fryer LG, Parbu-Patel A, Carling D (2002) Protein kinase inhibitors block the stimulation of the AMP-activated protein kinase by 5-amino-4-imidazolecarboxamide riboside. FEBS Lett 531(2):189–192
72. Ho RC, Alcazar O, Fujii N, Hirshman MF, Goodyear LJ (2004) p38gamma MAPK regulation of glucose transporter expression and glucose uptake in L6 myotubes and mouse skeletal muscle. Am J Physiol Regul Integr Comp Physiol 286(2):R342–R349. doi:10.1152/ajpregu.00563.2003
73. Antonescu CN, Huang C, Niu W, Liu Z, Eyers PA, Heidenreich KA et al (2005) Reduction of insulin-stimulated glucose uptake in L6 myotubes by the protein kinase inhibitor SB203580 is independent of p38MAPK activity. Endocrinology 146(9):3773–3781. doi:10.1210/en.2005-0404

74. Ribe D, Yang J, Patel S, Koumanov F, Cushman SW, Holman GD (2005) Endofacial competitive inhibition of glucose transporter-4 intrinsic activity by the mitogen-activated protein kinase inhibitor SB203580. Endocrinology 146(4):1713–1717. doi:10.1210/en.2004-1294
75. Akimoto T, Pohnert SC, Li P, Zhang M, Gumbs C, Rosenberg PB et al (2005) Exercise stimulates Pgc-1alpha transcription in skeletal muscle through activation of the p38 MAPK pathway. J Biol Chem 280(20):19587–19593. doi:10.1074/jbc.M408862200
76. Pogozelski AR, Geng T, Li P, Yin X, Lira VA, Zhang M et al (2009) p38gamma mitogen-activated protein kinase is a key regulator in skeletal muscle metabolic adaptation in mice. PLoS One 4(11):e7934. doi:10.1371/journal.pone.0007934
77. Perdiguero E, Ruiz-Bonilla V, Gresh L, Hui L, Ballestar E, Sousa-Victor P et al (2007) Genetic analysis of p38 MAP kinases in myogenesis: fundamental role of p38alpha in abrogating myoblast proliferation. EMBO J 26(5):1245–1256. doi:10.1038/sj.emboj.7601587
78. Davis RJ (2000) Signal transduction by the JNK group of MAP kinases. Cell 103(2):239–252
79. Sabio G, Davis RJ (2010) cJun NH2-terminal kinase 1 (JNK1): roles in metabolic regulation of insulin resistance. Trends Biochem Sci 35(9):490–496. doi:10.1016/j.tibs.2010.04.004
80. Bennett BL, Satoh Y, Lewis AJ (2003) JNK: a new therapeutic target for diabetes. Curr Opin Pharmacol 3(4):420–425
81. Hirosumi J, Tuncman G, Chang L, Gorgun CZ, Uysal KT, Maeda K et al (2002) A central role for JNK in obesity and insulin resistance. Nature 420(6913):333–336. doi:10.1038/nature01137
82. Sabio G, Kennedy NJ, Cavanagh-Kyros J, Jung DY, Ko HJ, Ong H et al (2010) Role of muscle c-Jun NH2-terminal kinase 1 in obesity-induced insulin resistance. Mol Cell Biol 30 (1):106–115. doi:10.1128/MCB.01162-09
83. Sabio G, Das M, Mora A, Zhang Z, Jun JY, Ko HJ et al (2008) A stress signaling pathway in adipose tissue regulates hepatic insulin resistance. Science 322(5907):1539–1543. doi:10.1126/science.1160794
84. Sabio G, Cavanagh-Kyros J, Ko HJ, Jung DY, Gray S, Jun JY et al (2009) Prevention of steatosis by hepatic JNK1. Cell Metab 10(6):491–498. doi:10.1016/j.cmet.2009.09.007
85. Martineau LC, Gardiner PF (2001) Insight into skeletal muscle mechanotransduction: MAPK activation is quantitatively related to tension. J Appl Physiol (1985) 91(2):693–702
86. Aronson D, Violan MA, Dufresne SD, Zangen D, Fielding RA, Goodyear LJ (1997) Exercise stimulates the mitogen-activated protein kinase pathway in human skeletal muscle. J Clin Invest 99(6):1251–1257. doi:10.1172/JCI119282
87. Aronson D, Dufresne SD, Goodyear LJ (1997) Contractile activity stimulates the c-Jun NH2-terminal kinase pathway in rat skeletal muscle. J Biol Chem 272(41):25636–25640
88. Fujii N, Boppart MD, Dufresne SD, Crowley PF, Jozsi AC, Sakamoto K et al (2004) Overexpression or ablation of JNK in skeletal muscle has no effect on glycogen synthase activity. Am J Physiol Cell Physiol 287(1):C200–C208. doi:10.1152/ajpcell.00415.2003
89. Aronson D, Boppart MD, Dufresne SD, Fielding RA, Goodyear LJ (1998) Exercise stimulates c-Jun NH2 kinase activity and c-Jun transcriptional activity in human skeletal muscle. Biochem Biophys Res Commun 251(1):106–110. doi:10.1006/bbrc.1998.9435
90. Wisdom R, Johnson RS, Moore C (1999) c-Jun regulates cell cycle progression and apoptosis by distinct mechanisms. EMBO J 18(1):188–197. doi:10.1093/emboj/18.1.188
91. Karin M, Gallagher E (2005) From JNK to pay dirt: jun kinases, their biochemistry, physiology and clinical importance. IUBMB Life 57(4–5):283–295. doi:10.1080/15216540500097111
92. Johnson GL, Nakamura K (2007) The c-jun kinase/stress-activated pathway: regulation, function and role in human disease. Biochim Biophys Acta 1773(8):1341–1348. doi:10.1016/j.bbamcr.2006.12.009
93. Ryder JW, Fahlman R, Wallberg-Henriksson H, Alessi DR, Krook A, Zierath JR (2000) Effect of contraction on mitogen-activated protein kinase signal transduction in skeletal

muscle. Involvement of the mitogen- and stress-activated protein kinase 1. J Biol Chem 275 (2):1457–1462

94. Hayashi T, Hirshman MF, Dufresne SD, Goodyear LJ (1999) Skeletal muscle contractile activity in vitro stimulates mitogen-activated protein kinase signaling. Am J Physiol 277(4 Pt 1):C701–C707
95. Yu M, Stepto NK, Chibalin AV, Fryer LG, Carling D, Krook A et al (2003) Metabolic and mitogenic signal transduction in human skeletal muscle after intense cycling exercise. J Physiol 546(Pt 2):327–335
96. Williamson D, Gallagher P, Harber M, Hollon C, Trappe S (2003) Mitogen-activated protein kinase (MAPK) pathway activation: effects of age and acute exercise on human skeletal muscle. J Physiol 547(Pt 3):977–987. doi:10.1113/jphysiol.2002.036673
97. Widegren U, Wretman C, Lionikas A, Hedin G, Henriksson J (2000) Influence of exercise intensity on ERK/MAP kinase signalling in human skeletal muscle. Pflugers Arch: Eur J Physiol 441(2–3):317–322
98. Zhou GX, Meier KE, Buse MG (1993) Sequential activation of two mitogen activated protein (MAP) kinase isoforms in rat skeletal muscle following insulin injection. Biochem Biophys Res Commun 197(2):578–584. doi:10.1006/bbrc.1993.2518
99. Hei YJ, McNeill JH, Sanghera JS, Diamond J, Bryer-Ash M, Pelech SL (1993) Characterization of insulin-stimulated seryl/threonyl protein kinases in rat skeletal muscle. J Biol Chem 268(18):13203–13213
100. Sherwood DJ, Dufresne SD, Markuns JF, Cheatham B, Moller DE, Aronson D et al (1999) Differential regulation of MAP kinase, p70 (S6K), and Akt by contraction and insulin in rat skeletal muscle. Am J Physiol 276(5 Pt 1):E870–E878
101. Virkamaki A, Ueki K, Kahn CR (1999) Protein-protein interaction in insulin signaling and the molecular mechanisms of insulin resistance. J Clin Invest 103(7):931–943. doi:10.1172/JCI6609
102. Daum G, Eisenmann-Tappe I, Fries HW, Troppmair J, Rapp UR (1994) The ins and outs of Raf kinases. Trends Biochem Sci 19(11):474–480
103. Krook A, Widegren U, Jiang XJ, Henriksson J, Wallberg-Henriksson H, Alessi D et al (2000) Effects of exercise on mitogen- and stress-activated kinase signal transduction in human skeletal muscle. Am J Physiol Regul Integr Comp Physiol 279(5):R1716–R1721
104. Widegren U, Ryder JW, Zierath JR (2001) Mitogen-activated protein kinase signal transduction in skeletal muscle: effects of exercise and muscle contraction. Acta Physiol Scand 172 (3):227–238. doi:10.1046/j.1365-201x.2001.00855.x
105. Raney MA, Turcotte LP (2006) Regulation of contraction-induced FA uptake and oxidation by AMPK and ERK1/2 is intensity dependent in rodent muscle. Am J Physiol Endocrinol Metab 291(6):E1220–E1227. doi:10.1152/ajpendo.00155.2006

Chapter 11
Mechanism of Skeletal Muscle Contraction: Role of Mechanical Muscle Contraction in Glucose Homeostasis

Yasuro Furuichi

Abstract Physical exercise has beneficial effects on whole-body glucose homeostasis and reduces the risk of metabolic diseases such as obesity, diabetes, and insulin resistance. Muscle contraction increases glucose uptake by skeletal muscle cells via an insulin-independent signaling mechanism. There is an increasing evidence that contraction-induced glucose uptake is mediated by AMP-activated protein kinase (AMPK), an energy sensor in skeletal muscle. Recent studies have identified another signaling pathway involving sucrose nonfermenting AMPK-related kinase that is activated by muscle contraction. Acute muscle contraction also activates insulin-induced glucose transport, and TBC1D4 has been identified as a regulator of insulin sensitization. Increased lipid oxidation and utilization resulting from chronic muscle contraction can stimulate insulin-induced glucose transport, since tissue accumulation of lipid metabolites—that is, lipotoxicity—is a basis for insulin resistance. Carnitine also normalizes intracellular lipid state by buffering excess accumulation of acetyl coenzyme A, a potent inhibitor of key enzymes in glucose metabolism. Finally, chronic exercise affects not only skeletal muscle but also pancreatic function and enhances insulin secretion. The current knowledge regarding the mechanism of glucose uptake induced by muscle contraction is summarized in this chapter.

Keywords AMPK • TBC1D4 • Insulin sensitivity • Lipotoxicity

11.1 Introduction

The skeletal muscle is the largest organ to take up blood glucose and accounts for 70 % of glucose disposal [1, 2]; thus, dysregulation of the glucose transport mechanism in skeletal muscle cells causes an elevation of blood glucose levels, leading to diabetes. Exercise is widely recognized as having beneficial effects for

Y. Furuichi (✉)
Department of Health Promotion Sciences, Graduate School of Human Health Sciences, Tokyo Metropolitan University, Minami-Osawa, Hachioji-city, Tokyo 192-0397, Japan
e-mail: furuichi@tmu.ac.jp

M. Inaba (ed.), *Musculoskeletal Disease Associated with Diabetes Mellitus*,
DOI 10.1007/978-4-431-55720-3_11

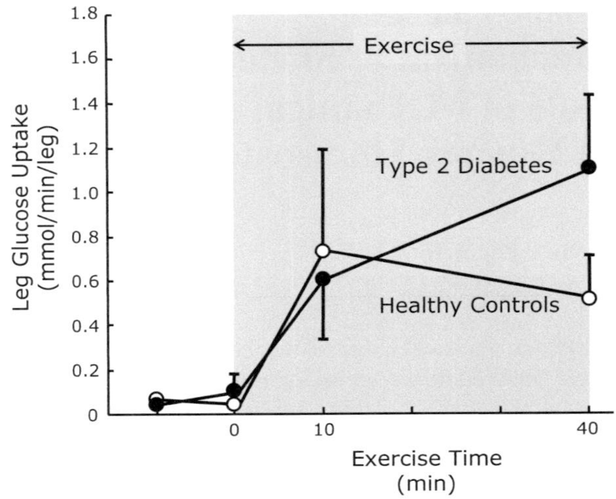

Fig. 11.1 Glucose uptake in the leg during a cycling exercise in type 2 diabetic patients and healthy controls (Modified from Martin et al. [3])

patients with diabetes mellitus because muscle contraction directly stimulates glucose uptake in skeletal muscle. This was first demonstrated two decades ago by a study that compared glucose uptake in skeletal muscle during cycling between insulin-resistant diabetic patients and healthy subjects, which found that glucose uptake in leg muscles was increased to a comparable degree in both groups [3] (Fig. 11.1). These results demonstrated that although insulin signaling is impaired in diabetic patients, the signaling mechanism for muscle contraction-induced glucose uptake remains intact, suggesting that it is independent of insulin signaling. Direct evidence for contraction-induced glucose transport was demonstrated in an in vitro muscle contraction model in which excised skeletal muscle was electrically stimulated [4], enabling the effect of muscle contraction on glucose transport in skeletal muscle to be examined independently of in vivo factors such as hormone and metabolite levels and blood flow. The role of muscle contraction as a stimulator of glucose uptake is now universally accepted, and much is known about the underlying signaling pathways.

Muscle contraction also improves whole-body glucose homeostasis, since a bout of muscle contraction can enhance insulin-induced signaling. Although insulin- and muscle contraction-induced glucose transport occur via independent mechanisms, muscle contraction affects molecules involved in the insulin cascade and is required to maintain intracellular lipid balance. Excess lipid accumulation in skeletal muscle cells caused by overfeeding potently inhibits insulin signaling, while chronic exercise increases the expression of proteins involved in glucose transport and mitochondrial biogenesis and improves pancreatic insulin secretion, suggesting that muscle contraction affects organs other than skeletal muscle. Understanding the mechanistic basis for improved glucose homeostasis resulting from muscle contraction is essential for developing effective drugs and optimizing exercise-based intervention strategies for disease. This chapter summarizes the current knowledge regarding the mechanism of glucose uptake induced by muscle contraction.

11.2 Regulation of Glucose Transport by Insulin- and Muscle Contraction-Induced Signaling

Glucose uptake by skeletal muscle cells is mediated by glucose transporters (GLUTs). Two of these, GLUT1 and GLUT4, are expressed in skeletal muscle; however, the latter is responsible for the acute regulation of glucose uptake. In the basal state, vesicles containing GLUT4 are pooled in the cytosol and translocated to the sarcolemma and T-tubules; glucose transport therefore depends on the presence of GLUT4 on the muscle cell surface, which is enhanced by insulin and muscle contraction via distinct signaling pathways. The current understanding of the molecular mechanisms of insulin- and contraction-induced glucose transport in skeletal muscle cells is summarized in Fig. 11.2.

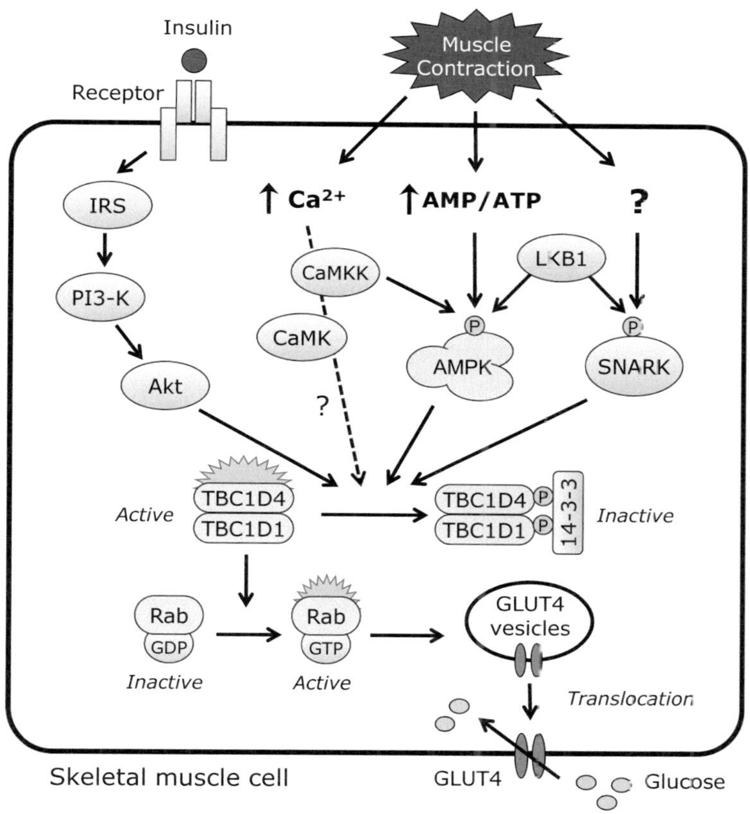

Fig. 11.2 Signaling pathways for insulin- and contraction-induced glucose uptake in skeletal muscle

11.2.1 Glucose Transport Mediated by Insulin Signaling

Insulin produced by beta cells in the pancreas is a potent stimulator of glucose transport into skeletal muscle cells. The regulation of glucose transport involving the insulin signaling pathway and the activation of various intracellular proteins has been summarized by recent review articles [5]. Briefly, the binding of insulin to its receptor triggers the activation of the associated tyrosine kinase, leading to tyrosine phosphorylation of insulin receptor substrate (IRS)-1 and activation of phosphatidylinositol 3-kinase (PI3K) followed by Akt, resulting in the translocation of GLUT4 to the muscle cell surface where glucose transport occurs via facilitative diffusion (Fig. 11.2). As described later, muscle contraction affects insulin signaling and increases insulin sensitivity.

11.2.2 Muscle Contraction Increases Glucose Transport via AMP-Activated Protein Kinase (AMPK) Activation

AMP-activated protein kinase (AMPK) is a heterotrimer composed of a catalytic α-subunit (α1 and α2) and regulatory β- (β1 and β2) and γ-subunits (γ1, γ2, and γ3). Only three combinations of these exist in skeletal muscle, namely, α1/β2/γ1, α2/β2/γ1, and α2/β2/γ3 [6]. The γ-subunit has a binding domain for ATP, ADP, and AMP and thereby acts as an energy sensor. Thr^{172} is the regulatory phosphorylation site of the α-subunit, and its phosphorylation is essential for catalytic activity [7, 8]. Liver kinase B1 (LKB1) was identified as an enzyme that phosphorylates Thr^{172} in the skeletal muscle [9] and is the major kinase regulating AMPKα: muscle-specific deletion of LKB1 abolishes AMPKα2 activity under basal and contraction-stimulated conditions [10].

A decrease in intracellular energy stores is a major trigger for contraction-induced glucose uptake. Intracellular ATP is consumed during muscle contraction, which increases AMP and ADP concentrations. This leads to the activation of AMPK, a serine/threonine kinase belonging to a family that is highly conserved among eukaryotic species and acting as a sensor of energy levels in the skeletal muscle [11]. Increases in AMP:ATP and ADP:ATP ratios cause conformational changes in the APMK complex, which induces AMPK phosphorylation by upstream kinases [12, 13].

Contraction-induced glucose uptake is mediated by AMPK activation. This was established by pharmacological experiments using the AMPK activator 5-aminoimidazole-4-carboxamide-1-β-4-ribofuranoside (AICAR), which was shown to stimulate glucose transport in skeletal muscle independently of the effects of insulin [14, 15]. AICAR is taken up by muscle cells and phosphorylated to yield 5-aminoimidazole-4-carboxamide ribonucleotide, a monophosphorylated derivative that mimics the effects of AMP on AMPK. The effect of AICAR treatment on glucose transport was comparable to that of muscle contraction, which was not inhibited by the PI3K inhibitor wortmannin [15]. These findings suggest that AICAR stimulates glucose transport via an insulin-independent signaling mechanism.

11.2.3 Sucrose Nonfermenting AMPK-Related Kinase (SNARK) Mediates Contraction-Induced Glucose Transport

Contraction-induced glucose uptake occurs via the LKB1/AMPK axis. The contribution of AMPK to glucose transport in skeletal muscle has been evaluated in transgenic mice that express a dominant-negative form of AMPKα in this tissue [16, 17]. As expected, AICAR- and contraction-induced AMPKα activity was completely abolished in these mice; however, AICAR- but not contraction-stimulated glucose uptake was inhibited [17]. These results suggest that AMPK regulates contraction-induced glucose transport but that other molecules are also likely to be involved.

While AMPKα2 mutant mice showed normal contraction-stimulated glucose transport [17], this was markedly reduced in muscle-specific LKB1 knockout mice lacking AMPKα2 activity [10], implying that one or more additional LKB1 substrates are involved. SNARK has been identified as a contraction-activated signal that mediates glucose transport in skeletal muscle [18]. Muscle contraction increased SNARK activity in skeletal muscles of normal mice but was abolished in LKB1 knockout mice, suggesting that SNARK is a downstream effector of LKB1 in the regulation of glucose transport [18].

11.2.4 Effect of Ca^{2+} Signaling on Skeletal Muscle Glucose Transport

Ca^{2+} released from the sarcoplasmic reticulum initiates muscle contraction and is thought to directly regulate glucose uptake. Skeletal muscle glucose uptake was increased in response to low concentrations of caffeine, a stimulator of sarcoplasmic reticulum Ca^{2+} release, in the absence of contractile activity and alternation of cellular energy status [19, 20]. These reports suggest that Ca^{2+} release is sufficient to increase glucose uptake in a signaling mechanism that is independent of AMPK. However, several studies have demonstrated that caffeine induces AMPK activation in the absence of muscle contraction [21, 22]; from this it was concluded that Ca^{2+} release per se does not regulate glucose transport [23, 24]. It has been proposed that increased cytosolic Ca^{2+} reuptake into the sarcoplasmic reticulum increases energy demand and results in AMPK activation [23].

Ca^{2+}-sensitive signaling molecules regulates glucose transport during muscle contraction. Ca^{2+}/calmodulin-dependent protein kinase kinases (CaMKKs) phosphorylate Thr^{172} of AMPK, potentially activating AMPK signaling [25, 26], and CaMKKα overexpression in mouse skeletal muscle increases AMPK Thr^{172} phosphorylation as well as glucose uptake [27]. Ca^{2+}/calmodulin-dependent protein kinase (CaMK)II is also considered as a regulator of contraction-induced glucose uptake in skeletal muscles: the transfection of a CaMKII-specific inhibitory peptide into mouse skeletal muscle in vivo reduced contraction-induced glucose transport [28]. However, it has been suggested that the contribution of CaMK-mediated glucose transport is relatively low and its role is now less certain [23].

11.2.5 Downstream Effectors of Glucose Transport During Muscle Contraction

Although insulin- and contraction-induced signaling pathways in glucose uptake are distinct, both stimuli induce the translocation of GLUT4. Recent studies have shown that the insulin- and contraction-induced signaling pathways converge on some molecules in skeletal muscle. The molecules at the nexus are Tre-2/Bub2-Cdc16 (TBC)1 and domain family TBC1D1 and TBC1D4 (also known as Akt substrate of 160 kDa or AS160), which are Rab GTPase-activating proteins (GAPs) that regulate GLUT4 traffic. When TBC1D1 and TBC1D4 are phosphorylated by upstream signaling, they bind 14-3-3 protein and inhibit GAP activity, leading to the conversion of inactive GDP-loaded to active GTP-loaded Rab. The active form recruits various effectors and allows the transport and fusion of GLUT4 storage vesicles to the plasma membrane [29]. TBC1D1 and TBC1D4 exhibit GAP activity toward a number of Rab proteins [30, 31], suggesting that these participate in GLUT4 translocation via their GTPase activities.

11.3 Exercise Increases Insulin Sensitivity in Skeletal Muscles

Another important beneficial effect of muscle contraction on glucose homeostasis is the improvement of insulin sensitivity in skeletal muscle. The direct effect of muscle contraction on glucose uptake declines within a few hours, but insulin-induced glucose uptake in exercised muscle remains elevated for several hours [32–35]. This insulin sensitization by muscle contraction was first reported in an investigation of the effect of one-legged exercise on glucose uptake in response to insulin infusion [36]. The results demonstrated that glucose uptake was significantly higher in exercised than in rested legs 4 h after exercise. In support of these findings, it was shown in both humans and rodents that acute muscle contraction is associated with increased insulin sensitivity for up to 72 h after the acute effect of exercise on glucose uptake has disappeared [32, 33, 35]. Insulin-stimulated glucose transport following several hours of exercise is accompanied by enhanced GLUT4 translocation without an associated increase in GLUT4 expression or proximal insulin signaling [37, 38]. Interestingly, insulin sensitization following pre-muscle contraction is observed in insulin-resistant muscle from mice fed with a high-fat diet [37]. Therefore, insulin sensitization by muscle contraction is gaining attention for its potential application in pharmaceutics for the treatment of obesity-related diabetes.

It is unknown which molecules are responsible for insulin sensitivity after muscle contraction, but recent studies have shown that acute contraction increased phosphorylation of GAPs [32]. In experiments on isolated rat skeletal muscles, site-specific phosphorylation of TBC1D4 was increased in exercise relative to rested muscle [37, 39, 40]. It was also reported the acute exercise increased insulin-stimulated glucose transport, which was correlated with TBC1D4 phosphorylation in healthy human subjects [41, 42], whereas insulin-stimulated phosphorylation of TBC1D1 remained unaffected by pre-exercise [40, 41]. Taken together, these data suggest that muscle contraction enhances insulin sensitivity via stimulation of TBC1D4 phosphorylation.

11.4 Chronic Exercise Improves Glucose Homeostasis

11.4.1 Effect of Chronic Exercise on Glucose Transport Mediated by Insulin Signaling in Skeletal Muscle

Physical activity is known to improve glucose homeostasis in healthy and diabetic individuals. Insulin sensitivity is correlated with degree of physical activity [43]; therefore, regular exercise is a therapeutic means of improving glucose metabolism. Various studies have shown that exercise training improves glucose tolerance and insulin action in insulin-resistant individuals [44] or type 2 diabetic patients [45]. The molecular mechanism underlying enhanced glucose uptake with chronic exercise may be linked to increased expression and activity of proteins involved in glucose uptake and metabolism in skeletal muscle: chronic exercise was shown to increase GLUT4 expression and enhance glucose uptake in resting and contracting muscles [46, 47].

Exercise training improves insulin-stimulated glucose uptake by enhancing insulin signaling, which is impaired in skeletal muscles of diabetic individuals [48]. Importantly, chronic exercise increased insulin-stimulated PI3K activity—a regulatory step in glucose uptake—in skeletal muscles with a concomitant increase in PI3K activity and IRS-1 expression [40–42], suggesting that IRS-1 is likely the predominant factor responsible for exercise-induced changes in insulin signaling to PI3K in skeletal muscles.

Another mechanism for the enhancement of insulin sensitivity following chronic exercise is the upregulation of TBC1D4 phosphorylation. Actually, chronic endurance training increased TBC1D4 protein expression and its phosphorylation induced by insulin stimulation [49, 50]. Recently, Consitt et al. showed that TBC1D4 phosphorylation by insulin signaling was impaired in insulin resistance subjects, and long-term chronic endurance exercise increased whole body insulin action and reversed the impairments in TBC1D4 phosphorylation [51]. These findings suggest that increases in insulin-induced glucose uptake can be explained by altered TBC1D4 signaling.

11.4.2 Effect of Chronic Exercise on Insulin Secretion by Pancreatic Islets

Chronic exercise can affect whole-body glucose metabolism by enhancing insulin secretion by the pancreas. In general, chronic exercise is associated with a reduction in blood-insulin concentration [52]. This does not reflect a decrease in the ability of the pancreas to secrete insulin, but results from an increase in insulin sensitivity in skeletal muscles due to exercise, which reduces the amount of insulin required to maintain glucose availability.

The effect of chronic exercise on insulin secretion by the pancreas has been extensively studied, but the findings remain controversial, likely due to differences in experimental models such as the in vivo model [53, 54], isolated islets [55, 56], and single beta cell assay [57, 58] that have been used to evaluate insulin secretion. To evaluate the ability of islets to secrete insulin without the influence of an extracellular environment, our group has used isolated pancreatic islets maintained by a perfusion system to examine insulin secretion in response to high-glucose stimulation, since pancreatic beta cells sense glucose levels in the circulation and consequently secrete insulin [59]. Chronic exercise on a treadmill enhanced glucose-induced insulin secretion while pancreatic insulin level and tissue weight were unaltered [60]. It is unclear how chronic exercise (i.e., muscle contraction) improves pancreatic function, but the cross talk between the skeletal muscle and the pancreas may be explained by activities of glucagon-like peptide (GLP)-1—which is a stimulator of insulin secretion—and interleukin (IL)-6, which was shown to enhance insulin secretion by stimulating GLP-1 secretion from intestinal L and pancreatic alpha cells [61]. IL-6 is a myokine whose concentration in blood increases markedly during exercise [62]; therefore, the exercise-induced improvement of islet function may be explained by IL-6 and GLP-1 signaling.

11.5 Muscle Contraction Improves Intracellular Lipid State

11.5.1 Effect of Muscle Contraction on Lipid-Induced Insulin Resistance

Lipids are important metabolic substrates in the maintenance of skeletal muscle contractile activity. During muscle contraction, skeletal muscle cells take up fatty acids as a source of ATP. However, an imbalance between lipid supply and demand—for instance, caused by excess accumulation of intracellular lipid metabolites—leads to various metabolic disorders such as insulin resistance, type 2 diabetes, and obesity [63, 64]. Intracellular lipids are used to synthesize complex lipids including diacylglycerol, which activates serine kinases such as protein kinase C and cJun terminal kinase and subsequently inhibits insulin signaling molecules such as insulin receptor and IRS-1 [65–67]. This lipid-induced dysregulation of glucose metabolism is referred to as lipotoxicity [68].

Lipid-induced insulin resistance in muscle results from an impaired lipid oxidation capacity in mitochondria [69], which was shown to be reduced in insulin-resistant subjects relative to controls [70, 71]. An impaired capacity for oxidizing fatty acids leads to intramyocellular fat accumulation and reduced insulin sensitivity. Muscle contraction is the most effective way of reducing lipid accumulation and preventing lipid-induced insulin resistance. Chronic exercise increases the oxidative capacity of skeletal muscle by inducing the upregulation of proteins involved in mitochondrial biogenesis such as peroxisome proliferator-activated receptor-γ coactivator [72]. Endurance training was shown to enhance insulin sensitivity via increased skeletal muscle fat oxidation [73], and muscle contraction induced by electrical stimulation in the rat hindlimb increased insulin-stimulated glucose transport, which was associated with reductions in diacylglycerol and ceramide levels [74].

11.5.2 Carnitine Relieves Acetyl-CoA-Induced Inhibition of Glucose Metabolism

Carnitine transports fatty acids across the mitochondrial membrane in skeletal muscle cells. Although it is primarily known for the translocation of acyl coenzyme A (CoA) into the mitochondrial matrix for beta oxidation, recent studies have shown that carnitine also buffers excess mitochondrial acetyl CoA, an intermediate metabolite of beta oxidation and glycolytic metabolism that enters the tricarboxylic acid (TCA) cycle and is oxidized to generate ATP [75]. However, excess accumulation of acetyl CoA inhibits pyruvate dehydrogenase (PDH), a rate-limiting enzyme for pyruvate entry into the TCA cycle [76], resulting in negative regulation

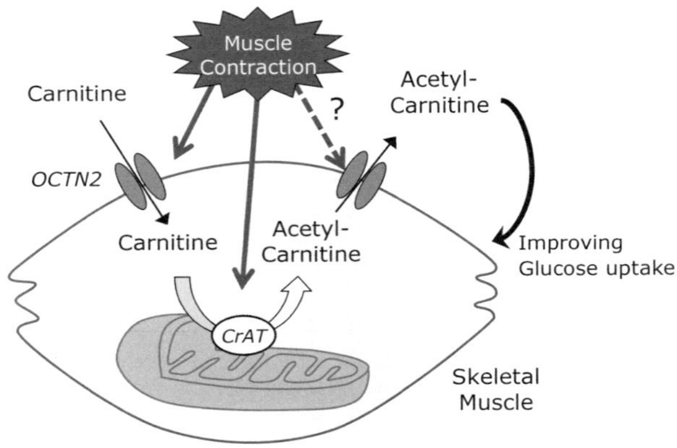

Fig. 11.3 Carnitine dynamics during muscle contraction in skeletal muscle

of glucose uptake; this occurs upon increased energy production, such as during exercise or after feeding [77, 78]. Under these conditions, acetyl CoA accumulation is reversed by carnitine acetyltransferase (CrAT) present in the mitochondrial matrix, which converts acetyl CoA to acetylcarnitine and free CoA, thereby buffering acetyl CoA and CoA levels (Fig. 11.3). Given that impaired mitochondrial function induces insulin resistance in skeletal muscle, CrAT has been proposed as a key regulator of glucose homeostasis in skeletal muscle [79]. Muscle-specific CrAT knockout mice showed glucose intolerance, insulin resistance, and metabolic inflexibility [80], and it is reported that skeletal muscle CrAT activity is impaired in obese and diabetic mice [81], providing evidence of a pathophysiological role for CrAT.

Carnitine metabolism changes during muscle contraction based on its role in energy production and maintenance of acetyl CoA concentration. Exercise causes a rapid decrease in the level of carnitine, which is converted to acetylcarnitine, in skeletal muscle [82, 83]. We recently visualized the distribution of endogenous acetylcarnitine in rat skeletal muscle by matrix-assisted laser desorption/ionization imaging mass spectrometry, which integrates microscopy and mass spectrometry [84]. Acetylcarnitine accumulation upon muscle contraction corresponded to regions of glycogen depletion, suggesting that carnitine acetylation occurs as a result of high metabolic demand during sustained muscle contraction.

In addition to its role in relieving PDH inhibition, it was hypothesized that acetylcarnitine is exported from skeletal muscle cells in response to an increase in intracellular acetylcarnitine concentration and serves as a biologically active substrate [79]. For example, acetylcarnitine inhibited tumor necrosis factor-α-induced insulin resistance via the AMPK pathway in cultured cells [85], and plasma acetylcarnitine concentration was found to increase during human exercise [86], suggesting that acetylcarnitine produced during muscle contraction may be exported to serve a different function. Muscle contraction also increased carnitine transport from the blood to skeletal muscle cells via the carnitine transporter OCTN2 [87, 88]; however, additional studies are needed to assess the physiological significance of this observation.

References

1. Shulman GI, Rothman DL, Jue T, Stein P, DeFronzo RA, Shulman RG (1990) Quantitation of muscle glycogen synthesis in normal subjects and subjects with non-insulin-dependent diabetes by 13C nuclear magnetic resonance spectroscopy. N Engl J Med 322:223–228
2. DeFronzo RA, Jacot E, Jequier E, Maeder E, Wahren J, Felber JP (1981) The effect of insulin on the disposal of intravenous glucose. Results from indirect calorimetry and hepatic and femoral venous catheterization. Diabetes 30:1000–1007
3. Martin IVAK, Katz A, Wahren J, Iva K (1995) Splanchnic and muscle metabolism during exercise in NIDDM patients. Am J Physiol Endocrinol Metab 269:583–590
4. Holloszy JO (2003) A forty-year memoir of research on the regulation of glucose transport into muscle. Am J Physiol Endocrinol Metab 284:E453–E467
5. Leto D, Saltiel AR (2012) Regulation of glucose transport by insulin: traffic control of GLUT4. Nat Rev Mol Cell Biol 13:383–396
6. Birk JB, Wojtaszewski JFP (2006) Predominant alpha2/beta2/gamma3 AMPK activation during exercise in human skeletal muscle. J Physiol 577:1021–1032
7. Hawley SA, Davison M, Woods A, Davies SP, Beri RK, Carling D, Hardie DG (1996) Characterization of the AMP-activated protein kinase kinase from rat liver and identification of threonine 172 as the major site at which it phosphorylates AMP-activated protein kinase. J Biol Chem 271:27879–27887
8. Stein SC, Woods A, Jones NA, Davison MD, Carling D (2000) The regulation of AMP-activated protein kinase by phosphorylation. Biochem J 345(Pt 3):437–443
9. Shaw RJ, Kosmatka M, Bardeesy N, Hurley RL, Witters LA, DePinho RA, Cantley LC (2004) The tumor suppressor LKB1 kinase directly activates AMP-activated kinase and regulates apoptosis in response to energy stress. Proc Natl Acad Sci U S A 101:3329–3335
10. Sakamoto K, McCarthy A, Smith D, Green KA, Grahame Hardie D, Ashworth A, Alessi DR (2005) Deficiency of LKB1 in skeletal muscle prevents AMPK activation and glucose uptake during contraction. EMBO J 24:1810–1820
11. Hardie DG, Scott JW, Pan DA, Hudson ER (2003) Management of cellular energy by the AMP-activated protein kinase system. FEBS Lett 546:113–120
12. Carling D (2004) The AMP-activated protein kinase cascade – a unifying system for energy control. Trends Biochem Sci 29:18–24
13. Hardie DG, Carling D, Carlson M (1998) The AMP-activated/SNF1 protein kinase subfamily: metabolic sensors of the eukaryotic cell? Annu Rev Biochem 67:821–855
14. Merrill GF, Kurth EJ, Hardie DG, Winder WW (1997) AICA riboside increases AMP-activated protein kinase, fatty acid oxidation, and glucose uptake in rat muscle. Am J Physiol 273:E1107–E1112
15. Hayashi T, Hirshman MF, Kurth EJ, Winder WW, Goodyear LJ (1998) Evidence for 5′ AMP-activated protein kinase mediation of the effect of muscle contraction on glucose transport. Diabetes 47:1369–1373
16. Mu J, Brozinick JT, Valladares O, Bucan M, Birnbaum MJ (2001) A role for AMP-activated protein kinase in contraction- and hypoxia-regulated glucose transport in skeletal muscle. Mol Cell 7:1085–1094
17. Fujii N, Hirshman MF, Kane EM, Ho RC, Peter LE, Seifert MM, Goodyear LJ (2005) AMP-activated protein kinase alpha2 activity is not essential for contraction- and hyperosmolarity-induced glucose transport in skeletal muscle. J Biol Chem 280:39033–39041
18. Koh H-J, Toyoda T, Fujii N et al (2010) Sucrose nonfermenting AMPK-related kinase (SNARK) mediates contraction-stimulated glucose transport in mouse skeletal muscle. Proc Natl Acad Sci U S A 107:15541–15546
19. Wright DC, Geiger PC, Holloszy JO, Han D-H (2005) Contraction- and hypoxia-stimulated glucose transport is mediated by a Ca^{2+}-dependent mechanism in slow-twitch rat soleus muscle. Am J Physiol Endocrinol Metab 288:E1062–E1066

20. Wright DC, Hucker KA, Holloszy JO, Han DH (2004) Ca^{2+} and AMPK both mediate stimulation of glucose transport by muscle contractions. Diabetes 53:330–335
21. Jensen TE, Rose AJ, Hellsten Y, Wojtaszewski JFP, Richter EA (2007) Caffeine-induced Ca^{2+} release increases AMPK-dependent glucose uptake in rodent soleus muscle. Am J Physiol Endocrinol Metab 293:E286–E292
22. Raney MA, Turcotte LP (2008) Evidence for the involvement of CaMKII and AMPK in Ca^{2+}-dependent signaling pathways regulating FA uptake and oxidation in contracting rodent muscle. J Appl Physiol 104:1366–1373
23. Richter EA, Hargreaves M (2013) Exercise, GLUT4, and skeletal muscle glucose uptake. Physiol Rev 93:993–1017
24. Jensen TE, Sylow L, Rose AJ, Madsen AB, Angin Y, Maarbjerg SJ, Richter EA (2014) Contraction-stimulated glucose transport in muscle is controlled by AMPK and mechanical stress but not sarcoplasmatic reticulum Ca^{2+} release. Mol Metab 3:742–753
25. Hurley RL, Anderson KA, Franzone JM, Kemp BE, Means AR, Witters LA (2005) The Ca^{2+}/calmodulin-dependent protein kinase kinases are AMP-activated protein kinase kinases. J Biol Chem 280:29060–29066
26. Hawley SA, Pan DA, Mustard KJ, Ross L, Bain J, Edelman AM, Frenguelli BG, Hardie DG (2005) Calmodulin-dependent protein kinase kinase-beta is an alternative upstream kinase for AMP-activated protein kinase. Cell Metab 2:9–19
27. Witczak CA, Fujii N, Hirshman MF, Goodyear LJ (2007) Ca2+/calmodulin-dependent protein kinase kinase-alpha regulates skeletal muscle glucose uptake independent of AMP-activated protein kinase and Akt activation. Diabetes 56:1403–1409
28. Witczak CA, Jessen N, Warro DM, Toyoda T, Fujii N, Anderson ME, Hirshman MF, Goodyear LJ (2010) CaMKII regulates contraction- but not insulin-induced glucose uptake in mouse skeletal muscle. Am J Physiol Endocrinol Metab 298:E1150–E1160
29. Sakamoto K, Holman GD (2008) Emerging role for AS160/TBC1D4 and TBC1D1 in the regulation of GLUT4 traffic. Am J Physiol Endocrinol Metab 295:E29–E37
30. Mîinea CP, Sano H, Kane S, Sano E, Fukuda M, Peränen J, Lane WS, Lienhard GE (2005) AS160, the Akt substrate regulating GLUT4 translocation, has a functional Rab GTPase-activating protein domain. Biochem J 391:87–93
31. Roach WG, Chavez JA, Mîinea CP, Lienhard GE (2007) Substrate specificity and effect on GLUT4 translocation of the Rab GTPase-activating protein Tbc1d1. Biochem J 403:353–358
32. Cartee GD (2015) Roles of TBC1D1 and TBC1D4 in insulin- and exercise-stimulated glucose transport of skeletal muscle. Diabetologia 58:19–30
33. Wojtaszewski JF, Hansen BF, Gade, Kiens B, Markuns JF, Goodyear LJ, Richter EA (2000) Insulin signaling and insulin sensitivity after exercise in human skeletal muscle. Diabetes 49:325–331
34. Jessen N, Pold R, Buhl ES, Jensen LS, Schmitz O, Lund S (2003) Effects of AICAR and exercise on insulin-stimulated glucose uptake, signaling, and GLUT-4 content in rat muscles. J Appl Physiol 94:1373–1379
35. Friedrichsen M, Mortensen B, Pehmøller C, Birk JB, Wojtaszewski JFP (2013) Exercise-induced AMPK activity in skeletal muscle: role in glucose uptake and insulin sensitivity. Mol Cell Endocrinol 366:204–214
36. Richter E, Mikines K, Galbo H, Kiens B (1989) Effect of exercise on insulin action in human skeletal muscle. J Appl Physiol 66:876–885
37. Castorena CM, Arias EB, Sharma N, Cartee GD (2014) Postexercise improvement in insulin-stimulated glucose uptake occurs concomitant with greater AS160 phosphorylation in muscle from normal and insulin-resistant rats. Diabetes 63:2297–2308
38. Hansen PA, Nolte LA, Chen MM, Holloszy JO (1998) Increased GLUT-4 translocation mediates enhanced insulin sensitivity of muscle glucose transport after exercise. J Appl Physiol 85:1218–1222

39. Schweitzer GG, Arias EB, Cartee GD (2012) Sustained postexercise increases in AS160 Thr642 and Ser588 phosphorylation in skeletal muscle without sustained increases in kinase phosphorylation. J Appl Physiol 113:1852–1861
40. Funai K, Schweitzer GG, Sharma N, Kanzaki M, Cartee GD (2009) Increased AS160 phosphorylation, but not TBC1D1 phosphorylation, with increased postexercise insulin sensitivity in rat skeletal muscle. Am J Physiol Endocrinol Metab 297:E242–E251
41. Pehmøller C, Brandt N, Birk JB, Høeg LD, Sjøberg KA, Goodyear LJ, Kiens B, Richter EA, Wojtaszewski JFP (2012) Exercise alleviates lipid-induced insulin resistance in human skeletal muscle-signaling interaction at the level of TBC1 domain family member 4. Diabetes 61:2743–2752
42. Treebak JT, Frøsig C, Pehmøller C et al (2009) Potential role of TBC1D4 in enhanced post-exercise insulin action in human skeletal muscle. Diabetologia 52:891–900
43. Seals DR, Hagberg JM, Allen WK, Hurley BF, Dalsky GP, Ehsani AA, Holloszy JO (1984) Glucose tolerance in young and older athletes and sedentary men. J Appl Physiol 56:1521–1525
44. Hughes VA, Fiatarone MA, Fielding RA, Kahn BB, Ferrara CM, Shepherd P, Fisher EC, Wolfe RR, Elahi D, Evans WJ (1993) Exercise increases muscle GLUT-4 levels and insulin action in subjects with impaired glucose tolerance. Am J Physiol 264:E855–E862
45. Schneider SH, Amorosa LF, Khachadurian AK, Ruderman NB (1984) Studies on the mechanism of improved glucose control during regular exercise in type 2 (non-insulin-dependent) diabetes. Diabetologia 26:355–360
46. Kawanaka K, Tabata I, Katsuta S, Higuchi M (1997) Changes in insulin-stimulated glucose transport and GLUT-4 protein in rat skeletal muscle after training. J Appl Physiol 83:2043–2047
47. Ivy JL (2004) Muscle insulin resistance amended with exercise training: role of GLUT4 expression. Med Sci Sports Exerc 36:1207–1211
48. Zierath JR (2002) Invited review: exercise training-induced changes in insulin signaling in skeletal muscle. J Appl Physiol 93:773–781
49. Frøsig C, Rose AJ, Treebak JT, Kiens B, Richter EA, Wojtaszewski JFP (2007) Effects of endurance exercise training on insulin signaling in human skeletal muscle: interactions at the level of phosphatidylinositol 3-kinase, Akt, and AS160. Diabetes 56:2093–2102
50. Vind BF, Pehmøller C, Treebak JT, Birk JB, Hey-Mogensen M, Beck-Nielsen H, Zierath JR, Wojtaszewski JFP, Højlund K (2011) Impaired insulin-induced site-specific phosphorylation of TBC1 domain family, member 4 (TBC1D4) in skeletal muscle of type 2 diabetes patients is restored by endurance exercise-training. Diabetologia 54:157–167
51. Consitt LA, van Meter J, Newton CA, Collier DN, Dar MS, Wojtaszewski JFP, Treebak JT, Tanner CJ, Houmard JA (2013) Impairments in site-specific AS160 phosphorylation and effects of exercise training. Diabetes 62:3437–3447
52. Bradley RL, Jeon JY, Liu F-F, Maratos-Flier E (2008) Voluntary exercise improves insulin sensitivity and adipose tissue inflammation in diet-induced obese mice. Am J Physiol Endocrinol Metab 295:E586–E594
53. Park S, Hong SM, Lee JE, Sung SR (2007) Exercise improves glucose homeostasis that has been impaired by a high-fat diet by potentiating pancreatic beta-cell function and mass through IRS2 in diabetic rats. J Appl Physiol 103:1764–1771
54. Farrell PA, Caston AL, Rodd D (1991) Changes in insulin response to glucose after exercise training in partially pancreatectomized rats. J Appl Physiol 70:1563–1568
55. Huang H-H, Farmer K, Windscheffel J, Yost K, Power M, Wright DE, Stehno-Bittel L (2011) Exercise increases insulin content and basal secretion in pancreatic islets in type 1 diabetic mice. Exp Diabetes Res 2011:481427
56. Calegari VC, Zoppi CC, Rezende LF, Silveira LR, Carneiro EM, Boschero AC (2011) Endurance training activates AMP-activated protein kinase, increases expression of uncoupling protein 2 and reduces insulin secretion from rat pancreatic islets. J Endocrinol 208:257–264

57. Farrell PA, Caston AL, Rodd D, Engdahl J (1992) Effect of training on insulin secretion from single pancreatic beta cells. Med Sci Sports Exerc 24:426–433
58. Lamontagne J, Masiello P, Marcil M, Delghingaro-Augusto V, Burelle Y, Prentki M, Nolan CJ (2007) Circulating lipids are lowered but pancreatic islet lipid metabolism and insulin secretion are unaltered in exercise-trained female rats. Appl Physiol Nutr Metab 32:241–248
59. Takagi M, Manabe Y (2014) Mechanisms underlying alterations in glucose metabolism due to exercise. J Phys Fit Sport Med 3:423–427
60. Tsuchiya M, Manabe Y, Yamada K, Furuichi Y, Hosaka M, Fujii NL (2012) Chronic exercise enhances insulin secretion ability of pancreatic islets without change in insulin content in non-diabetic rats. Biochem Biophys Res Commun 430:676–682
61. Ellingsgaard H, Hauselmann I, Schuler B et al (2011) Interleukin-6 enhances insulin secretion by increasing glucagon-like peptide-1 secretion from L cells and alpha cells. Nat Med 17:1481–1489
62. Pedersen BK, Febbraio MA (2008) Muscle as an endocrine organ: focus on muscle-derived interleukin-6. Physiol Rev 88:1379–1406
63. Pan DA, Lillioja S, Kriketos AD, Milner MR, Baur LA, Bogardus C, Jenkins AB, Storlien LH (1997) Skeletal muscle triglyceride levels are inversely related to insulin action. Diabetes 46:983–988
64. Muoio DM, Koves TR (2007) Lipid-induced metabolic dysfunction in skeletal muscle. Novartis Found Symp 286:24–38, discussion 38–46, 162–3, 196–203
65. Shulman GI (2000) Cellular mechanisms of insulin resistance. J Clin Invest 106:171–176
66. Samuel VT, Petersen KF, Shulman GI (2010) Lipid-induced insulin resistance: unravelling the mechanism. Lancet 375:2267–2277
67. Yu C, Chen Y, Cline GW et al (2002) Mechanism by which fatty acids inhibit insulin activation of insulin receptor substrate-1 (IRS-1)-associated phosphatidylinositol 3-kinase activity in muscle. J Biol Chem 277:50230–50236
68. Unger RH (2002) Lipotoxic diseases. Annu Rev Med 53:319–336
69. Morino K, Petersen KF, Shulman GI (2006) Molecular mechanisms of insulin resistance in humans and their potential links with mitochondrial dysfunction. Diabetes 55(Suppl 2):S9–S15
70. Petersen KF, Dufour S, Befroy D, Garcia R, Shulman GI (2004) Impaired mitochondrial activity in the insulin-resistant offspring of patients with type 2 diabetes. N Engl J Med 350:664–671
71. Befroy DE, Petersen KF, Dufour S, Mason GF, de Graaf RA, Rothman DL, Shulman GI (2007) Impaired mitochondrial substrate oxidation in muscle of insulin-resistant offspring of type 2 diabetic patients. Diabetes 56:1376–1381
72. Adhihetty PJ, Irrcher I, Joseph A-M, Ljubicic V, Hood DA (2003) Plasticity of skeletal muscle mitochondria in response to contractile activity. Exp Physiol 88:99–107
73. Goodpaster BH, Katsiaras A, Kelley DE (2003) Enhanced fat oxidation through physical activity is associated with improvements in insulin sensitivity in obesity. Diabetes 52:2191–2197
74. Holloway GP, Han XX, Jain SS, Bonen A, Chabowski A (2014) Chronic muscle stimulation improves insulin sensitivity while increasing subcellular lipid droplets and reducing selected diacylglycerol and ceramide species in obese Zucker rats. Diabetologia 57:832–840
75. Furuichi Y, Goto-Inoue N, Fujii NL (2014) Role of carnitine acetylation in skeletal muscle. J Phys Fit Sport Med 3:163–168
76. Sugden MC, Holness MJ (2003) Recent advances in mechanisms regulating glucose oxidation at the level of the pyruvate dehydrogenase complex by PDKs. Am J Physiol Endocrinol Metab 284:E855–E862
77. Koves TR, Ussher JR, Noland RC et al (2008) Mitochondrial overload and incomplete fatty acid oxidation contribute to skeletal muscle insulin resistance. Cell Metab 7:45–56

78. Thyfault JP, Cree MG, Tapscott EB, Bell JA, Koves TR, Ilkayeva O, Wolfe RR, Dohm GL, Muoio DM (2010) Metabolic profiling of muscle contraction in lean compared with obese rodents. Am J Physiol Regul Integr Comp Physiol 299:R926–R934
79. Noland RC, Koves TR, Seiler SE, Lum H, Lust RM, Ilkayeva O, Stevens RD, Hegardt FG, Muoio DM (2009) Carnitine insufficiency caused by aging and overnutrition compromises mitochondrial performance and metabolic control. J Biol Chem 284:22840–22852
80. Muoio DM, Noland RC, Kovalik J-P et al (2012) Muscle-specific deletion of carnitine acetyltransferase compromises glucose tolerance and metabolic flexibility. Cell Metab 15:764–777
81. Seiler SE, Martin OJ, Noland RC, Slentz DH, Debalsi KL, Ilkayeva OR, An J, Newgard CB, Koves TR, Muoio DM (2014) Obesity and lipid stress inhibit carnitine acetyltransferase activity. J Lipid Res 55:635–644
82. Hiatt WR, Regensteiner JG, Wolfel EE, Ruff L, Brass EP (1989) Carnitine and acylcarnitine metabolism during exercise in humans. Dependence on skeletal muscle metabolic state. J Clin Invest 84:1167–1173
83. Foster CV, Harris RC (1987) Formation of acetylcarnitine in muscle of horse during high intensity exercise. Eur J Appl Physiol Occup Physiol 56:639–642
84. Furuichi Y, Goto-Inoue N, Manabe Y, Setou M, Masuda K, Fujii NL (2014) Imaging mass spectrometry reveals fiber-specific distribution of acetylcarnitine and contraction-induced carnitine dynamics in rat skeletal muscles. Biochim Biophys Acta 1837:1699–1706
85. Zhang Z, Zhao M, Li Q, Zhao H, Wang J, Li Y (2009) Acetyl-l-carnitine inhibits TNF-alpha-induced insulin resistance via AMPK pathway in rat skeletal muscle cells. FEBS Lett 583:470–474
86. Vukovich MD, Costill DL, Fink WJ (1994) Carnitine supplementation: effect on muscle carnitine and glycogen content during exercise. Med Sci Sports Exerc 26:1122–1129
87. Furuichi Y, Sugiura T, Kato Y, Shimada Y, Masuda K (2010) OCTN2 is associated with carnitine transport capacity of rat skeletal muscles. Acta Physiol (Oxf) 200:57–64
88. Furuichi Y, Sugiura T, Kato Y, Takakura H, Hanai Y, Hashimoto T, Masuda K (2012) Muscle contraction increases carnitine uptake via translocation of OCTN2. Biochem Biophys Res Commun 418:774–779

Chapter 12
Ectopic Fat Accumulation and Glucose Homeostasis: Ectopic Fat Accumulation in Muscle

Katsuhito Mori, Tomoaki Morioka, Koka Motoyama, and Masanori Emoto

Abstract Adipocytes can serve as energy storage reservoirs against calorie overload. Beyond its capacity, the spillover of stored energy from adipose tissue results in ectopic fat accumulation in tissues, including skeletal muscle. The development of medical technology has enabled the quantification of intramyocellular lipid (IMCL) content. IMCL levels may be regulated by the balance between lipid influx and its mitochondrial oxidation. Therefore, it is plausible that increased IMCL content is strongly associated with insulin resistance, possibly through excessive lipid overload accompanied by obesity and/or mitochondrial dysfunction due to aging and inherited abnormalities such as type 2 diabetes. However, it is known that trained athletes with high insulin sensitivity paradoxically display high levels of IMCL. Therefore, in addition to the quantity of IMCLs, lipid moieties (quality), including diacylglycerol, should be considered to discuss IMCLs and insulin resistance. Recent emerging evidence suggests that intramyocellular enzymes such as diacylglycerol acyltransferase 1 and stearoyl-CoA desaturase-1 can regulate muscle insulin sensitivity regardless of the amount of IMCLs. In this chapter, we focus on IMCLs and insulin resistance considering intramyocellular lipid moieties and insulin signaling.

Keywords Intramyocellular lipid • Insulin resistance • Skeletal muscle • Fatty acid

12.1 Introduction

Insulin resistance plays a major role in onset and progression of type 2 diabetes. Although the precise underlying mechanisms remain unclear, obesity is believed to be deeply involved in these processes. In simple terms, an overload of calorie intake can cause adiposity. Adipocytes can serve as energy storage reservoirs against a

K. Mori, M.D. (✉) • T. Morioka • K. Motoyama • M. Emoto
The Department of Metabolism, Endocrinology and Molecular Medicine, Osaka City University Graduate School of Medicine, 1-4-3, Asahi-machi, Abeno-ku, Osaka 545-8585, Japan
e-mail: ktmori@med.osaka-cu.ac.jp

M. Inaba (ed.), *Musculoskeletal Disease Associated with Diabetes Mellitus*,
DOI 10.1007/978-4-431-55720-3_12

certain level of caloric overload. However, excess intake beyond the capacity of adipocytes might lead to lipid overflow from adipose tissue into other organs, such as the liver and skeletal muscle. As these organs are not equipped to store excess fat, it is hypothesized that ectopic fat accumulation induced by lipid overload could provoke their dysfunction. In addition to simple vision, recent intensive research has provided substantial knowledge and information such as the concepts of 'adipokines', 'visceral adiposity', and 'intramyocellular lipids' (IMCLs) or 'intramyocellular triglycerides' [1]. In this chapter, we discuss the inseparable association between adiposity and insulin resistance based on glucose and lipid metabolism. Moreover, we focus on ectopic fat accumulation in skeletal muscle, which could not be clarified previously. I defined the term 'lipid' as fatty acids (FAs) in the following sections.

12.2 Overview of Carbohydrate and Lipid Metabolism

To maintain homeostasis, dietary intake is necessary. For example, digested carbohydrates are distributed throughout the body as glucose, which are the most common monosaccharide and primary energy source in humans. Under physiological conditions, glucose that enters into cells is aerobically metabolized by the tricarboxylic acid (TCA) cycle via glycolysis, resulting in efficient ATP synthesis. Regarding glycolysis, three rate-limiting enzymes exist. Hexokinase (HK), phosphofructokinase (PFK), and pyruvate kinase irreversibly catalyze their own substrates. Pyruvate, the end product of aerobic glycolysis, is further converted by pyruvate dehydrogenase (PDH) into acetyl-CoA, which is a major fuel for the TCA cycle (Fig. 12.1). PDH is regulated by elevated levels of acetyl-CoA and nicotinamide adenine dinucleotide (reducing form) NADH via negative feedback (Fig. 12.2: left side). The remaining glucose is stored as glycogen (glycogen synthesis) mainly in the liver and skeletal muscle. Glycogen stored in muscle provides a source of ATP during muscle contraction, whereas that stored in the liver helps to maintain blood glucose levels, especially during the early stages of fasting (Fig. 12.1). Thus, against energy demand, glycogenolysis is rapidly engaged. Excess amounts of carbohydrates (glucose) are converted to FAs, which are stored as triacylglycerol (TG), via acetyl-CoA (Fig. 12.1). TG is the most concentrated source of energy, especially in adipocytes.

Concerning lipids, diet-originated FAs are transported in the circulation as either TG in lipoprotein and hydrolyzed by lipoprotein lipase or bound to albumin [2]. After uptake into cells, a CoA moiety is ligated to FA by acyl-CoA synthase. Fatty acyl-CoA enters mitochondria for oxidation or the TG synthesis pathway for energy storage, especially in adipocytes (Fig. 12.1). Against energy demand, FAs from TG in lipid droplets are catalyzed by three lipases. Adipose triglyceride lipase, hormone-sensitive lipase, and monoacylglycerol lipase degrade TG, diacylglycerol (DG), and monoacylglycerol, respectively. Finally, the generated FAs and glycerol are released into the bloodstream for transport to other tissues (Fig. 12.1) [2, 3].

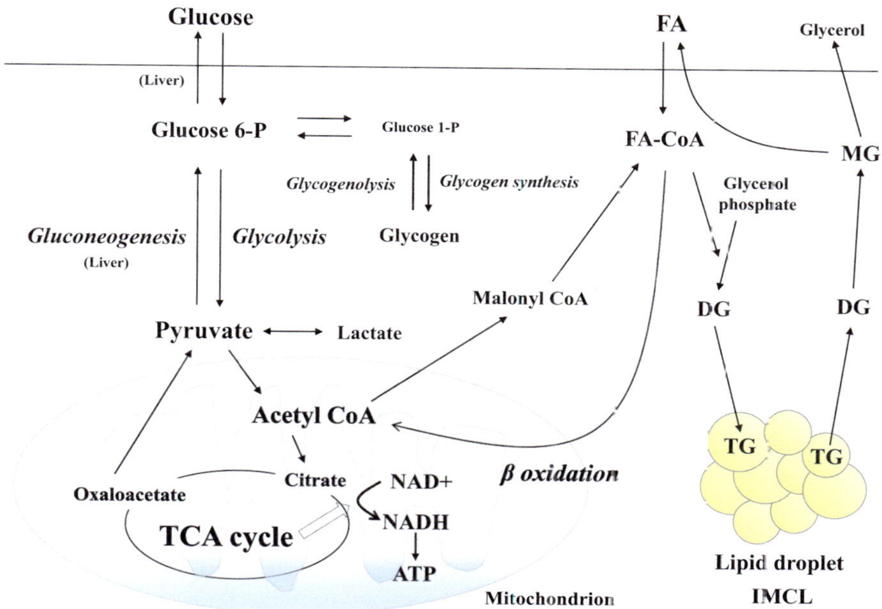

Fig. 12.1 Overview of carbohydrate and lipid metabolism. Glycolysis is utilized by all tissues for the catabolism of glucose to provide energy in the form of ATP. Pyruvate dehydrogenase irreversibly converts pyruvate, the end product of glycolysis, into acetyl-CoA. This compound is a primary fuel for the TCA cycle and the platform for FA synthesis. The major function of the TCA cycle is the oxidation of acetyl-CoA to CO_2 and H_2O. In this process, NAD+ is reduced to NADH, resulting in the generation of ATP. Glucose is stored as glycogen in an easily metabolizable form. Glycogen is rapidly degraded in contracting muscle. Excess amounts of glucose are converted to FAs through acetyl-CoA and acyl-CoA. Dietary FA enters cells and forms FA-CoA. When needed as fuel, FA is subjected to β oxidation in mitochondria. For storage, FA is esterified as TG and then incorporated into lipid droplets. When energy is needed, TG is reversely degraded into FA and glycerol. *Glucose 6-P* glucose 6-phosphate, *FA* fatty acid, *FA-CoA* fatty acyl-CoA, *MG* monoacylglycerol, *DG* diacylglycerol, *TG* triacylglycerol, *TCA cycle* tricarboxylic acid cycle, *NAD+* nicotinamide adenine dinucleotide, *IMCL* intramyocellular lipid

12.3 Intramyocellular Lipid Metabolism and Insulin Resistance

12.3.1 Insulin Resistance and Ectopic Fat Accumulation in Skeletal Muscle

As opposed to adipose tissue, which can be visualized as obesity under high calorie intake, it has been difficult to quantify IMCLs. Through muscle biopsy, it has been reported that TG content of skeletal muscle is usually less than 0.5 % volume density in a lean subject and can increase to more than 1.5 % in obese individuals [4]. However, proton nuclear magnetic resonance spectroscopy (1H-MRS) has made it possible to noninvasively measure IMCLs consisting primarily of TG [5]. Recent findings suggest that IMCLs are strongly associated with insulin resistance in skeletal muscle [6, 7]. Diet- and exercise-induced reduction of IMCL levels resulted in improvement of muscle insulin resistance [8]. Therefore, IMCLs appear to be a causal factor for obesity-related insulin resistance. However, trained athletes with high insulin sensitivity display relatively high levels of IMCLs. This phenomenon is known as 'the athlete's paradox' [9], as we will discuss later. To solve this mystery, both IMCLs (intramyocellular fat accumulation) and extracellular and/or intracellular lipid (FAs) should be considered. The complicated interactions among these factors could induce insulin resistance as a consequence. Insulin resistance is defined as a failure of insulin-stimulated glucose uptake into skeletal muscle through the glucose transporter 4 (GLUT4). Therefore, we attempt to discuss the mechanism by which either an extracellular or intracellular lipid could interrupt intracellular insulin signaling, considering the following connection with intracellular lipids (IMCLs).

12.3.2 Extramyocellular FAs and Insulin Resistance

12.3.2.1 The Glucose-FA Cycle Described by Randle et al.

It has long been known that FAs can induce insulin resistance. Randle et al. proposed a hypothesis considering the link between intracellular glucose and lipid metabolism [10]. High concentrations of extracellular FAs could increase its influx into cells. Consequently, enhanced β oxidation of FAs occurs in mitochondria, resulting in increased ratios of acetyl-CoA to CoA and NADH to NAD+ (Fig. 12.2: left side). As lipid oxidation (increase of acetyl-CoA content) provides a sufficient energy supply for the TCA cycle, PDH is inactivated, and glucose oxidation is reduced. The accumulation of citrate resulting from the increased β oxidation of FAs inhibits PFK, which is one of the rate-limiting enzymes of glycolysis. Then, an increase of glucose 6-phosphate (glucose 6-P) levels results in additional negative feedback and HK inhibition. Therefore, an increase in intracellular glucose levels could inhibit insulin-stimulated glucose uptake as a negative feedback mechanism of energy balance (Fig. 12.2: left side). This hypothesis is attractive and apparently theoretical. In this case, increased intracellular concentrations of glucose and glucose 6-P as well as glycogen are expected in skeletal muscle. However, it has been extremely difficult to prove this hypothesis in humans without repeated muscle biopsies. Even if a sample can be obtained, short-term hypoxia induces changes in metabolite concentrations.

12.3.2.2 Revision of the Traditional Hypothesis

To overcome these difficulties, Shulman's group adopted carbon-13 (13C) and phosphorus-31 (31P) MRS. This state-of-the-art technique has enabled non-invasive measurements of intramyocellular G6P, glycogen, and glucose levels. Insulin-stimulated glucose uptake and intracellular glucose metabolism were evaluated in the presence of high FA levels under a euglycemic hyperinsulinemic clamp using 13C-MRS and 31P-MRS combined with muscle biopsy samples. Surprisingly, reductions in intramyocellular glucose 6-P and glucose concentrations and decreased glycogen synthesis were observed, suggesting that insulin-stimulated glucose transport activity was inhibited by FA [11]. Therefore, the traditional hypothesis that impaired insulin-stimulated glucose uptake due to negative feedback of FA-induced inhibition of glycolysis has been revised [12, 13].

The next question is at what point is insulin signaling inhibited in FA-induced insulin resistance. Although the detailed mechanism of insulin-stimulated glucose uptake via GLUT4 translocation to the plasma membrane is unclear, FAs appear to inhibit a relatively proximal step of insulin signaling [14]. Examination using muscle biopsy samples unveiled reduced insulin receptor substrate-1 (IRS-1) – associated phosphatidylinositol 3-kinase (PI3K) activity as described in subsequent sections.

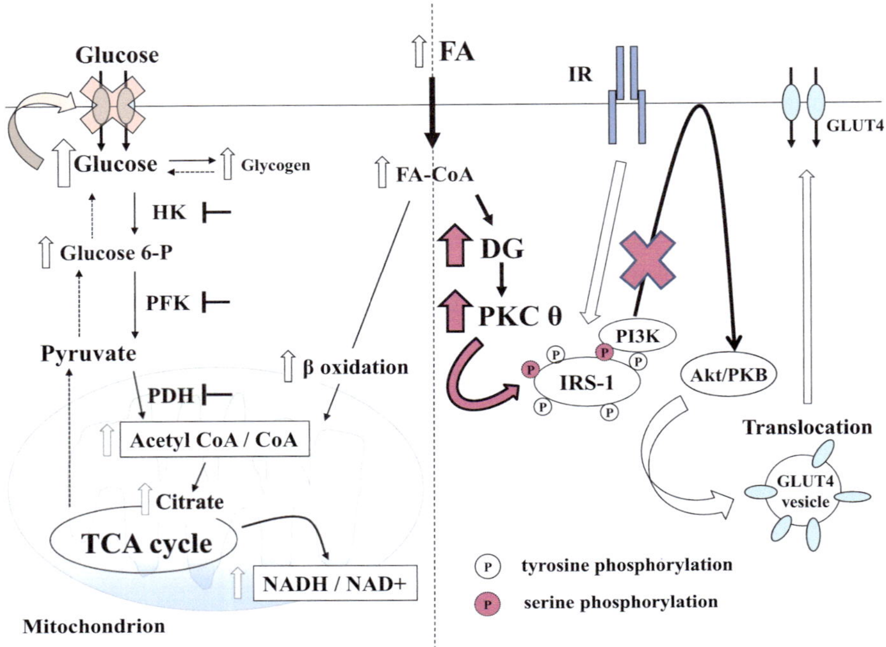

Fig. 12.2 FA-induced insulin resistance (hypothesis and revision). Intracellular FA influx causes β oxidation, resulting in increased ratios of acetyl-CoA to CoA and NADH to NAD+ in mitochondria. As a result, PDH is inactivated. Simultaneously, the accumulation of citrate inhibits PFK and the subsequent increase of glucose 6-P levels, inhibition of HK, and promotion of glycogen synthesis. Therefore, intracellular glucose accumulation inhibits glucose uptake (*left side*). However, recent findings suggest that both intracellular glucose 6-P and glucose levels are decreased in FA-induced insulin-resistant skeletal muscle. Alternatively, it has been hypothesized that FA-induced impairment of insulin stimulates glucose uptake. Increased transport of FA transiently increases DG content, leading to PKC-θ activation. Stimulated PKC-θ induces serine phosphorylation in IRS-1, which antagonizes the insulin-stimulated tyrosine phosphorylation in IRS-1. Thus, the binding of IRS-1 to PI3K is blocked, resulting in the inhibition of downstream insulin signaling, including the final step of GLUT4 translocation (*right side*). *Glucose 6-P* glucose 6-phosphate, *HK* hexokinase, *PFK* phosphofructokinase, *PDH* pyruvate dehydrogenase, *TCA cycle* tricarboxylic acid cycle, *NAD+* nicotinamide adenine dinucleotide, *FA* fatty acid, *FA-CoA* fatty acyl-CoA, *DG* diacylglycerol, *TG* triacylglycerol, *PKC-θ* protein kinase C θ, *IR* insulin receptor, *IRS-1* insulin receptor substrate-1, *PI3K* phosphatidylinositol 3 kinase, *GLUT4* glucose transporter 4

12.3.3 Intramyocellular Lipid and Insulin Resistance

Excess circulating FAs are taken up into skeletal muscle by passive diffusion and protein-mediated transport [15]. Excess intramyocellular FAs are oxidized or esterified as TG and then incorporated into lipid droplets for storage. As described previously, because IMCL content is strongly associated with insulin resistance, it appears to partly explain obesity-related insulin resistance in skeletal muscle. However, based on this concept, 'the athlete's paradox' is not fully understood [16].

12.3.3.1 IMCL and Diacylglycerol Acyltransferase 1 (DGAT1)

One of the key factors for explaining this discrepancy may be DGAT1, which transfers FAs from fatty acyl-CoA to DG to create TG (Fig. 12.3). In other words, DG but not TG appears capable of playing a central role in insulin resistance. For example, mice overexpressing DGAT1 in skeletal muscle display a dissociation of DG and TG content. These mice accumulate TG with low DG content in skeletal muscle, but they are protected against fat-induced insulin resistance in skeletal muscle [17]. In addition, a single session of exercise increased muscle DGAT1 expression accompanied by increased TG, reduced DG, and improved FA-induced insulin resistance in humans. In turn, activation of the pro-inflammatory JNK/NF-κB pathway was suppressed regardless of IMCL accumulation [18]. These findings suggest that DG but not TG can cause insulin resistance. TG may be metabolically 'inactive.'

Focusing on the function of DGAT1 in skeletal muscle, it could act as a protector against insulin resistance. On the contrary, DGAT1-null mice are resistant to diet-induced obesity and insulin resistance. Interestingly, transplantation of adipose tissue from DGAT1-null mice to wild-type mice results in decreased adiposity and increased insulin sensitivity [19]. Contrary to skeletal muscle, SCD1 deficiency in adipose tissue may be favorable. We must always consider the organ being discussed and the links among organs.

12.3.3.2 IMCLs and Stearoyl-CoA Desaturase-1 (SCD1)

Another factor may be stearoyl-CoA desaturase-1 (SCD1), which converts saturated fatty acids (SFAs) into monounsaturated fatty acids (MUFAs). SCD1 introduces cis-double bonds between the 9th and 10th carbons of acyl-CoA, mainly in stearoyl-CoA (18:0) or palmitoyl-CoA (16:0) to generate oleoyl-CoA (18:1 (9)) or palmitoleoyl-CoA (16:1 (9)), respectively [20, 21] (Fig. 12.3). Regarding the SCD1 and SCD5 isoforms in humans, SCD1 is highly expressed in skeletal muscle [21]. It is known that SFAs, such as stearic acid (18:0), are generally toxic. In comparison, MUFAs, such as oleic acid (18:1), are cytoprotective [22]. Similarly, SFAs can more readily induce insulin resistance compared to MUFAs [23]. Moreover, SCD1 contributes to lipid bilayer fluidity by adjusting the appropriate ratio of MUFAs/SFAs in the cell membrane through the conversion of SFAs to MUFAs [21].

Thus, it is expected that higher SCD1 expression could be beneficial with regard to metabolic disorders. In fact, both acute bouts of aerobic exercise [18] and chronic endurance exercise [4] can increase SCD1 expression in skeletal muscle. SCD1 expression is higher in athletes than that in sedentary subjects [4], although both groups display increased IMCL levels. Elevated SCD1 may promote increased

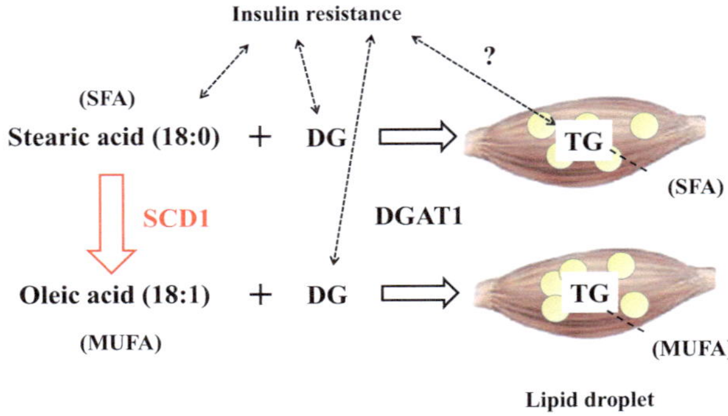

Fig. 12.3 DGAT1, SCD-1, and IMCLs. IMCLs, which reflect TG content in skeletal muscle, are not always associated with insulin resistance. For example, endurance athletes with high insulin sensitivity exhibit high IMCL levels. DGAT1 and SCD1 may be involved in this discrepancy. DGAT1 transfers FAs to DG to form TG, which is metabolically inactive. Thus, DGAT1 appears to improve insulin resistance induced by DG through the formation of TG. SFAs display lipotoxic and pro-inflammatory properties compared with MUFAs. Because SCD1 converts SFAs into MUFAs, it appears to protect against FA-induced insulin resistance in skeletal muscle. *IMCL* intramyocellular lipid, *DGAT1* diacylglycerol acyltransferase 1, *SCD1* stearoyl-CoA desaturase-1, *SFA* saturated fatty acid, *MUFA* monounsaturated fatty acid, *DG* diacylglycerol, *TG* triacylglycerol

MUFA content in IMCLs, which may result in higher lipid quality. Again, SCD1 may explain 'the athlete's paradox' [21].

However, as previously noted in DGAT1-null mice, whole-body SCD1-deficient mice adversely exhibit enhanced energy expenditure and improved insulin signaling [24, 25]. Unfortunately, data from skeletal muscle-specific SCD1 deficient mice are not available at present. Regardless, further studies will be needed to clarify the role of SCD1 in skeletal muscle.

12.3.3.3 DG and Protein Kinase C (PKC)-θ

The next issue is the mechanism by which DG, a substrate of DGAT1, induces insulin resistance in skeletal muscle. Recent intensive research suggested the involvement of the PKC family. The PKC family, a group of serine-threonine kinases, consists of conventional, novel, and atypical PKCs [26]. Among them, novel PKCs (δ, ε, η, and θ) intrinsically have high affinity for DG [27]. Compared to the importance of PKC-ε in hepatic insulin resistance [12], PKC-θ appears to play a critical role in muscle insulin resistance (Fig. 12.2: right side).

Acute elevation of circulating FAs induced skeletal muscle insulin resistance in rats. In this process, insulin-stimulated phosphorylation of IRS-1 was inhibited in association with PKC-θ activation [28]. An increase in circulating FA levels increased intracellular acyl-CoA and DG levels, resulting in PKC-θ stimulation in rats. Activated PKC-θ antagonizes the insulin-stimulated tyrosine phosphorylation of IRS-1 through an increase of serine phosphorylation of IRS-1 (Fig. 12.2: right side) [29]. The central role of PKC-θ in lipid-induced insulin resistance was identified using mice lacking PKC-θ. Fat-induced insulin resistance was prevented in these mice [30]. Moreover, it was confirmed whether PKC-θ – mediated serine phosphorylation of IRS-1 could inhibit fat-induced inhibition of insulin signaling. For this purpose, transgenic mice in which serines in IRS-1 were mutated to alanines in a muscle-specific manner were generated. Expectedly, these transgenic mice exhibited a significant increase in insulin-stimulated IRS-1 – associated PI3K activity and downstream Akt phosphorylation in skeletal muscle under high-fat diet feeding compared with wild-type mice [31]. These findings suggest that serine phosphorylation of IRS-1 induced by PKC-θ is critical in FA-induced insulin resistance in skeletal muscle.

Another question is whether these phenomena are observed in humans. In response, a recent study performed serial muscle biopsies before and during lipid infusion in healthy subjects. In this process, intramyocellular DG levels transiently increased within 2.5 h and subsequently decreased at 4 h after the lipid infusion. The transient rise of DG content preceded myocellular PKC-θ activation, which was observed at 4 h. Increased serine phosphorylation in IRS-1 and inhibited Akt phosphorylation in response to insulin stimulation were also observed simultaneously. This study uncovered a similar significant association between intramyocellular DG content and PKC-θ activation in subjects who were obese and who had type 2 diabetic and muscle insulin resistance [32]. These findings suggest that DG-induced PKC-θ activation plays a critical role in lipid-induced insulin resistance in human skeletal muscle.

12.3.4 Mitochondrial FA Oxidation and Insulin Resistance

In addition to FA uptake into cells, the intracellular oxidative disposal of FAs in mitochondria also regulates IMCL levels (Fig. 12.4). To assess mitochondrial oxidative and phosphorylation activity, 13C and 31P MRS, respectively, have been adopted. Using these methods, it has been reported that both mitochondrial TCA flux and mitochondrial ATP synthesis rates were reduced in elderly subjects compared to young subjects with similar body constitution, suggesting aging-induced mitochondrial dysfunction. This acquired defect in mitochondria was inversely associated with IMCL content [33]. Moreover, inherited mitochondrial defects were also identified. Mitochondrial rates of ATP production were reduced in the young, lean, insulin-resistant offspring of type 2 diabetic subjects compared with matched control subjects without insulin resistance [34]. Increased IMCL levels were also found in subjects whose parents have diabetes, which may be due to diminished mitochondrial activity. These findings suggest that acquired and/or inherited mitochondrial disorders can lead to decreased fat oxidation, resulting in insulin resistance via the intracellular accumulation of DG and TG [13, 35].

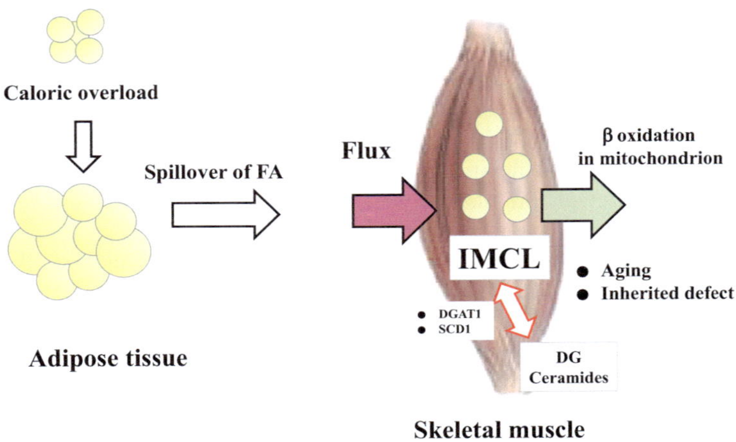

Fig. 12.4 IMCL depends on the net balance of FA influx and oxidation. The input of FA into skeletal muscle may depend on caloric intake. Mitochondrial oxidation contributes to FA consumption. This balance might regulate IMCL content. Apart from its amount, the quality of intracellular lipid (moieties) affects insulin resistance in skeletal muscle. *IMCL* intramyocellular lipid, *FA* fatty acid

The link between impaired mitochondrial FA oxidation and insulin resistance may be acceptable. However, it remains controversial which type of lipid is critical in inducing insulin resistance, although DG is one of the likely candidates, as described previously. A recent study focused on IMCL metabolites using comprehensive mass spectrometry-based lipidomics to qualify individual molecular species of sphingolipids including ceramide, DG, and acyl-CoA. Intriguingly, sphingolipids, and not DGs, were significantly elevated within the skeletal muscle of severe obese women, accompanied by lower mitochondrial contents and capacities [36].

12.4 Summary and Future Directions

The measurement of IMCLs has been a breakthrough in the research fields of diabetes and obesity. The quantification of TG in skeletal muscle has provided many clues regarding the mechanism of insulin resistance. However, many questions that are not solved by a simple story remain, such as the athlete's paradox. We should consider IMCL components (quality) in addition to lipid content (quantity). Although DGAT1 and SCD1 in skeletal muscle were discussed in this chapter, the exact role of these enzymes in insulin resistance has not been completely elucidated, especially in the whole body. Another remaining problem may be IMCL moieties such as DG, fatty acyl-CoA, and ceramide. In particular, ceramide is the 'hub' lipid in sphingolipid metabolism. Ceramide is a precursor for the sphingomyelin and glycosphingolipid families. It is also generated from dihydroceramide or the breakdown of sphingomyelin [37]. Further studies are necessary to address dynamically controlled IMCLs considering the complexity of lipid moieties.

References

1. Hocking S, Samocha-Bonet D, Milner KL, Greenfield JR, Chisholm DJ (2013) Adiposity and insulin resistance in humans: the role of the different tissue and cellular lipid depots. Endocr Rev 34:463–500. doi:10.1210/er.2012-1041
2. Watt MJ, Hoy AJ (2012) Lipid metabolism in skeletal muscle: generation of adaptive and maladaptive intracellular signals for cellular function. Am J Physiol Endocrinol Metab 302: E1315–E1328. doi:10.1152/ajpendo.00561.2011
3. Young SG, Zechner R (2013) Biochemistry and pathophysiology of intravascular and intracellular lipolysis. Genes Dev 27:459–484. doi:10.1101/gad.209296.112
4. Amati F, Dube JJ, Alvarez-Carnero E, Edreira MM, Chomentowski P, Coen PM et al (2011) Skeletal muscle triglycerides, diacylglycerols, and ceramides in insulin resistance: another paradox in endurance-trained athletes? Diabetes 60:2588–2597. doi:10.2337/db10-1221
5. Yokoyama H, Mori K, Emoto M, Araki T, Teramura M, Mochizuki K et al (2008) Non-oxidative glucose disposal is reduced in type 2 diabetes, but can be restored by aerobic exercise. Diabet Obes Metab 10:400–407. doi:10.1111/j.1463-1326.2007.00716.x
6. Krssak M, Falk Petersen K, Dresner A, DiPietro L, Vogel SM, Rothman DL et al (1999) Intramyocellular lipid concentrations are correlated with insulin sensitivity in humans: a 1H NMR spectroscopy study. Diabetologia 42:113–116. doi:10.1007/s001250051123
7. Perseghin G, Scifo P, De Cobelli F, Pagliato E, Battezzati A, Arcelloni C et al (1999) Intramyocellular triglyceride content is a determinant of in vivo insulin resistance in humans: a 1H-13C nuclear magnetic resonance spectroscopy assessment in offspring of type 2 diabetic parents. Diabetes 48:1600–1606
8. Tamura Y, Tanaka Y, Sato F, Choi JB, Watada H, Niwa M et al (2005) Effects of diet and exercise on muscle and liver intracellular lipid contents and insulin sensitivity in type 2 diabetic patients. J Clin Endocrinol Metab 90:3191–3196. doi:10.1210/jc.2004-1959
9. Goodpaster BH, He J, Watkins S, Kelley DE (2001) Skeletal muscle lipid content and insulin resistance: evidence for a paradox in endurance-trained athletes. J Clin Endocrinol Metab 86:5755–5761. doi:10.1210/jcem.86.12.8075
10. Randle PJ, Garland PB, Hales CN, Newsholme EA (1963) The glucose fatty-acid cycle. Its role in insulin sensitivity and the metabolic disturbances of diabetes mellitus. Lancet 1 (7285):785–789
11. Roden M, Price TB, Perseghin G, Petersen KF, Rothman DL, Cline GW et al (1996) Mechanism of free fatty acid-induced insulin resistance in humans. J Clin Invest 97:2859–2865. doi:10.1172/JCI118742
12. Samuel VT, Petersen KF, Shulman GI (2010) Lipid-induced insulin resistance: unraveling the mechanism. Lancet 375(9733):2267–2277. doi:10.1016/S0140-6736(10)60408-4
13. Shulman GI (2014) Ectopic fat in insulin resistance, dyslipidemia, and cardiometabolic disease. N Engl J Med 371:1131–1141. doi:10.1056/NEJMra1011035
14. Dresner A, Laurent D, Marcucci M, Griffin ME, Dufour S, Cline GW et al (1999) Effects of free fatty acids on glucose transport and IRS-1-associated phosphatidylinositol 3-kinase activity. J Clin Invest 103:253–259. doi:10.1172/JCI5001
15. Saini-Chohan HK, Mitchell RW, Vaz FM, Zelinski T, Hatch GM (2012) Delineating the role of alterations in lipid metabolism to the pathogenesis of inherited skeletal and cardiac muscle

disorders: thematic review series: genetics of human lipid diseases. J Lipid Res 53:4–27. doi:10.1194/jlr.R012120
16. Stannard SR, Johnson NA (2004) Insulin resistance and elevated triglyceride in muscle: more important for survival than "thrifty" genes? J Physiol 554:595–607. doi:10.1113/jphysiol.2003.053926
17. Liu L, Zhang Y, Chen N, Shi X, Tsang B, Yu YH (2007) Upregulation of myocellular DGAT1 augments triglyceride synthesis in skeletal muscle and protects against fat-induced insulin resistance. J Clin Invest 117:1679–1689. doi:10.1172/JCI30565
18. Schenk S, Horowitz JF (2007) Acute exercise increases triglyceride synthesis in skeletal muscle and prevents fatty acid-induced insulin resistance. J Clin Invest 117:1690–1698. doi:10.1172/JCI30566
19. Chen HC, Jensen DR, Myers HM, Eckel RH, Farese RV Jr (2003) Obesity resistance and enhanced glucose metabolism in mice transplanted with white adipose tissue lacking acyl CoA: diacylglycerol acyltransferase 1. J Clin Invest 111:1715–1722. doi:10.1172/JCI15859
20. Kusunoki J, Kanatani A, Moller DE (2006) Modulation of fatty acid metabolism as a potential approach to the treatment of obesity and the metabolic syndrome. Endocrine 29:91–100. doi:10.1385/ENDO:29:1:91
21. Stamatikos AD, Paton CM (2013) Role of stearoyl-CoA desaturase-1 in skeletal muscle function and metabolism. Am J Physiol Endocrinol Metab 305:E767–E775. doi:10.1152/ajpendo.00268.2013
22. Nolan CJ, Larter CZ (2009) Lipotoxicity: why do saturated fatty acids cause and monounsaturates protect against it? J Gastroenterol Hepatol 24:703–706. doi:10.1111/j.1440-1746.2009.05823.x
23. Hunnicutt JW, Hardy RW, Williford J, McDonald JM (1994) Saturated fatty acid-induced insulin resistance in rat adipocytes. Diabetes 43:540–545
24. Rahman SM, Dobrzyn A, Dobrzyn P, Lee SH, Miyazaki M, Ntambi JM (2003) Stearoyl-CoA desaturase 1 deficiency elevates insulin-signaling components and down-regulates protein-tyrosine phosphatase 1B in muscle. Proc Natl Acad Sci U S A 100:11110–11115. doi:10.1073/pnas.1934571100
25. Dobrzyn P, Jazurek M, Dobrzyn A (1797) Stearoyl-CoA desaturase and insulin signaling – what is the molecular switch? Biochim Biophys Acta 2010:1189–1194. doi:10.1016/j.bbabio.2010.02.007
26. Newton AC (2003) Regulation of the ABC kinases by phosphorylation: protein kinase C as a paradigm. Biochem J 370:361–371. doi:10.1042/BJ20021626
27. Dries DR, Gallegos LL, Newton AC (2007) A single residue in the C1 domain sensitizes novel protein kinase C isoforms to cellular diacylglycerol production. J Biol Chem 282:826–830. doi:10.1074/jbc.C600268200
28. Griffin ME, Marcucci MJ, Cline GW, Bell K, Barucci N, Lee D et al (1999) Free fatty acid-induced insulin resistance is associated with activation of protein kinase C theta and alterations in the insulin signaling cascade. Diabetes 48:1270–1274
29. Yu C, Chen Y, Cline GW, Zhang D, Zong H, Wang Y et al (2002) Mechanism by which fatty acids inhibit insulin activation of insulin receptor substrate-1 (IRS-1)-associated phosphatidylinositol 3-kinase activity in muscle. J Biol Chem 277:50230–50236. doi:10.1074/jbc.M200958200
30. Kim JK, Fillmore JJ, Sunshine MJ, Albrecht B, Higashimori T, Kim DW et al (2004) PKC-theta knockout mice are protected from fat-induced insulin resistance. J Clin Invest 114:823–827. doi:10.1172/JCI22230
31. Morino K, Neschen S, Bilz S, Sono S, Tsirigotis D, Reznick RM et al (2008) Muscle-specific IRS-1 Ser->Ala transgenic mice are protected from fat-induced insulin resistance in skeletal muscle. Diabetes 57:2644–2651. doi:10.2337/db06-0454
32. Szendroedi J, Yoshimura T, Phielix E, Koliaki C, Marcucci M, Zhang D et al (2014) Role of diacylglycerol activation of PKCtheta in lipid-induced muscle insulin resistance in humans. Proc Natl Acad Sci U S A 111:9597–9602. doi:10.1073/pnas.1409229111

33. Petersen KF, Befroy D, Dufour S, Dziura J, Ariyan C, Rothman DL et al (2003) Mitochondrial dysfunction in the elderly: possible role in insulin resistance. Science 300:1140–1142. doi:10.1126/science.1082889
34. Petersen KF, Dufour S, Befroy D, Garcia R, Shulman GI (2004) Impaired mitochondrial activity in the insulin-resistant offspring of patients with type 2 diabetes. N Engl J Med 350:664–671. doi:10.1056/NEJMoa031314
35. Befroy DE, Petersen KF, Dufour S, Mason GF, de Graaf RA, Rothman DL et al (2007) Impaired mitochondrial substrate oxidation in muscle of insulin-resistant offspring of type 2 diabetic patients. Diabetes 56:1376–1381. doi:10.2337/db06-0783
36. Coen PM, Hames KC, Leachman EM, DeLany JP, Ritov VB, Menshikova EV et al (2013) Reduced skeletal muscle oxidative capacity and elevated ceramide but not diacylglycerol content in severe obesity. Obesity 21:2362–2371. doi:10.1002/oby.20381
37. Hannun YA, Obeid LM (2011) Many ceramides. J Biol Chem 286:27855–27862. doi:10.1074/jbc.R111.254359

Chapter 13
Ectopic Fat Accumulation in the Liver and Glucose Homeostasis

Toshinari Takamura, Hirofumi Misu, and Shuichi Kaneko

Abstract Liver fat is associated not only with enhanced hepatic glucose production but also with skeletal muscle insulin resistance, supporting a central role of fatty liver in systemic insulin resistance and existence of a network between the liver and skeletal muscle. Palmitate and cholesterol act as toxic lipids to cause hepatic insulin resistance via mitochondria-derived oxidative stress. Obesity-mediated disruption in crosstalk among protein-, glucose- and lipid-metabolism pathways results in hepatic insulin resistance, enhanced gluconeogenesis and liver steatosis by impairing proteasome function. The liver plays as an endocrine organ to produce functional hepatokines and thereby mediates fatty liver-associated skeletal muscle insulin resistance through unique mechanisms. Selenoprotein P is upregulated through FoxOs and hyperglycemia and causes resistance to insulin, angiogenesis and exercise through reductive stress. LECT2 is upregulated in satiety through AMPK inactivation and contributes to the development of muscle insulin resistance and obesity by activating JNK and by impairing myogenesis, respectively.

Therefore, overnutrition evokes remodeling of nutrient homeostasis by toxic lipids and proteasome dysfunction in the liver. The remodeling also results in the overproduction of hepatokines that disrupt inter-organ network leading to pathology of diabetes.

Keywords Fatty liver • Insulin resistance • Hepatokine • Selenoprotein P • LECT2

T. Takamura (✉) • H. Misu
Department of Comprehensive Metabology, Kanazawa University Graduate School of Medical Sciences, 13-1 Takara-machi, Kanazawa, Ishikawa 920-8640, Japan
e-mail: ttakamura@m-kanazawa.jp

S. Kaneko
Department of Disease Control and Homeostasis, Kanazawa University Graduate School of Medical Sciences, 13-1 Takara-machi, Kanazawa 920-8640, Ishikawa, Japan

M. Inaba (ed.), *Musculoskeletal Disease Associated with Diabetes Mellitus*,
DOI 10.1007/978-4-431-55720-3_13

13.1 Introduction

Insulin resistance is a core pathology of type 2 diabetes mellitus, nonalcoholic fatty liver disease (NAFLD) and cardiovascular diseases. The severity of insulin resistance may differ among the major insulin-target organs, the liver, skeletal muscle and adipose tissue, suggesting that these organs crosstalk each other to keep whole body energy homeostasis. Disruption of inter-organ networks leads to insulin resistance. Over-nutrition is one of the major environmental factors that disrupt the inter-organ networks [1]. Although obesity is less common [2], diabetes is a huge and growing problem in Asia [3], suggesting that Asian people may be feasible to obesity-associated metabolic dysregulation. Accumulating evidence suggests that ectopic fat accumulation in insulin-target organs leads to the development of insulin resistance in each organ by altering oxidative stress [4, 5] and gene expression profiles [6, 7]. Specifically, the liver functions as a center to maintain whole body energy homeostasis by sensing nutrient stimuli and by producing a variety of nutrients and bioactive substances.

In this review, we show the clinical evidence for significance of liver fat in whole body glucose homeostasis, remodeling of nutrient homeostasis in the liver and interorgan networks via liver-derived hormone hepatokines.

13.2 Ectopic Fat Accumulation and Organ-Specific Insulin Resistance

Disruption of hepatic insulin signaling in liver-specific insulin receptor knockout (LIRKO) mice results in fasting and postprandial hyperglycemia and the subsequent development of peripheral (muscle) insulin resistance [8], whereas glucose homeostasis remains normal in mice of disrupted insulin signaling both in the skeletal muscle and adipose tissue [9]. These observations suggest that hepatic insulin resistance is the primary event leading to diabetes and the subsequent development of peripheral tissue insulin resistance. Indeed, liver steatosis is associated with whole-body insulin resistance, independently of body mass index (BMI), in Japanese patients with NAFLD [10]. However, the role of intramyocellular fat accumulation in insulin sensitivity is also on debate, and no previous studies have demonstrated the association among the insulin-targeting organs comprehensively and simultaneously. Therefore, to understand organ networks that sense excessive energy and regulate insulin action, elucidating the association between fat accumulation and organ-specific insulin resistance among the liver, skeletal muscle and adipose tissue, is important, especially in humans.

We have addressed the association of ectopic fat accumulation with organ-specific insulin resistance among the liver, skeletal muscle and adipose tissue in Japanese patients with NAFLD, systematically using reliable methods including liver biopsy, assessment of glucose metabolism measured by an euglycemic hyperinsulinemic clamp study with stable-isotope-labeled glucose, bioelectrical impedance analysis and proton magnetic resonance spectroscopy (^{1}H-MRS) [11]. As shown in Fig. 13.1, both histological liver steatosis score and intrahepatic lipid (IHL) are significantly correlated negatively with a muscle insulin sensitivity index Rd and positively with a hepatic insulin resistance index HGP × fasting plasma insulin (FPI) (Fig. 13.1). In the multiple regression analysis, liver steatosis score is significantly correlated with both HGP × FPI ($\beta = 0.284$, $P < 0.05$) and Rd ($\beta = -0.300$, $P < 0.01$) after adjusted with age, sex and BMI. Unexpectedly, intramyocellular lipid (IMCL) is not associated with any of organ-specific insulin resistance indices (Fig. 13.1). Adipose tissue mass is correlated with HGP × FPI and Rd, but not with % suppression of free fatty acids, an adipose tissue insulin sensitivity index (Fig. 13.1) [11]. Therefore, indices of fat accumulation in the skeletal muscle and adipose tissue are not associated with their own organ-specific insulin resistance (Fig. 13.2). It is known that IMCL is increased not only with obesity but also by enhanced physical fitness [12]. Therefore, absolute fat contents do not always predict insulin resistance in the skeletal muscle. Rather, toxic lipids that cause insulin resistance in the skeletal muscle should be further researched. On the other hand, hepatic steatosis per se is central surrogate pathology indicative of insulin resistance in both liver and skeletal muscle in patients with NAFLD (Fig. 13.2). There may be a network between the liver and skeletal muscle to maintain whole body energy homeostasis (Fig. 13.2). To date, whether hepatic steatosis is a consequence or cause of skeletal muscle insulin resistance remains uncertain because a longitudinal observation of the relationship is lacking. However, some possibilities are assumed for the link as follows: (1) Skeletal muscle insulin resistance causes obesity and subsequent hepatic steatosis as experimentally shown in mice with muscle-selective insulin resistance [13]. Indeed, Flannery et al. reported that skeletal muscle insulin resistance promotes increased hepatic de novo lipogenesis and hepatic steatosis in the elderly [14]. (2) The neuronal pathway from the liver might modulate peripheral insulin sensitivity [15]. (3) Some nutrients, such as fatty acids and amino acids, might link hepatic steatosis and skeletal muscle insulin resistance [16]. (4) A liver-derived hormone named as hepatokine affects the distant organ insulin sensitivity [17]. Molecular mechanisms underlying the link between liver fat and altered glucose metabolism are discussed in the following sections.

13.3 Possible Molecular Mechanisms Underlying Mystery of the Selective Insulin Resistance in the Type 2 Diabetic Liver

In the liver, insulin suppresses glucose production and enhances lipogenesis. Indeed, total insulin resistance in the liver observed in the LIRKO mice present hyperglycemia without fatty liver [8]. However, in the liver with type 2 diabetes,

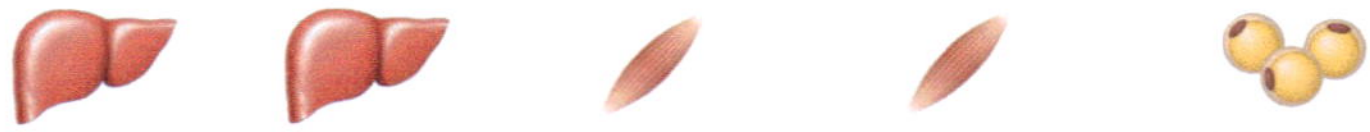

	HGP × FPI		%HGP		Rd		Rd/SSPI		%FFA	
	r	*p*	*r*	*p*	*r*	*p*	*r*	*p*	*r*	*p*
Steatosis	0.401**	0.001	-0.161	0.187	-0.495***	<0.001	-0.460***	<0.001	-0.086	0.483
Grade	0.397**	0.001	-0.151	0.214	-0.359**	0.002	-0.361**	0.003	-0.061	0.616
Stage	0.227	0.060	-0.109	0.371	-0.300*	0.012	-0.248*	0.042	-0.001	0.991
IHL	0.245	0.089	-0.114	0.436	-0.315*	0.028	-0.271	0.062	-0.135	0.356
IMCL	0.250	0.065	-0.215	0.115	-0.156	0.256	-0.183	0.185	-0.060	0.662
Fat-free mass	0.031	0.801	-0.117	0.347	-0.216	0.079	-0.211	0.090	-0.433***	<0.001
Total fat mass	0.495***	<0.001	-0.147	0.235	-0.594***	<0.001	-0.536***	<0.001	-0.205	0.096
Body fat percentage	0.481***	<0.001	-0.115	0.355	-0.518***	<0.001	-0.478***	<0.001	-0.001	0.994
VO_2	-0.129	0.342	0.191	0.158	0.418**	0.001	0.405**	0.002	0.115	0.397

Fig. 13.1 Univariate correlation between ectopic fat and organ-specific insulin resistance HGP, hepatic glucose production; FPI, fasting plasma insulin; SSPI, steady state plasma insulin; IHL, intrahepatic lipid; IMCL, intramyocellular lipid; VO_2, basal oxygen consumption rate per body weight. $*p < 0.05$, $**p < 0.01$, $***p < 0.001$ (Modified from Ref. [11])

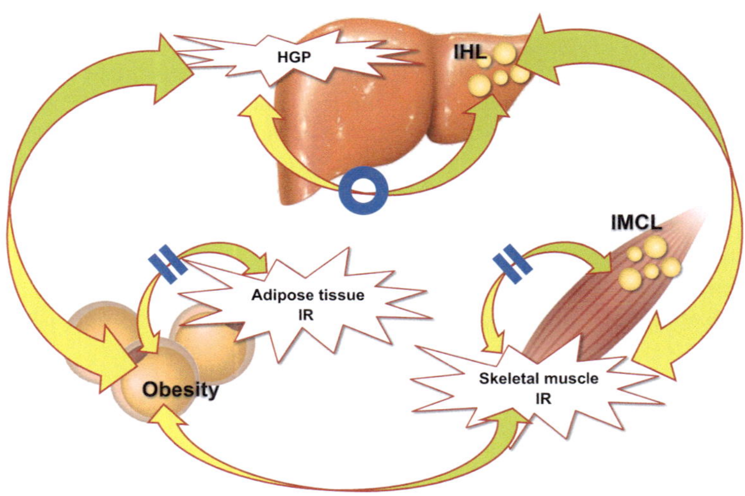

Fig. 13.2 Relationship between intracellular lipid accumulation and organ-specific insulin resistance among three major insulin-targeting organs, the liver, skeletal muscle and adipose tissue Skeletal muscle insulin resistance is not associated with intramyocellular lipid accumulation, but with hepatic steatosis, suggesting that there is inter-organ network between the liver and skeletal muscle in human (Modified from Ref. [11])

insulin fails to suppress gluconeogenesis but still activates lipogenesis, the pathology of which is regarded as a 'selective insulin resistance'-like phonotype [18] (Fig. 13.3). Notably, the indices for hepatic fat accumulation are associated with HGP × FPI, but not with % suppression of HGP during the hyperinsulinemic clamp (Fig. 13.1) [11], suggesting that the liver fat is associated with basal HGP itself, possibly independently of insulin resistance. Indeed, HGP is not solely regulated by insulin, but also by other hormones such as glucagon and glucocorticoid. Transcription factors such as forkhead box protein O (FoxO), cAMP response element-binding protein (CREB), peroxisome proliferator-activated receptor gamma coactivator 1-alpha (PGC-1α), hepatocyte nuclear factor 4α (HNF4α) and glucocorticoid receptors are involved in the regulation of gluconeogenesis by the hormones and nutrients. In addition, hepatic steatosis also occurs independently of insulin resistance. Of the triacylglycerol accumulated in the liver of patients with NAFLD, 59.0 % arises from non-esterified fatty acids mainly derived from the adipose tissue and 14.9 % from the diet, whereas only 26.1 % from *de novo* lipogenesis [19]. Transcription factors such as liver X receptor (LXR), sterol regulatory element-binding protein-1c (SREBP-1c) and carbohydrate response element binding protein (ChREBP) are involved in the *de novo* lipogenesis. Of these, SREBP-1c is a master regulator of hepatic *de novo* synthesis of fatty acids and is activated not only by insulin but also by glucose, fatty acids, amino acids, SREBP-1c itself, LXR, mechanistic target of rapamycin complex 1 (mTORC1) and endoplasmic reticulum (ER) stress [20].

Triglyceride itself is not a toxic lipid and rather may be protective to prevent toxic effects of free fatty acids. Rather, free cholesterol and saturated free fatty acid palmitate are regarded as toxic lipids that cause hepatic insulin resistance via oxidative stress [17] as follows:

1. Mice fed an atherogenic diet rich in cholesterol and cholate show steatohepatitis, oxidative stress and hepatic insulin resistance [4]. In the liver of this model, *SREBP-1c* is upregulated possibly via cholesterol-mediated LXR activation,

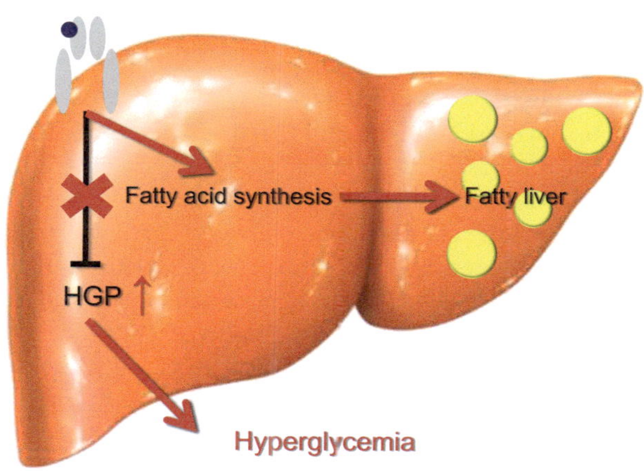

Fig. 13.3 Selective insulin resistance-like phenotype in the liver with type 2 diabetes
In the liver with type 2 diabetes, insulin fails to suppress gluconeogenesis but continues to activate lipogenesis, which is regarded as a 'selective insulin resistance'-like phonotype

leading to *de novo* lipogenesis in the liver. In addition, hepatic expression of insulin receptor substrate (IRS)-2 was downregulated by cholesterol diet. Shimano et al. discovered that SREBP-1c binds to E-box in the promoter of *IRS-2* competitively with TFE3 and FoxO1, and thus downregulates *IRS-2* [21]. These findings may link lipogenesis and insulin resistance in the liver.

2. In an *in vitro* fatty liver system using H4IIEC3 hepatocytes, a saturated fatty acid palmitate, but not an unsaturated fatty acid oleate, inhibits insulin-stimulated tyrosine phosphorylation of insulin receptor substrate 2 and serine phosphorylation of Akt, through c-Jun NH_2-terminal kinase (JNK) activation [5]. In this model, mitochondrial β oxidation-derived reactive oxygen species (ROS) play a causal role in the palmitate-induced JNK activation [5]. Therefore, toxic lipid-induced mitochondrial ROS may also underlie the link between steatosis and insulin resistance in the liver. Indeed, in human, genes involved in mitochondrial oxidative phosphorylation (OXPHOS) are coordinately upregulated and positively correlated with those involved in a ROS-related pathway in the livers of obese type 2 diabetic patients compared with those of non-obese type 2 diabetic patients [7]. These findings in toxic lipids-induced hepatic steatosis also contribute to the selective insulin resistance-like phonotype in type 2 diabetic livers [18].

13.4 Crosstalk Among Glucose, Protein and Lipid Metabolic Pathways in the Liver

Growing evidence suggests that chronic endoplasmic reticulum (ER) stress in the liver is a major contributor to obesity-induced insulin resistance [22, 23]. ER is responsible for protein quality control [24]. The burden of unfolded proteins in the ER lumen is identified as an ER stress by several ER stress sensors, known as ATF6, PERK and IRE-1. The ER stress sensors trigger cellular adaptation for unfolded protein accumulation to restore normal function of the cell, which is called as the unfolded protein response (UPR). Chronic UPRs are causally linked to the pathogenesis of human metabolic diseases such as obesity and type 2 diabetes. Accumulating evidence suggests that obesity promotes ER stress, which is detected as an enhanced UPR signaling, that activates JNK and impairs insulin signaling at the level of IRSs in the liver and adipose tissue [25]. However, the molecular mechanisms linking obesity and ER stress were not fully understood.

In searching for metabolic pathways that are significantly altered by obesity in the livers of people with type 2 diabetes, we found that genes involved in ubiquitin-proteasome pathways are coordinately upregulated in obese individuals [7]. Proteasomes play fundamental roles in processes that are essential for cell viability by degrading misfolded proteins [26]. Unexpectedly from the expression data, liver proteasome activity was reduced by approximately 30–40 % in mouse models of obesity, such as genetically obese ob/ob mice, diabetic db/db mice and C57BL/6 mice fed a high fat diet (HFD) [27]. As a consequence, ubiquitinated proteins were accumulated in the liver of these obese model mice. These results suggest that liver proteasome activity is reduced in animal models of obesity. Thus, coordinate upregulation of the genes involved in the ubiquitin-proteasome pathway in obese patients and mouse models of obesity may compensate for impaired proteasome function. Therefore, we hypothesized that proteasome dysregulation in the liver is involved in the development of hepatic insulin resistance in obesity and type 2 diabetes. To test this hypothesis, we generated PA28α-PA28β-PA28γ triple-knockout (PA28 KO) mice, the genes of which are up-regulated in the livers of patients with obesity and in those of mice fed HFD [27], as a model of impaired proteasome function and investigated their metabolic phenotypes as follows: (1) Hepatic proteasome activity in PA28 KO mice fed a standard chow is reduced by 35 % as compared with wild-type mice. As expected, ubiquitinated proteins are accumulated in the liver of the PA28 KO mice. (2) Electron micrographs reveals massive expansion of the ER in the livers of PA28 KO mice, suggestive of UPR. Indeed, the liver in PA28 KO mice show the evidence of ER stress, such as increased levels of Grp78, CHOP, p-PERK, p-eIF2α and p-IRE-1α, as well as ER stress-inducible mRNAs encoding CHOP and the spliced form of XBP-1 (XBP-1s), as compared with wild-type mice. (3) Phosphorylation of JNK and its downstream target c-Jun are significantly increased in the livers of PA28 KO mice as compared with those of wild-type mice. (4) Although body weight is not altered, PA28 KO mice fed the standard chow present glucose intolerance. Hyperinsulinemic-euglycemic clamp experiments and western blot analysis of the insulin signaling pathway reveal that PA28 deficiency impairs insulin signaling mainly in the liver, but not in the skeletal muscle, and thereby induces systemic glucose intolerance in vivo. These findings illustrate that proteasome dysfunction causes ER stress, JNK activation and thereby cause insulin resistance in the liver (Fig. 13.4). Yang et al. reported that hepatic autophagy is downregulated in the livers of ob/ob mice and that defective autophagy in Atg7 KO mice causes ER stress and hepatic insulin resistance [28]. Therefore, it is possible that both proteasome- and autophagy-mediated protein degradation are impaired in the livers of obese individuals, further exacerbating ER stress.

(5) PA28 KO mice show hepatic steatosis associated with upregulated *Srebf1* and *Acc1* and increased cleaved/active SREBP-1c (Fig. 13.4). SREBP-1c is activated by ER stress [20]. In addition, proteasome dysfunction results in increased protein levels of SREBP-1c because proteasome is responsible for the degradation of SREBP-1c [29].

(6) FoxO1 protein amounts dramatically increase in both cytoplasmic and nuclear fractions, probably due to proteasome dysfunction in the liver of PA28 KO mice (Fig. 13.4). Spliced XBP-1 directly binds FoxO1 and promotes its protein degradation via the proteasome [30]. In the liver of PA28 KO mice, spliced XBP1 protein is increased, probably due to increased phosphorylation of IRE1α, an endonuclease for *XBP1* gene. In addition, hepatic insulin resistance caused by ER stress/JNK pathway and increased SREBP-1c that downregulates IRS-2 further accumulates FoxO1 in the nucleus, leading to induction of genes involved in gluconeogenesis such as *Pepck1*.

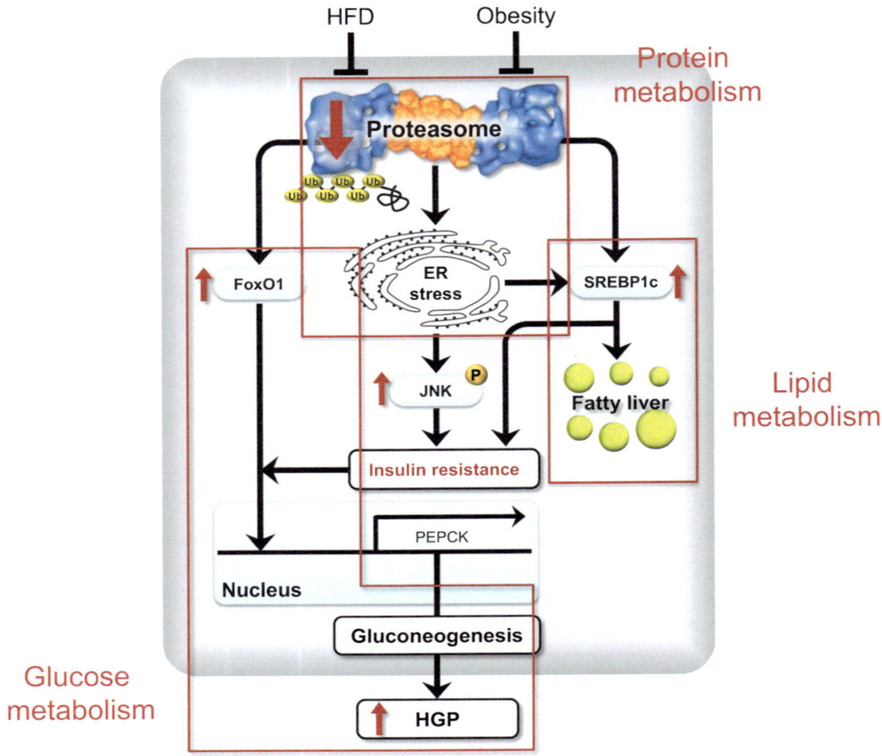

Fig. 13.4 Crosstalk among protein, glucose and lipid metabolic pathways
Proteasome function is impaired in the state of obesity, followed by endoplasmic reticulum (ER) stress, JNK activation and insulin resistance in the liver. Proteasome dysfunction also results in increased protein levels of FoxO1 and SREBP-1c because proteasome is responsible for the degradation of FoxO1 and SREBP-1c, which are master transcription factors for gluconeogenesis and lipogenesis, respectively. SREBP-1c is also activated by ER stress. Such activation of these factors occurs independently of insulin resistance and may mimic so-called 'selective insulin resistance' in the liver with type 2 diabetes, that is, coexistence of fatty liver and enhanced gluconeogenesis (Modified from Ref. [27])

These findings suggest that proteasome dysfunction may be a primary event linking obesity and ER stress-induced insulin resistance in the liver. In addition, there seems to be a crosstalk among protein-, glucose- and lipid-metabolism pathways (Fig. 13.3). Notably, the activation of SREBP-1c and FoxO1 occurred independently of insulin resistance, and may mimic so-called 'selective insulin resistance' in the liver with type 2 diabetes, that is, coexistence of fatty liver and enhanced gluconeogenesis (Fig. 13.2).

Proteasome function seems to be altered differently in different tissues. Insulinopenic hyperglycemia impairs proteasome activity in the liver and kidney [31, 32], whereas proteasome activity is enhanced in the wasted muscle of obese diabetic db/db mice [33]. Taken together, these findings indicate that obesity predominantly induces proteasome dysfunction in the liver. This clarifies the previous finding that ER stress causes insulin resistance in the liver together with the adipose tissue [22] and brain [34]. Significance of enhanced proteasome activity in the skeletal muscle of obese model mice should be investigated in future.

13.5 Role of Hepatokines that Mediate Inter-Organ Network During Remodeling of Energy Homeostasis

As described above, we hypothesized that a liver-derived hormone, hepatokine, affects the distant organ insulin sensitivity. Human hepatic gene expression information accumulated by using serial analysis of gene expression (SAGE) technique and DNA chip methods [35, 36] were used to identify genes with signal peptides whose hepatic expression levels were significantly correlated with glycemic control (HbA1c), obesity (BMI) or insulin resistance (HOMA-R and metabolic clearance rate). Expression of the candidates hepatokine genes were further referred to the various animal models of diabetes, obesity and fatty liver [4, 37–39]. Based on these approaches, we isolated 62 candidate genes for hepatokines associated with insulin resistance, hyperglycemia and obesity [35].

13.5.1 Selenoprotein P

Of these, we identified a gene encoding selenoprotein P, the expression levels of which were positively correlated with insulin resistance and hyperglycemia [40]. Indeed, serum levels of selenoprotein P are elevated in people with type 2 diabetes and significantly correlated with fasting plasma glucose and HbA1c levels [40]. Selenoprotein P (in humans encoded by the *SEPP1* gene) is upregulated through FoxOs (Fig. 13.5). Insulin downregulates *SEPP1* by phosphorylating and inactivating FoxO1 [41], whereas antidiabetic metformin activates AMP-activated protein kinase (AMPK), phosphorylates and inactivates FoxO3a, and thereby downregulates *SEPP1* in hepatocytes [42].

Selenoprotein P causes insulin resistance in the liver at least in part by inactivating AMPK [40] (Fig. 13.5). Selenoproein P also impairs angiogenesis by inducing VEGF resistance in vascular endothelial cells [43].

Specifically, selenoprotein P acts as a redox protein by activating glutathione peroxidase. Unexpectedly in the large-scale intervention study, selenium supplementation was paradoxically associated with an increased risk for diabetes in humans [44]. Also, in our previous study in a cultured hepatocyte cell line, antioxidant reagents, N-acetyl-L-cysteine, rescued palmitate-induced insulin resistance only partly, whereas it effectively suppressed palmitate-induced activation of

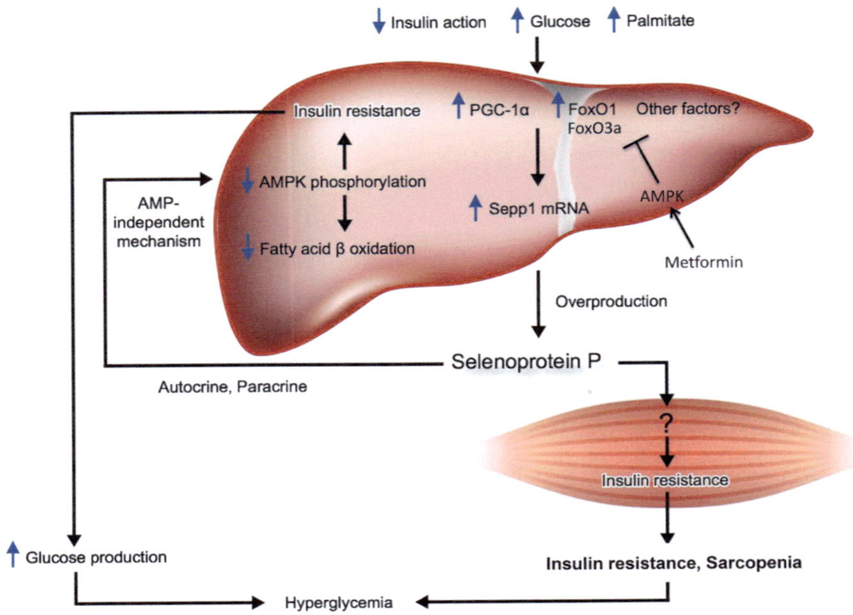

Fig. 13.5 Selenoprotein P causes insulin resistance in the liver and skeletal muscle. *SEPP1* is upregulated through FoxOs
Insulin downregulates *SEPP1* by inactivating FoxO1, whereas antidiabetic metformin activates AMPK, inactivates FoxO3a and thereby downregulates *SEPP1* in hepatocytes. Selenoprotein P causes hepatic insulin resistance at least partly by inactivating AMPK (Modified from Ref. [48])

JNK [5]. To solve this paradox, we addressed the concentration-dependent effects of ROS on insulin signaling in hepatocytes. Treatment with high concentrations of H_2O_2 reduced insulin-stimulated Akt phosphorylation by activating JNK, whereas lower concentrations of H_2O_2 enhanced insulin-stimulated phosphorylation of Akt by suppressing PTP1B activity [45]. Therefore, depending on its concentration, H_2O_2 exerts positive or negative effect on insulin signal transduction in hepatocytes. It might be possible that selenoprotein P deprives a physiologic ROS burst that is required for insulin signal transduction and thereby causes insulin resistance, the condition referred to a reductive stress. Indeed, similar to the selenoprotein P KO mice, mice lacking one of the selenoproteins involved in the elimination of physiological ROS, glutathione peroxidase 1, are reported to be protected from high-fat-diet-induced insulin resistance [46].

Interestingly, supplementation with antioxidants precludes health-promoting effects of physical exercise in humans [47]. Consistent with the concept of mitohormesis, exercise-induced oxidative stress ameliorates insulin resistance and causes an adaptive response promoting endogenous antioxidant defense capacity. In this regard, we recently identified a putative skeletal muscle receptor for selenoprotein P. Molecular mechanisms how selenoprotein P causes skeletal muscle insulin resistance are under investigation through investigating the skeletal muscle-specific selenoprotein P KO mice (Fig. 13.5).

Serum levels of selenoprotein P are inversely associated with those of adiponectin [48] that enhances skeletal muscle insulin sensitivity [49]. Therefore, overproduction of selenoprotein P in association with hepatic steatosis, by directly or indirectly lowering adiponectin levels, causes skeletal muscle insulin resistance.

13.5.2 LECT2

Our second hepatokine is leukocyte cell-derived chemotaxin 2 (LECT2), the gene of which is most correlated with BMI [50]. LECT2 is a 16 kDa secretory protein originally identified from cultured supernatant of human T-cell line as a neutrophil chemotactic factor [51]. LECT2 (in humans encoded by the *LECT2* gene) is expressed preferentially by human adult and fetal liver cells and is secreted into the blood stream [52]. LECT2 enhances macrophage function via the CD209a/DC-SIGN receptor and improves immunity in bacterial sepsis [53]. More recently, it has been reported that LECT2 suppresses hepatocellular carcinoma by direct binding and inactivating hepatocyte growth factor (HGF) receptor MET [54]. However, the role of LECT2 in the development of obesity and insulin resistance was unknown. We characterized molecular aspects of LECT2 as follows: (1) Serum LECT2 levels are correlated positively with BMI, waist circumference, HOMA-R and HbA1c, and negatively with insulin sensitivity Matsuda index [50]. These data indicate that the serum levels of LECT2 are positively associated with both adiposity and the severity of insulin resistance in humans. (2) *Lect2* is upregulated in HFD (vs. standard chow) feeding, fed (vs. fasted) state and resting (vs. exercise) state. In these experimental conditions, AMPK phosphorylation is impaired. Indeed, *Lect2* expression in H4 hepatocytes is upregulated by dominant negative-AMPK infection, whereas downregulated by constitutive active-AMPK transfection. These findings indicate that AMPK downregulates LECT2 expression in hepatocytes (Fig. 13.6). (3) Glucose or insulin loading test reveals that *Lect2* KO mice show lower blood glucose levels after glucose or insulin injection. (4) Hyperinsulinemic-euglycemic clamp studies show that glucose infusion rate and peripheral glucose disposal are increased in *Lect2* KO mice, whereas endogenous glucose production EGP is unaffected. These results indicate that *Lect2* KO mice have better insulin sensitivity in skeletal muscle but not in the liver. (5) In vitro in C2C12 myocytes, recombinant LECT2 protein phosphorylates JNK and decreases insulin-stimulated Akt phosphorylation, which is rescued by double knockdown of JNK1 and JNK2. (6) To further elucidate the role of LECT2 in the development of obesity-associated insulin resistance, we feed *Lect2* KO mice a 60 % HFD. *Lect2* KO mice are protected from the HFD-induced weight gain. Serum levels of insulin decrease in the KO mice in both fasting and fed conditions. (7) *Lect2* KO mice present higher heat production in both light and dark phases. This may be caused by enhanced myogenesis, because all of the subsets of myosin heavy chain are upregulated in the

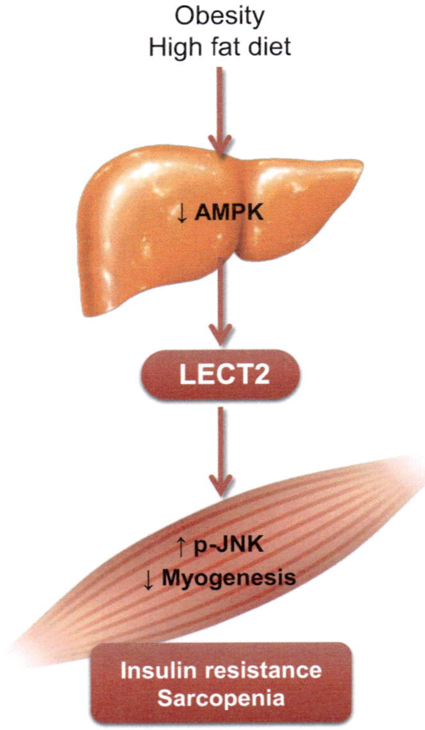

Fig. 13.6 A satiety-associated LECT2 causes skeletal muscle insulin resistance. LECT2 is a satiety-associated hepatokine that is induced by inactivating AMPK in the liver. Overproduction of LECT2 contributes to the development of muscle insulin resistance and obesity by activating JNK and by impairing myogenesis, respectively (Modified from Ref. [50])

Lect2 KO mice. As a consequence, physical-exercise-assessed muscle endurance was significantly higher in *Lect2* KO mice than wild-type mice. These findings suggest that LECT2 decreases energy expenditure by inhibiting myogenesis (Fig. 13.6).

In conclusion, LECT2 is a satiety-associated hepatokine that is induced by inactivating AMPK in the liver. Overproduction of LECT2 contributes to the development of muscle insulin resistance and obesity by activating JNK and by impairing myogenesis, respectively (Fig. 13.6).

References

1. Yamada T, Katagiri H (2007) Avenues of communication between the brain and tissues/organs involved in energy homeostasis. Endocr J 54(4):497–505. PubMed Epub 2007/05/19. eng
2. (OECD) TOfEC-oaD. OBESITY Update. 2014.
3. (IDF) IDF. IDF DIABETES ATLAS (2014) 6: Available from: http://www.idf.org/diabetesatlas

4. Matsuzawa N, Takamura T, Kurita S, Misu H, Ota T, Ando H et al (2007) Lipid-induced oxidative stress causes steatohepatitis in mice fed an atherogenic diet. Hepatology 46 (5):1392–1403. PubMed eng
5. Nakamura S, Takamura T, Matsuzawa-Nagata N, Takayama H, Misu H, Noda H et al (2009) Palmitate induces insulin resistance in H4IIEC3 hepatocytes through reactive oxygen species produced by mitochondria. J Biol Chem 284(22):14809–14818. PubMed eng
6. Mootha VK, Lindgren CM, Eriksson KF, Subramanian A, Sihag S, Lehar J et al (2003) PGC-1alpha-responsive genes involved in oxidative phosphorylation are coordinately downregulated in human diabetes. Nat Genet 34(3):267–273. PubMed
7. Takamura T, Misu H, Matsuzawa-Nagata N, Sakurai M, Ota T, Shimizu A et al (2008) Obesity upregulates genes involved in oxidative phosphorylation in livers of diabetic patients. Obesity (Silver Spring) 16(12):2601–2609. PubMed Epub 2008/10/11. eng
8. Michael MD, Kulkarni RN, Postic C, Previs SF, Shulman GI, Magnuson MA et al (2000) Loss of insulin signaling in hepatocytes leads to severe insulin resistance and progressive hepatic dysfunction. Mol Cell 6(1):87–97. PubMed
9. Lauro D, Kido Y, Castle AL, Zarnowski MJ, Hayashi H, Ebina Y et al (1998) Impaired glucose tolerance in mice with a targeted impairment of insulin action in muscle and adipose tissue. Nat Genet 20(3):294–298. PubMed Epub 1998/11/07. eng
10. Sakurai M, Takamura T, Ota T, Ando H, Akahori H, Kaji K et al (2007) Liver steatosis, but not fibrosis, is associated with insulin resistance in nonalcoholic fatty liver disease. J Gastroenterol 42(4):312–317. PubMed eng
11. Kato K, Takamura T, Takeshita Y, Ryu Y, Misu H, Ota T et al (2014) Ectopic fat accumulation and distant organ-specific insulin resistance in Japanese people with nonalcoholic fatty liver disease. PLoS One 9(3):e92170. PubMed Pubmed Central PMCID: 3961287
12. Thamer C, Machann J, Bachmann O, Haap M, Dahl D, Wietek B et al (2003) Intramyocellular lipids: anthropometric determinants and relationships with maximal aerobic capacity and insulin sensitivity. J Clin Endocrinol Metab 88(4):1785–1791. PubMed
13. Kim JK, Michael MD, Previs SF, Peroni OD, Mauvais-Jarvis F, Neschen S et al (2000) Redistribution of substrates to adipose tissue promotes obesity in mice with selective insulin resistance in muscle. J Clin Invest 105(12):1791–1797. PubMed Pubmed Central PMCID: 378504
14. Flannery C, Dufour S, Rabol R, Shulman GI, Petersen KF (2012) Skeletal muscle insulin resistance promotes increased hepatic de novo lipogenesis, hyperlipidemia, and hepatic steatosis in the elderly. Diabetes 61(11):2711–2717. PubMed Pubmed Central PMCID: 3478531
15. Uno K, Katagiri H, Yamada T, Ishigaki Y, Ogihara T, Imai J et al (2006) Neuronal pathway from the liver modulates energy expenditure and systemic insulin sensitivity. Science 312 (5780):1656–1659. PubMed eng
16. Newgard CB (2012) Interplay between lipids and branched-chain amino acids in development of insulin resistance. Cell Metab 15(5):606–614. PubMed Pubmed Central PMCID: 3695706
17. Takamura T, Misu H, Ota T, Kaneko S (2012) Fatty liver as a consequence and cause of insulin resistance: lessons from type 2 diabetic liver. Endocr J 59(9):745–763. PubMed
18. Brown MS, Goldstein JL (2008) Selective versus total insulin resistance: a pathogenic paradox. Cell Metab 7(2):95–96. PubMed
19. Donnelly KL, Smith CI, Schwarzenberg SJ, Jessurun J, Boldt MD, Parks EJ (2005) Sources of fatty acids stored in liver and secreted via lipoproteins in patients with nonalcoholic fatty liver disease. J Clin Invest 115(5):1343–1351. PubMed Pubmed Central PMCID: 1087172
20. Rutkowski DT, Wu J, Back SH, Callaghan MU, Ferris SP, Iqbal J et al (2008) UPR pathways combine to prevent hepatic steatosis caused by ER stress-mediated suppression of transcriptional master regulators. Dev Cell 15(6):829–840. PubMed Pubmed Central PMCID: 2923556
21. Shimano H (2007) SREBP-1c and TFE3, energy transcription factors that regulate hepatic insulin signaling. J Mol Med 85(5):437–444. PubMed

22. Ozcan U, Cao Q, Yilmaz E, Lee AH, Iwakoshi NN, Ozdelen E et al (2004) Endoplasmic reticulum stress links obesity, insulin action, and type 2 diabetes. Science 306(5695):457–461. PubMed
23. Ozcan U, Yilmaz E, Ozcan L, Furuhashi M, Vaillancourt E, Smith RO et al (2006) Chemical chaperones reduce ER stress and restore glucose homeostasis in a mouse model of type 2 diabetes. Science 313(5790):1137–1140. PubMed
24. Walter P, Ron D (2011) The unfolded protein response: from stress pathway to homeostatic regulation. Science 334(6059):1081–1086. PubMed
25. Yalcin A, Hotamisligil GS (2013) Impact of ER protein homeostasis on metabolism. Diabetes 62(3):691–693. PubMed Pubmed Central PMCID: 3581203
26. Voges D, Zwickl P, Baumeister W (1999) The 26S proteasome: a molecular machine designed for controlled proteolysis. Annu Rev Biochem 68:1015–1068. PubMed
27. Otoda T, Takamura T, Misu H, Ota T, Murata S, Hayashi H et al (2013) Proteasome dysfunction mediates obesity-induced endoplasmic reticulum stress and insulin resistance in the liver. Diabetes 62(3):811–824. PubMed Pubmed Central PMCID: 3581221
28. Yang L, Li P, Fu S, Calay ES, Hotamisligil GS (2010) Defective hepatic autophagy in obesity promotes ER stress and causes insulin resistance. Cell Metab 11(6):467–478. PubMed Pubmed Central PMCID: 2881480
29. Hirano Y, Yoshida M, Shimizu M, Sato R (2001) Direct demonstration of rapid degradation of nuclear sterol regulatory element-binding proteins by the ubiquitin-proteasome pathway. J Biol Chem 276(39):36431–36437. PubMed
30. Zhou Y, Lee J, Reno CM, Sun C, Park SW, Chung J et al (2011) Regulation of glucose homeostasis through a XBP-1-FoxO1 interaction. Nat Med 17(3):356–365. PubMed Pubmed Central PMCID: 3897616
31. Queisser MA, Yao D, Geisler S, Hammes HP, Lochnit G, Schleicher ED et al (2010) Hyperglycemia impairs proteasome function by methylglyoxal. Diabetes 59(3):670–678. PubMed Pubmed Central PMCID: 2828656
32. Portero-Otin M, Pamplona R, Ruiz MC, Cabiscol E, Prat J, Bellmunt MJ (1999) Diabetes induces an impairment in the proteolytic activity against oxidized proteins and a heterogeneous effect in nonenzymatic protein modifications in the cytosol of rat liver and kidney. Diabetes 48(11):2215–2220. PubMed
33. Wang X, Hu Z, Hu J, Du J, Mitch WE (2006) Insulin resistance accelerates muscle protein degradation: Activation of the ubiquitin-proteasome pathway by defects in muscle cell signaling. Endocrinology 147(9):4160–4168. PubMed
34. Ozcan L, Ergin AS, Lu A, Chung J, Sarkar S, Nie D et al (2009) Endoplasmic reticulum stress plays a central role in development of leptin resistance. Cell Metab 9(1):35–51. PubMed
35. Takamura T, Misu H, Yamashita T, Kaneko S (2008) SAGE application in the study of diabetes. Curr Pharm Biotechnol 9(5):392–399. PubMed Epub 2008/10/16. eng
36. Misu H, Takamura T, Matsuzawa N, Shimizu A, Ota T, Sakurai M et al (2007) Genes involved in oxidative phosphorylation are coordinately upregulated with fasting hyperglycaemia in livers of patients with type 2 diabetes. Diabetologia 50(2):268–277. PubMed
37. Ota T, Takamura T, Kurita S, Matsuzawa N, Kita Y, Uno M et al (2007) Insulin resistance accelerates a dietary rat model of nonalcoholic steatohepatitis. Gastroenterology 132 (1):282–293. PubMed eng
38. Matsuzawa-Nagata N, Takamura T, Ando H, Nakamura S, Kurita S, Misu H et al (2008) Increased oxidative stress precedes the onset of high-fat diet-induced insulin resistance and obesity. Metabolism 57(8):1071–1077. PubMed eng
39. Ando H, Takamura T, Matsuzawa-Nagata N, Shima KR, Nakamura S, Kumazaki M et al (2009) The hepatic circadian clock is preserved in a lipid-induced mouse model of non-alcoholic steatohepatitis. Biochem Biophys Res Commun 380(3):684–688. PubMed Epub 2009/03/17. eng

40. Misu H, Takamura T, Takayama H, Hayashi H, Matsuzawa-Nagata N, Kurita S et al (2010) A liver-derived secretory protein, selenoprotein P, causes insulin resistance. Cell Metab 12 (5):483–495. PubMed Epub 2010/11/03. eng
41. Speckmann B, Walter PL, Alili L, Reinehr R, Sies H, Klotz LO et al (2008) Selenoprotein P expression is controlled through interaction of the coactivator PGC-1alpha with FoxO1a and hepatocyte nuclear factor 4alpha transcription factors. Hepatology 48(6):1998–2006. PubMed
42. Takayama H, Misu H, Iwama H, Chikamoto K, Saito Y, Murao K et al (2014) Metformin suppresses expression of the selenoprotein P gene via an AMP-activated kinase (AMPK)/FoxO3a pathway in H4IIEC3 hepatocytes. J Biol Chem 289(1):335–345. PubMed Pubmed Central PMCID: 3879556
43. Ishikura K, Misu H, Kumazaki M, Takayama H, Matsuzawa-Nagata N, Tajima N et al (2014) Selenoprotein P as a diabetes-associated hepatokine that impairs angiogenesis by inducing VEGF resistance in vascular endothelial cells. Diabetologia 57(9):1968–1976. PubMed
44. Stranges S, Marshall JR, Natarajan R, Donahue RP, Trevisan M, Combs GF et al (2007) Effects of long-term selenium supplementation on the incidence of type 2 diabetes: a randomized trial. Ann Intern Med 147(4):217–223. PubMed Epub 2007/07/11. eng
45. Iwakami S, Misu H, Takeda T, Sugimori M, Matsugo S, Kaneko S et al (2011) Concentration-dependent dual effects of hydrogen peroxide on insulin signal transduction in H4IIEC hepatocytes. PLoS One 6(11):e27401, PubMed Pubmed Central PMCID: 3216925. Epub 2011/11/22. eng
46. Loh K, Deng H, Fukushima A, Cai X, Boivin B, Galic S et al (2009) Reactive oxygen species enhance insulin sensitivity. Cell Metab 10(4):260–272. PubMed Epub 2009/10/08. eng
47. Ristow M, Zarse K, Oberbach A, Kloting N, Birringer M, Kiehntopf M et al (2009) Antioxidants prevent health-promoting effects of physical exercise in humans. Proc Natl Acad Sci U S A 106(21):8665–8670, PubMed Pubmed Central PMCID: 2680430. Epub 2009/05/13. eng
48. Misu H, Ishikura K, Kurita S, Takeshita Y, Ota T, Saito Y et al (2012) Inverse correlation between serum levels of selenoprotein P and adiponectin in patients with type 2 diabetes. PLoS One 7(4):e34952. PubMed Pubmed Central PMCID: 3319626. Epub 2012/04/13. eng
49. Iwabu M, Yamauchi T, Okada-Iwabu M, Sato K, Nakagawa T, Funata M et al (2010) Adiponectin and AdipoR1 regulate PGC-1alpha and mitochondria by Ca(2+) and AMPK/SIRT1. Nature 464(7293):1313–1319. PubMed
50. Lan F, Misu H, Chikamoto K, Takayama H, Kikuchi A, Mohri K et al (2014) LECT2 functions as a hepatokine that links obesity to skeletal muscle insulin resistance. Diabetes 63 (5):1649–1664. PubMed
51. Yamagoe S, Yamakawa Y, Matsuo Y, Minowada J, Mizuno S, Suzuki K (1996) Purification and primary amino acid sequence of a novel neutrophil chemotactic factor LECT2. Immunol Lett 52(1):9–13. PubMed
52. Yamagoe S, Mizuno S, Suzuki K (1998) Molecular cloning of human and bovine LECT2 having a neutrophil chemotactic activity and its specific expression in the liver. Biochim Biophys Acta 1396(1):105–113. PubMed
53. Lu XJ, Chen J, Yu CH, Shi YH, He YQ, Zhang RC et al (2013) LECT2 protects mice against bacterial sepsis by activating macrophages via the CD209a receptor. J Exp Med 210(1):5–13. PubMed Pubmed Central PMCID: 3549712
54. Chen CK, Yang CY, Hua KT, Ho MC, Johansson G, Jeng YM et al (2014) Leukocyte cell-derived chemotaxin 2 antagonizes MET receptor activation to suppress hepatocellular carcinoma vascular invasion by protein tyrosine phosphatase 1B recruitment. Hepatology 59 (3):974–985. PubMed

Chapter 14
Ectopic Fat Accumulation and Glucose Homeostasis: Role of Leptin in Glucose and Lipid Metabolism and Mass Maintenance in Skeletal Muscle

Tomoaki Morioka, Katsuhito Mori, Koka Motoyama, and Masanori Emoto

Abstract Skeletal muscle plays a major role in glucose homeostasis. Ectopic lipid accumulation in non-adipose tissue, including skeletal muscle, is an important feature of insulin resistance and type 2 diabetes. Leptin, an adipocyte-derived hormone, regulates glucose and lipid metabolism in skeletal muscle, independent of its central effects on food intake and energy expenditure. While in vitro evidence shows that leptin interacts with insulin signaling to enhance glucose uptake in skeletal muscle, in vivo studies indicate that enhanced insulin sensitivity and glucose uptake induced by leptin in skeletal muscle are mediated by a central mechanism. On the other hand, a direct effect of leptin on skeletal muscle lipid metabolism has been demonstrated in mice. Leptin stimulates mitochondrial fatty acid oxidation by directly activating 5′-AMP-activated protein kinase, through which it depletes the lipid content and reduces lipotoxicity in skeletal muscle. In a mouse model of obesity and diabetes, the regenerative capacity of skeletal muscle is impaired, causing sarcopenia. Evidence from several mouse studies indicates that leptin signaling regulates not only the lipid content of muscle but also muscle mass by inhibiting protein degradation and enhancing myoblast proliferation and differentiation. Thus, impaired leptin action might be a key factor in the negative regulation of skeletal muscle regeneration and the development of sarcopenia in obesity and diabetes. In this chapter, we discuss the current understanding of leptin's effects on glucose and lipid metabolism in skeletal muscle and on muscle mass maintenance and regeneration in the context of obesity and type 2 diabetes.

Keywords Leptin • AMPK • Intramyocellular lipid • Sarcopenia • Satellite cell

---

T. Morioka, M.D., Ph.D. (✉) • K. Mori • K. Motoyama • M. Emoto
Department of Metabolism, Endocrinology and Molecular Medicine, Osaka City University Graduate School of Medicine, 1-4-3, Asahi-machi, Abeno-ku, Osaka 545-8585, Japan
e-mail: m-tomo@med.osaka-cu.ac.jp

M. Inaba (ed.), *Musculoskeletal Disease Associated with Diabetes Mellitus*,
DOI 10.1007/978-4-431-55720-3_14

14.1 Effects of Leptin on Skeletal Muscle Glucose and Lipid Metabolism

14.1.1 Leptin and Its Effects on Peripheral Tissues

Leptin is a 16-kDa peptide hormone produced by adipose tissue that plays a pivotal role in the regulation of food intake and energy expenditure [1]. Many of leptin's effects are attributable to its actions in the central nervous system (CNS), especially in the basomedial hypothalamus, which expresses high levels of a long form of the leptin receptor (Ob-Rb) [2]. However, the short and long isoforms of the leptin receptor are widely distributed throughout peripheral organs, including the adipose tissue [3], skeletal muscle [4], pancreas [5], and liver [6], and leptin exerts its physiological effects on hematopoiesis, angiogenesis, reproduction, glucose metabolism, and lipid metabolism independent of its effects on the CNS [2, 7–9]. Indeed, in leptin-deficient *ob/ob* mice, administration of low-dose leptin normalized glycemia and insulinemia, even though body weight and food intake were not reduced [10], indicating that the metabolic effects of leptin are independent of its effects on appetite and body weight.

14.1.2 Effects of Leptin on Glucose Metabolism in Skeletal Muscle

Skeletal muscle contributes to insulin-stimulated glucose disposal and whole-body fatty acid oxidation. It is one of the primary tissues responsible for insulin resistance in obesity and type 2 diabetes [11, 12]. Although the mechanism by which leptin affects glucose metabolism has not been fully determined, crosstalk between leptin and insulin signaling pathways at the level of insulin receptor substrate (IRS) and phosphatidylinositol-3 kinase (PI3-kinase) has been observed in cultured muscle cells [13–16]. Studies using C2C12 myotubes have demonstrated that leptin activates Janus kinase (JAK) 2, which induces the tyrosine phosphorylation of IRS-2, leading to activation of PI3-kinase [16] and stimulation of glucose transport and glycogen synthesis [15]. Leptin has also been shown to increase glucose uptake and glucose transporter 4 translocation by enhancing the DNA-binding activity of signal transducer and activator of transcription (STAT) 3 and the activity of extracellular signal-regulated kinase (ERK) 2 in C2C12 myotubes [14]. PI3-kinase, but not JAK-2, is also involved in leptin-stimulated glucose uptake in rat L6 muscle cells [13]. However, studies using isolated muscle have produced conflicting results regarding the effect of leptin on glucose uptake in skeletal muscle. Leptin acutely increased glucose uptake in isolated soleus muscles from rat [17] and mouse [18] without an additive effect of insulin. However, in another study, acute leptin treatment did not alter glycogen synthesis or insulin-stimulated glycogen synthesis in isolated mouse soleus and extensor digitorum longus (EDL) muscles [19]. These conflicting results might derive from differences in the duration of leptin treatment, concentration of leptin, or type of muscle fiber. Several studies have investigated the in vivo effect of leptin on glucose metabolism in skeletal muscle [20, 21]. Acute intravenous leptin infusion in leptin-deficient *ob/ob* mice increased whole-body glucose turnover and stimulated glucose uptake in the brown adipose tissue, brain, and heart, but not in the skeletal muscle or white adipose tissue [20]. Kamohara et al. [21] found that acute intravenous leptin infusion into wild-type mice increased whole-body glucose turnover and glucose uptake in the brown fat, EDL, and soleus muscle. Similar effects were observed after both intravenous and intracerebroventricular infusion of leptin, and leptin-induced glucose uptake was blunted in denervated muscles, suggesting that the CNS mediates the leptin-induced increase in glucose metabolism. These in vivo studies indicate that leptin regulates glucose metabolism via pathways independent of skeletal muscle.

14.1.3 Leptin Directly Regulates Skeletal Muscle Lipid Metabolism

Ectopic lipid accumulation in non-adipose tissues, including the skeletal muscle, liver, heart, and pancreas, is an important feature of obesity and is closely associated with insulin resistance and glucose intolerance [11, 22]. Skeletal muscle from obese individuals has an increased triacylglycerol (TAG) content, which is strongly associated with decreased insulin sensitivity [11, 23, 24]. The mechanisms by which skeletal muscle TAG storage increases in obesity have not been fully elucidated, but increased fatty acid uptake into muscle from the circulation or reduced fatty acid oxidation in muscle mitochondria could play a role [11, 24]. Fatty acid metabolism in resting skeletal muscle is regulated by several hormones, such as leptin, insulin, and epinephrine [24].

Previous studies have shown that in vivo leptin treatment improves insulin sensitivity partly through its extraneural effects, through which the fat content of adipose and non-adipose tissues, including skeletal muscle, is depleted [10, 25, 26]. Direct and acute effects of leptin on fatty acid partitioning toward oxidation and away from storage have been shown in skeletal muscle isolated from mice [19, 27] and humans [24] and in C2C12 myotubes [28]. Muoio et al. [19] found that leptin promoted fatty acid oxidation and decreased fatty acid incorporation into TAG in soleus muscles isolated from C57BL/6J mice and that leptin attenuated the antioxidative and lipogenic effects of insulin by 50 % when both hormones were present. Importantly, the oxidative and anti-lipogenic actions of leptin on skeletal muscle fatty acid metabolism are mediated by a direct mechanism, while the stimulatory effects of leptin on glucose metabolism are mediated by a central mechanism, indicating a critical role of skeletal muscle in mediating leptin's effects on adiposity. However, the molecular mechanisms that mediate leptin's effects on skeletal muscle lipid metabolism remain to be elucidated.

14.1.4 AMPK Mediates Leptin Signaling in Skeletal Muscle

Recent studies have shown that leptin directly activates 5′-AMP-activated protein kinase (AMPK) in skeletal muscle [29, 30]. AMPK is a heterotrimeric enzyme that senses cellular energy levels to maintain the balance between ATP production and consumption in all eukaryotic cells [31]. AMPK switches off anabolic pathways and activates catabolism in response to a decrease in the ATP/AMP ratio by phosphorylating key enzymes involved in intermediate metabolism [31]. Activation of AMPK is involved in glucose transport in skeletal muscle induced by metabolic stress, such as contraction and hypoxia [32–34]. Therefore, direct AMPK activation by leptin in skeletal muscle could partly explain leptin-induced glucose uptake and metabolism [35].

The AMPK pathway also activates fatty acid oxidation and prevents fatty acids from accumulating in skeletal muscle cells as TAG [35, 36]. When activated during exercise and skeletal muscle contraction, AMPK inhibits acetyl-CoA carboxylase (ACC) to reduce the malonyl-CoA concentration and the entry of long-chain acyl-CoA into the mitochondria for β-oxidation, thereby restoring energy balance [36]. Olsen et al. [37] observed that activation of AMPK by 5-aminoimidazole-4-carboxamide ribonucleotide ameliorated fatty acid-induced insulin resistance in isolated rat EDL muscles; the effect was abolished by an AMPK-specific inhibitor. Minokoshi et al. [30] found that leptin selectively stimulated the phosphorylation and activation of the α2 catalytic subunit of AMPK in mouse skeletal muscle. They examined AMPK activity in skeletal muscle after intrahypothalamic and intravenous injection of leptin in mice. Leptin acted directly on muscle to activate AMPK at an early time point (15 min), whereas leptin acted through the hypothalamic-sympathetic nervous system axis to activate AMPK at a later time point (6 h) [30]. In parallel with its activation of AMPK, leptin phosphorylated and inactivated ACC, thereby stimulating fatty acid oxidation in skeletal muscle. AMPK inactivation by dominant-negative AMPK inhibited the leptin-induced phosphorylation of ACC [30]. Thus, the direct activation of AMPK might be a critical pathway through which leptin promotes fatty acid oxidation and prevents the deleterious effects of intramyocellular lipid accumulation.

14.1.5 Leptin Resistance and Skeletal Muscle Lipid Accumulation

In most forms of obesity, circulating leptin levels are elevated and the effect of leptin on appetite and body weight is diminished, a phenomenon referred to as leptin resistance [38, 39]. A number of mechanisms have been proposed to explain leptin resistance, including alterations in the transport of leptin across the blood-brain barrier, alterations in cellular leptin receptor signaling, and perturbations in developmental programing [38, 39]. Although a defect in leptin action in the CNS is considered a determinant of leptin resistance, little is known about whether leptin resistance occurs in peripheral tissues, including skeletal muscle. Steinberg et al. demonstrated that leptin treatment increased the partitioning of fatty acids toward oxidation and away from storage in skeletal muscle from lean controls, whereas the effects were absent in skeletal muscle from obese individuals [24] and rats fed a high-fat diet [40]. Dulloo et al. [41] found that leptin failed to stimulate thermogenesis in soleus muscles from diet-induced obese mice, but not in those from lean mice. These experimental observations suggest that leptin resistance in skeletal muscle contributes to myocellular lipid accumulation and underlies the pathogenesis of insulin resistance in obesity and type 2 diabetes.

14.2 Leptin Regulates Skeletal Muscle Mass and Regeneration

14.2.1 Sarcopenia and Insulin Resistance

In addition to the dysregulation of glucose and lipid metabolism in skeletal muscle, an age-related decline in muscle mass and strength, a process named sarcopenia [42], also contributes to insulin resistance and type 2 diabetes, especially in the elderly [43, 44]. Conversely, insulin resistance and/or obesity might underlie the development of sarcopenia [43, 45]. The combination of sarcopenia and obesity, termed sarcopenic obesity, produces important age-related changes in body composition. Sarcopenic obesity is more closely associated with insulin resistance [44], metabolic syndrome [46], atherosclerosis [47], functional decline, and mortality than obesity or sarcopenia alone [43, 45, 48]. Therefore, sarcopenic obesity is a growing concern in the elderly population [43].

Several mechanisms might underlie sarcopenic obesity: impaired secretion and/or action of anabolic hormones, including growth hormone, insulin, and insulin-like growth factor-I; secretion of pro-inflammatory factors or cytokines, including tumor necrosis factor-α, interleukin (IL)-6, and C-reactive protein; secretion of bioactive proteins from adipocytes (adipocytokines), including adiponectin and leptin; and production of anti-inflammatory cytokines, including IL-10 and IL-15 [49].

14.2.2 Leptin Might Link Obesity to Sarcopenia

Obesity and insulin resistance are often accompanied by elevated levels of circulating leptin and leptin resistance, in which the effects of leptin on energy and glucose are impaired [38, 39]. In addition, sarcopenia contributes to the development of age-related insulin resistance and type 2 diabetes [43, 44]. Therefore, elevated leptin levels in the circulation or leptin resistance might play an important role in sarcopenic obesity. A few studies have investigated the clinical association between leptin and sarcopenia and/or obesity [50–52]. In a study of elderly patients over 80 years old who required continuing inpatient care ($n = 30$), Hubbard et al. [50] reported that frail patients had lower serum leptin levels than those who were not frail, probably because of their low body fat. In a study of healthy elderly subjects ($n = 45$, mean 77.6 years old), Waters et al. [52] found that subjects with sarcopenic obesity had higher serum leptin levels than sarcopenic, obese, or normal lean subjects and that the appendicular skeletal muscle mass was independently and negatively correlated with leptin levels in all groups. Kohara et al. [51] used computed tomography to measure the thigh muscle cross-sectional area and visceral fat area in middle-aged and elderly subjects in the general population ($n = 782$) and found that the thigh muscle mass was negatively associated with plasma leptin levels independent of other parameters, including visceral fat area and C-reactive protein. They also found that plasma leptin levels were higher in subjects with sarcopenic visceral obesity than in those with sarcopenia or visceral obesity alone. The clinical findings indicate that high leptin levels or leptin resistance plays an important role in the development of sarcopenia and in the link between obesity and sarcopenia. Although the mechanisms require further investigation, leptin or leptin resistance might contribute directly to sarcopenia through the activation of immune cells to produce pro-inflammatory cytokines [53], the negative interaction between leptin and the growth hormone/insulin-like growth factor-I axis [54, 55], a reduction in skeletal muscle protein synthesis [56], and impairment of the regenerative capacity of skeletal muscle [57].

14.2.3 Impaired Skeletal Muscle Regeneration in Obesity

Recent advances in stem cell research have shown that skeletal muscle has tissue-resident stem cells, called satellite cells, that are mainly responsible for the regenerative activity in skeletal muscle. The satellite cells are required for early postnatal muscle growth and for the repair of muscle injury throughout adult life [58]. Pathological dysregulation of satellite cell function appears to play an important role in the age-dependent decline of muscle function and in muscle dystrophic diseases; it is also tightly related to metabolism [59]. Indeed, alterations in the metabolic state, such as those that occur with exercise [60] and calorie restriction [61], directly affect the activity of satellite cells. Several lines of evidence suggest that regeneration is impaired following muscle injury in rodent models of obesity and diabetes, possibly because of impaired muscle progenitor cell function [57, 59, 62]. Although the mechanisms underlying the impaired muscle regeneration in obesity remain elusive, recent experimental findings suggest that lipid overload in skeletal muscle under conditions of obesity affects not only insulin sensitivity but also muscle maintenance and regeneration through multiple factors, including toxic lipid metabolites, low-grade inflammation, and insulin/leptin resistance [57, 63].

14.2.4 Leptin Regulates Skeletal Muscle Mass and Regeneration

Previous studies have shown that *ob/ob* mice [64] and obese Zucker rats [65], lacking leptin or a functional leptin receptor, respectively, exhibit reduced skeletal muscle mass with decreased proliferative activity of muscle satellite cells when compared to their lean controls. More recently, Nguyen et al. [66] demonstrated that muscle injury induced by cardiotoxin injection resulted in delayed skeletal muscle regeneration in *ob/ob* and *db/db* mice, but not wild-type mice fed a high-fat diet as a less severe model of obesity. These findings indicate an important role of leptin signaling in skeletal muscle regeneration. The study also suggested that impaired muscle regeneration in *ob/ob* and *db/db* mice was associated with reduced macrophage accumulation, angiogenesis, and myoblast activity [66]. Leptin-specific regulation of skeletal muscle mass in mice has also been investigated in several recent studies. Arounleut et al. [67] reported that primary myoblasts from aged mice lacking all functional leptin receptor isoforms (POUND mice) exhibited impaired proliferation and decreased MyoD and myogenin expression when compared to control mice; leptin treatment attenuated these defects. Saintz et al. [68] also reported that administration of recombinant leptin in leptin-deficient *ob/ob* mice increased skeletal muscle mass and fiber size; the effects were associated with the inhibition of factors that promote protein catabolism (FoxO3, MAFbx, MuRF) in a pathway involving AMPK and PGC-1α, enhancement of muscle growth (reduced myostatin), and cell cycle progression (PCNA, cyclin D1). Moreover, alterations in the expression of skeletal muscle microRNAs have been associated specifically with age-related muscle atrophy in mice [69] and humans [70]. Hamnrick et al. [69] recently found that leptin treatment increased hind limb muscle mass and EDL fiber size in aged mice by modulating the expression of atrophy-related microRNAs in aging skeletal muscle. The experimental findings from mice, albeit not all mammalian species [71], indicate that leptin directly regulates skeletal muscle mass by inhibiting myofibrillar protein degradation and by promoting satellite cell proliferation and differentiation, thus adding a new mechanism for the regulation of insulin sensitivity and glucose metabolism by leptin. Because leptin resistance is commonly observed in obesity and type 2 diabetes [38, 39], a lack of leptin signaling could negatively impact skeletal muscle regeneration by impairing macrophage activity, angiogenesis, and satellite cell proliferation and differentiation.

14.3 Conclusions

Growing evidence indicates that adipocyte-derived leptin, in addition to acting centrally, acts directly on skeletal muscle to regulate whole-body glucose homeostasis. Although leptin increases glucose uptake in cultured myotubes and isolated

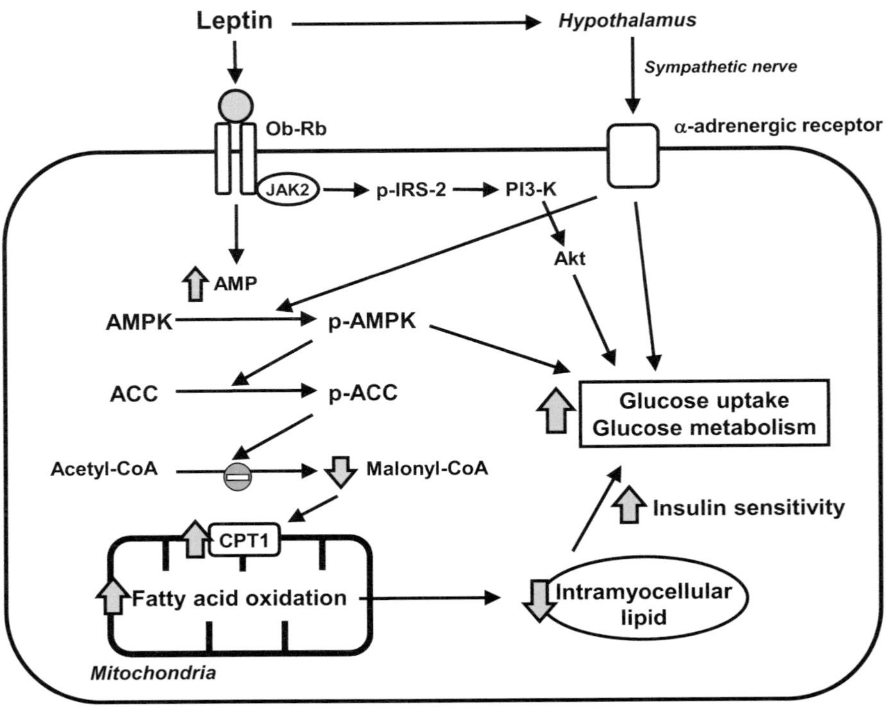

Fig. 14.1 Schematic representation of the leptin's effects on glucose and lipid metabolism in skeletal muscle

murine skeletal muscle at least partly by interacting with insulin signaling, in vivo studies have shown that leptin enhances glucose uptake and metabolism through a central mechanism, not through skeletal muscle [20, 21]. On the other hand, recent studies have provided evidence that leptin acts directly on skeletal muscle to deplete the intramyocellular lipid content and improve insulin sensitivity [10, 25, 26]. Direct activation of AMPK with inhibition of ACC is a critical pathway through which leptin promotes fatty acid oxidation and prevents the toxic effects of intramyocellular lipid accumulation in skeletal muscle [29, 30]. Because elevated circulating leptin levels are commonly observed in obesity, leptin insensitivity to fatty acid oxidation in skeletal muscle might cause intramyocellular lipid accumulation and thereby contribute to the pathogenesis of insulin resistance and diabetes (Fig. 14.1).

Recent studies have extended our understanding of the role of leptin in obesity and diabetes. The findings suggest there is a close association between leptin and the age-related changes in body composition that occur with sarcopenia or sarcopenic obesity, a condition that involves deteriorating insulin resistance and diabetes [43, 44]. Several studies have indicated that elevated leptin levels are associated with sarcopenia independent of obesity in adult humans [51, 52]. In a

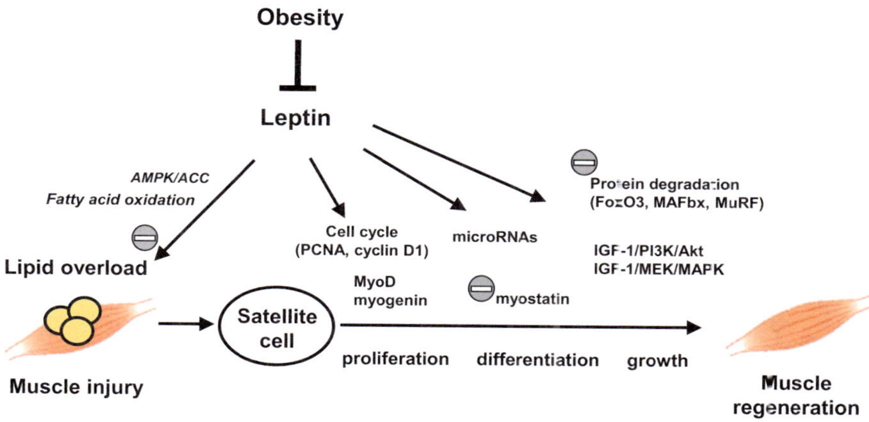

Fig. 14.2 Mechanisms by which leptin signaling regulates skeletal muscle mass. Leptin reduces intramyocellular lipid that impairs the activity of satellite cells. Leptin also directly promotes skeletal muscle regeneration through the regulation of several proteins and microRNAs linked to satellite cell proliferation/differentiation, muscle growth, and protein catabolism. Impaired leptin signaling in obesity might negatively impact skeletal muscle regeneration and contribute to sarcopenia

rodent model of obesity and diabetes, muscle regeneration was impaired following muscle injury because of the diminished proliferation and differentiation of satellite cells, tissue-resident stem cells in skeletal muscle [57, 59, 62]. Several studies in rodents have indicated that leptin signaling plays an important role in promoting skeletal muscle regeneration through the regulation of several proteins [56–68] and microRNAs [69] linked to muscle growth, cell cycle progression, and protein catabolism. Thus, the loss of functional leptin signaling might negatively impact skeletal muscle regeneration and contribute to sarcopenia in obesity and diabetes (Fig. 14.2).

Despite marked progress in recent years toward understanding the regulatory role of leptin in skeletal muscle lipid accumulation and glucose homeostasis, several questions pertaining to leptin's potential therapeutic use in patients with obesity and/or diabetes remain to be answered. For example, does leptin resistance occur at the local level of skeletal muscle, and, if so, how does it develop in skeletal muscle during obesity? The fact that impairment of the regenerative capacity of muscle satellite cells has been observed only in extremely obese mice in which leptin activity was genetically ablated (*ob*/*ob* and *db*/*db*) is another important issue [66–68]. Further investigation is warranted to elucidate whether moderate impairment of leptin action, commonly observed in diet-induced obesity, affects the regenerative capacity of skeletal muscle in humans and to identify factors or signaling pathways that link muscle lipid accumulation and impaired satellite cell function in the context of leptin resistance. Given the information currently available, exercise [60] and caloric restriction [61, 72] might be promising ways to enhance skeletal muscle fatty acid oxidation and promote skeletal muscle mass maintenance via the regeneration of satellite cells in obese and diabetic patients with leptin resistance. Continued advances are expected to improve our understanding of leptin's effects on glucose/lipid metabolism and skeletal muscle mass maintenance and to facilitate the therapeutic use of leptin in the treatment of human obesity and diabetes.

References

1. Ahima RS, Flier JS (2000) Leptin. Annu Rev Physiol 62:413–437
2. Myers MG Jr (2004) Leptin receptor signaling and the regulation of mammalian physiology. Recent Prog Horm Res 59:287–304
3. Kielar D, Clark JS, Ciechanowicz A, Kurzawski G, Sulikowski T, Naruszewicz M (1998) Leptin receptor isoforms expressed in human adipose tissue. Metab Clin Exp 47(7):844–847
4. Guerra B, Santana A, Fuentes T, Delgado-Guerra S, Cabrera-Socorro A, Dorado C et al (2007) Leptin receptors in human skeletal muscle. J Appl Physiol 102(5):1786–1792
5. Kieffer TJ, Heller RS, Habener JF (1996) Leptin receptors expressed on pancreatic beta-cells. Biochem Biophys Res Commun 224(2):522–527
6. Bjorbaek C, Kahn BB (2004) Leptin signaling in the central nervous system and the periphery. Recent Prog Horm Res 59:305–331
7. Denroche HC, Huynh FK, Kieffer TJ (2012) The role of leptin in glucose homeostasis. J Diabetes Investig 3(2):115–129
8. Margetic S, Gazzola C, Pegg GG, Hill RA (2002) Leptin: a review of its peripheral actions and interactions. Int J Obes Relat Metab Disord 26(11):1407–1433
9. Morioka T, Asilmaz E, Hu J, Dishinger JF, Kurpad AJ, Elias CF et al (2007) Disruption of leptin receptor expression in the pancreas directly affects beta cell growth and function in mice. J Clin Invest 117(10):2860–2868
10. Pelleymounter MA, Cullen MJ, Baker MB, Hecht R, Winters D, Boone T et al (1995) Effects of the obese gene product on body weight regulation in ob/ob mice. Science 269 (5223):540–543
11. Goodpaster BH, Wolf D (2004) Skeletal muscle lipid accumulation in obesity, insulin resistance, and type 2 diabetes. Pediatr Diabetes 5(4):219–226
12. Kahn BB, Flier JS (2000) Obesity and insulin resistance. J Clin Invest 106(4):473–481
13. Bates SH, Gardiner JV, Jones RB, Bloom SR, Bailey CJ (2002) Acute stimulation of glucose uptake by leptin in l6 muscle cells. Horm Metab Res 34(3):111–115
14. Berti L, Gammeltoft S (1999) Leptin stimulates glucose uptake in C2C12 muscle cells by activation of ERK2. Mol Cell Endocrinol 157(1–2):121–130
15. Berti L, Kellerer M, Capp E, Haring HU (1997) Leptin stimulates glucose transport and glycogen synthesis in C2C12 myotubes: evidence for a P13-kinase mediated effect. Diabetologia 40(5):606–609
16. Kellerer M, Koch M, Metzinger E, Mushack J, Capp E, Haring HU (1997) Leptin activates PI-3 kinase in C2C12 myotubes via janus kinase-2 (JAK-2) and insulin receptor substrate-2 (IRS-2) dependent pathways. Diabetologia 40(11):1358–1362
17. Ceddia RB, William WN Jr, Curi R (1999) Comparing effects of leptin and insulin on glucose metabolism in skeletal muscle: evidence for an effect of leptin on glucose uptake and decarboxylation. Int J Obes Relat Metab Disord 23(1):75–82
18. Harris RB (1998) Acute and chronic effects of leptin on glucose utilization in lean mice. Biochem Biophys Res Commun 245(2):502–509
19. Muoio DM, Dohm GL, Fiedorek FT Jr, Tapscott EB, Coleman RA (1997) Leptin directly alters lipid partitioning in skeletal muscle. Diabetes 46(8):1360–1363

20. Burcelin R, Kamohara S, Li J, Tannenbaum GS, Charron MJ, Friedman JM (1999) Acute intravenous leptin infusion increases glucose turnover but not skeletal muscle glucose uptake in ob/ob mice. Diabetes 48(6):1264–1269
21. Kamohara S, Burcelin R, Halaas JL, Friedman JM, Charron MJ (1997) Acute stimulation of glucose metabolism in mice by leptin treatment. Nature 389(6649):374–377
22. Unger RH, Clark GO, Scherer PE, Orci L (2010) Lipid homeostasis, lipotoxicity and the metabolic syndrome. Biochim Biophys Acta 1801(3):209–214
23. Kelley DE, Goodpaster BH (2001) Skeletal muscle triglyceride. An aspect of regional adiposity and insulin resistance. Diabetes Care 24(5):933–941
24. Steinberg GR, Parolin ML, Heigenhauser GJ, Dyck DJ (2002) Leptin increases FA oxidation in lean but not obese human skeletal muscle: evidence of peripheral leptin resistance. Am J Physiol Endocrinol Metab 283(1):E187–E192
25. Levin N, Nelson C, Gurney A, Vandlen R, de Sauvage F (1996) Decreased food intake does not completely account for adiposity reduction after ob protein infusion. Proc Natl Acad Sci U S A 93(4):1726–1730
26. Shimabukuro M, Koyama K, Chen G, Wang MY, Trieu F, Lee Y et al (1997) Direct antidiabetic effect of leptin through triglyceride depletion of tissues. Proc Natl Acad Sci U S A 94(9):4637–4641
27. Muoio DM, Dohm GL, Tapscott EB, Coleman RA (1999) Leptin opposes insulin's effects on fatty acid partitioning in muscles isolated from obese ob/ob mice. Am J Physiol 276(5 Pt 1): E913–E921
28. Suzuki A, Okamoto S, Lee S, Saito K, Shiuchi T, Minokoshi Y (2007) Leptin stimulates fatty acid oxidation and peroxisome proliferator-activated receptor alpha gene expression in mouse C2C12 myoblasts by changing the subcellular localization of the alpha2 form of AMP-activated protein kinase. Mol Cell Biol 27(12):4317–4327
29. Minokoshi Y, Kahn BB (2003) Role of AMP-activated protein kinase in leptin-induced fatty acid oxidation in muscle. Biochem Soc Trans 31(Pt 1):196–201
30. Minokoshi Y, Kim YB, Peroni OD, Fryer LG, Muller C, Carling D et al (2002) Leptin stimulates fatty-acid oxidation by activating AMP-activated protein kinase. Nature 415 (6869):339–343
31. Hardie DG (2007) AMP-activated/SNF1 protein kinases: conserved guardians of cellular energy. Nat Rev Mol Cell Biol 8(10):774–785
32. Hayashi T, Hirshman MF, Fujii N, Habinowski SA, Witters LA, Goodyear LJ (2000) Metabolic stress and altered glucose transport: activation of AMP-activated protein kinase as a unifying coupling mechanism. Diabetes 49(4):527–531
33. Hayashi T, Hirshman MF, Kurth EJ, Winder WW, Goodyear LJ (1998) Evidence for 5′ AMP-activated protein kinase mediation of the effect of muscle contraction on glucose transport. Diabetes 47(8):1369–1373
34. Mu J, Brozinick JT Jr, Valladares O, Bucan M, Birnbaum MJ (2001) A role for AMP-activated protein kinase in contraction- and hypoxia-regulated glucose transport in skeletal muscle. Mol Cell 7(5):1085–1094
35. Winder WW, Hardie DG (1999) AMP-activated protein kinase, a metabolic master switch: possible roles in type 2 diabetes. Am J Physiol 277(1 Pt 1):E1–E10
36. Long YC, Zierath JR (2006) AMP-activated protein kinase signaling in metabolic regulation. J Clin Invest 116(7):1776–1783
37. Olsen GS, Hansen BF (2002) AMP kinase activation ameliorates insulin resistance induced by free fatty acids in rat skeletal muscle. Am J Physiol Endocrinol Metab 283(5):E965–E970
38. Munzberg H, Myers MG Jr (2005) Molecular and anatomical determinants of central leptin resistance. Nat Neurosci 8(5):566–570
39. Myers MG, Cowley MA, Munzberg H (2008) Mechanisms of leptin action and leptin resistance. Annu Rev Physiol 70:537–556
40. Steinberg GR, Dyck DJ (2000) Development of leptin resistance in rat soleus muscle in response to high-fat diets. Am J Physiol Endocrinol Metab 279(6):E1374–E1382

41. Dulloo AG, Stock MJ, Solinas G, Boss O, Montani JP, Seydoux J (2002) Leptin directly stimulates thermogenesis in skeletal muscle. FEBS Lett 515(1–3):109–113
42. Cruz-Jentoft AJ, Baeyens JP, Bauer JM, Boirie Y, Cederholm T, Landi F et al (2010) Sarcopenia: European consensus on definition and diagnosis: report of the European working group on sarcopenia in older people. Age Ageing 39(4):412–423
43. Kohara K (2014) Sarcopenic obesity in aging population: current status and future directions for research. Endocrine 45(1):15–25
44. Srikanthan P, Hevener AL, Karlamangla AS (2010) Sarcopenia exacerbates obesity-associated insulin resistance and dysglycemia: findings from the National Health and Nutrition Examination Survey III. PLoS One 5(5):e10805
45. Stenholm S, Harris TB, Rantanen T, Visser M, Kritchevsky SB, Ferrucci L (2008) Sarcopenic obesity: definition, cause and consequences. Curr Opin Clin Nutr Metab Care 11(6):693–700
46. Lim S, Kim JH, Yoon JW, Kang SM, Choi SH, Park YJ et al (2010) Sarcopenic obesity: prevalence and association with metabolic syndrome in the Korean Longitudinal Study on Health and Aging (KLoSHA). Diabetes Care 33(7):1652–1654
47. Abbatecola AM, Chiodini P, Gallo C, Lakatta E, Sutton-Tyrrell K, Tylavsky FA et al (2012) Pulse wave velocity is associated with muscle mass decline: health ABC study. Age 34 (2):469–478
48. Zamboni M, Mazzali G, Fantin F, Rossi A, Di Francesco V (2008) Sarcopenic obesity: a new category of obesity in the elderly. Nutr Metab Cardiovasc Dis 18(5):388–395
49. Sakuma K, Yamaguchi A (2013) Sarcopenic obesity and endocrinal adaptation with age. Int J Endocrinol 2013:204164
50. Hubbard RE, O'Mahony MS, Calver BL, Woodhouse KW (2008) Nutrition, inflammation, and leptin levels in aging and frailty. J Am Geriatr Soc 56(2):279–284
51. Kohara K, Ochi M, Tabara Y, Nagai T, Igase M, Miki T (2011) Leptin in sarcopenic visceral obesity: possible link between adipocytes and myocytes. PLoS One 6(9):e24633
52. Waters DL, Qualls CR, Dorin RI, Veldhuis JD, Baumgartner RN (2008) Altered growth hormone, cortisol, and leptin secretion in healthy elderly persons with sarcopenia and mixed body composition phenotypes. J Gerontol A: Biol Med Sci 63(5):536–541
53. Dubey L, Hesong Z (2006) Role of leptin in atherogenesis. Exp Clin Cardiol 11(4):269–275
54. Casanueva FF, Dieguez C (1998) Interaction between body composition, leptin and growth hormone status. Bailliere Clin Endocrinol Metab 12(2):297–314
55. Dieguez C, Carro E, Seoane LM, Garcia M, Camina JP, Senaris R et al (2000) Regulation of somatotroph cell function by the adipose tissue. Int J Obes Relat Metab Disord 24(Suppl 2): S100–S103
56. Carbo N, Ribas V, Busquets S, Alvarez B, Lopez-Soriano FJ, Argiles JM (2000) Short-term effects of leptin on skeletal muscle protein metabolism in the rat. J Nutr Biochem 11 (9):431–435
57. Akhmedov D, Berdeaux R (2013) The effects of obesity on skeletal muscle regeneration. Front Physiol 4:371
58. Wagers AJ, Conboy IM (2005) Cellular and molecular signatures of muscle regeneration: current concepts and controversies in adult myogenesis. Cell 122(5):659–667
59. Jang YC, Sinha M, Cerletti M, Dall'Osso C, Wagers AJ (2011) Skeletal muscle stem cells: effects of aging and metabolism on muscle regenerative function. Cold Spring Harb Symp Quant Biol 76:101–111
60. Snijders T, Verdijk LB, van Loon LJ (2009) The impact of sarcopenia and exercise training on skeletal muscle satellite cells. Ageing Res Rev 8(4):328–338
61. Cerletti M, Jang YC, Finley LW, Haigis MC, Wagers AJ (2012) Short-term calorie restriction enhances skeletal muscle stem cell function. Cell Stem Cell 10(5):515–519
62. Vignaud A, Ramond F, Hourde C, Keller A, Butler-Browne G, Ferry A (2007) Diabetes provides an unfavorable environment for muscle mass and function after muscle injury in mice. Pathobiol: J Immunopathol Mol Cell Biol 74(5):291–300

63. Tamilarasan KP, Temmel H, Das SK, Al Zoughbi W, Schauer S, Vesely PW et al (2012) Skeletal muscle damage and impaired regeneration due to LPL-mediated lipotoxicity. Cell Death Dis 3:e354
64. Purchas RW, Romsos DR, Allen RE, Merkel RA (1985) Muscle growth and satellite cell proliferative activity in obese (OB/OB) mice. J Anim Sci 60(3):644–651
65. Peterson JM, Bryner RW, Alway SE (2008) Satellite cell proliferation is reduced in muscles of obese Zucker rats but restored with loading. Am J Physiol Cell Physiol 295(2):C521–C528
66. Nguyen MH, Cheng M, Koh TJ (2011) Impaired muscle regeneration in ob/ob and db/db mice. Sci World J 11:1525–1535
67. Arounleut P, Bowser M, Upadhyay S, Shi XM, Fulzele S, Johnson MH et al (2013) Absence of functional leptin receptor isoforms in the POUND (Lepr(db/lb)) mouse is associated with muscle atrophy and altered myoblast proliferation and differentiation. PLoS One 8(8):e72330
68. Sainz N, Rodriguez A, Catalan V, Becerril S, Ramirez B, Gomez-Ambrosi J et al (2009) Leptin administration favors muscle mass accretion by decreasing FoxO3a and increasing PGC-1alpha in ob/ob mice. PLoS One 4(9):e6808
69. Hamrick MW, Herberg S, Arounleut P, He HZ, Shiver A, Qi RQ et al (2010) The adipokine leptin increases skeletal muscle mass and significantly alters skeletal muscle miRNA expression profile in aged mice. Biochem Biophys Res Commun 400(3):379–383
70. Drummond MJ, McCarthy JJ, Fry CS, Esser KA, Rasmussen BB (2008) Aging differentially affects human skeletal muscle microRNA expression at rest and after an anabolic stimulus of resistance exercise and essential amino acids. Am J Physiol Endocrinol Metab 295(6):E1333–E1340
71. Will K, Kalbe C, Kuzinski J, Losel D, Viergutz T, Palin MF et al (2012) Effects of leptin and adiponectin on proliferation and protein metabolism of porcine myoblasts. Histochem Cell Biol 138(2):271–287
72. Anderson RM, Weindruch R (2010) Metabolic reprogramming, caloric restriction and aging. Trends Endocrinol Metab 21(3):134–141

Chapter 15
Evaluation of Insulin Resistance in Diabetes: Standard Protocol for a Euglycemic-Hyperinsulinemic Clamp Using an Artificial Pancreas

Masanori Emoto, Tomoaki Morioka, Hisayo Yokoyama, Yuko Sawada-Yamazaki, Koka Motoyama, Katsuhito Mori, Kiyoshi Maekawa, Yoshiki Nishizawa, and Masaaki Inaba

Abstract Insulin resistance plays a pivotal pathognomonic role in various pathophysiological states, including diabetes, obesity, and metabolic syndromes. A euglycemic-hyperinsulinemic (EH) clamp, the gold-standard method for evaluating insulin resistance in humans, has been performed according to the original protocol for each hospital or institute, which makes it difficult to compare the findings of different studies. We have established a standard protocol for the EH clamp using an artificial pancreas (AP, models STG-22 and STG-55, Nikkiso Co. Ltd. Tokyo), which has been widely used in Japan since 1987. Among the 351 Japanese subjects, 301 were type 2 diabetics, 12 were impaired glucose tolerance with obesity, and 38 had normal glucose tolerance. In this chapter, the standard protocol using the AP and the insulin resistance data are described in detail. By using an AP for the clamp, stable steady-state euglycemia and glucose infusion rates (GIR, metabolizable glucose [M] value) were achieved with high precision. The insulin resistance index, M/I, in type 2 diabetics was approximately 49 % lower than in patients with normal glucose tolerance and had a strong inverse correlation with body mass index. Furthermore, the validity and clinical implications of insulin resistance were clarified and reported according to the standard protocol for an EH clamp using an AP. In conclusion, a standard protocol for using an AP for an EH clamp would allow us to evaluate insulin resistance in detail and with high precision in various pathological states/diseases.

M. Emoto (✉) • T. Morioka • Y. Sawada-Yamazaki • K. Motoyama • K. Mori • K. Maekawa • M. Inaba
Metabolism, Endocrinology and Molecular Medicine, Osaka City University Graduate School of Medicine, 1-4-3, Asahi-machi, Abeno-ku, Osaka 545-8585, Japan
e-mail: memoto@med.osaka-cu.ac.jp

H. Yokoyama
Research Center for Urban Health and Sports, Osaka City University, Osaka, Japan

Y. Nishizawa
Osaka City University, Osaka, Japan

M. Inaba (ed.), *Musculoskeletal Disease Associated with Diabetes Mellitus*,
DOI 10.1007/978-4-431-55720-3_15

Keywords Insulin resistance • Euglycemic-hyperinsulinemic clamp • Artificial pancreas • Diabetes • Japanese

15.1 Introduction: Evaluation of Insulin Resistance in Humans

Insulin resistance is the predominant pathognomonic state for hyperglycemia in type 2 diabetes, the incidence of which is rapidly increasing in Japan and the Asian region. Furthermore, hyperinsulinemia due to insulin resistance is an underlying condition in hypertension, dyslipidemia, hyperuricemia, and atherosclerotic cardiovascular diseases in obesity and metabolic syndromes. Some oral antidiabetic drugs used in clinical practice have the potential to improve insulin resistance. In Japan, metformin, a biguanide, and pioglitazone, a thiazolidinedione, are usually prescribed for type 2 diabetes with obesity and/or insulin resistance. Other drugs such as glimepiride, a sulfonylurea drug, and some angiotensin-converting enzyme/angiotensin II receptor blocker inhibitors can also improve insulin resistance in addition to their main antihypertensive effects. Therefore, it is important and critical to evaluate insulin resistance in a practical clinical setting in patients with various lifestyle-related diseases as well as type 2 diabetes.

To date, various indexes and methods for evaluating insulin resistance in humans have been reported. The direct indexes for representing insulin resistance include the insulin tolerance test and the insulin suppression test, while indirect indexes include the homeostasis model assessment (HOMA-R), quantitative insulin sensitivity check index (QUICKI), Matsuda index, etc. In order to validate the precision of these indexes, a gold-standard index is needed for the evaluation of insulin resistance in humans. Since a proposal by DeFronzo in 1979, the euglycemic-hyperinsulinemic clamp technique, a glucose clamp technique, has been established and used as the gold-standard technique for the evaluation of insulin resistance in humans [1]. In this chapter, the standard protocol for a euglycemic-hyperinsulinemic clamp using an artificial pancreas for evaluating insulin resistance in Japan and its clinical implications are described in detail.

15.2 The Euglycemic-Hyperinsulinemic Clamp as a Gold-Standard Technique

15.2.1 Glucose Clamp Technique

In 1979, DeFronzo et al. proposed the glucose clamp technique, a method to quantitatively measure insulin sensitivity and insulin secretion in humans [1]. The glucose clamp technique includes two techniques: a euglycemic-hyperinsulinemic clamp and a hyperglycemic clamp. The former measures insulin sensitivity in the whole body, mainly in the muscle, in steady physiological and/or supraphysiological hyperinsulinemic conditions, while the latter measures insulin secretion capacity from the pancreas in response to a steady hyperglycemic physiological state. In the euglycemic-hyperinsulinemic clamp, metabolized glucose uptake in the whole body, in a steady hyperinsulinemic state within the physiological range, is measured quantitatively, which mainly represents the insulin sensitivity in the muscle.

15.2.2 The Principle of the Glucose Clamp Technique

The main actions of insulin in glucose metabolism in vivo are the increase of glucose uptake in the muscle, adipose tissue, and liver and a decrease of hepatic glucose production. In view of a hormone's dose-response curve, the maximum glucose uptake in the whole body is regarded as the *responsiveness of insulin*, and 50 % of the maximum glucose uptake is the *sensitivity of insulin* [2]. In the narrow sense, *insulin resistance* is a state of decreased insulin sensitivity, which is strictly different from *insulin unresponsiveness*, a decrease of insulin responsiveness.

In healthy subjects, the maximum glucose uptake in the whole body is achieved when the plasma immunoreactive insulin level (IRI) is around several hundred μU/mL (~500 μU/mL), while 50 % of the maximum is achieved for an IRI around 100 μU/mL. In a euglycemic-hyperinsulinemic clamp, the insulin sensitivity is represented by the metabolized glucose uptake (*M value*) in the whole body, when the IRI is around 100 μU/mL, which is when it is equal to 50 % of the maximum glucose uptake. In this physiological hyperinsulinemic state, insulin completely inhibits hepatic glucose production, and infused glucose is necessary to maintain euglycemia (around 90 mg/dL). The amount of infused glucose is equal to that of metabolized glucose uptake in the muscle and adipose tissue, because urinary glucose excretion is neglected. It has been reported that approximately 80 % of the glucose uptake by the whole body in a hyperinsulinemic state is metabolized in the muscle, while some glucose is also metabolized in the adipose tissue [3, 4]. Furthermore, metabolized glucose (*M value*) is regarded as an index of insulin sensitivity in the muscle.

In DeFronzo's original technique [1], a small polyethylene catheter was inserted under local Xylocaine anesthesia into a brachial artery for blood sampling. In the contralateral forearm vein, insulin was infused at a constant rate (40 $mU/min/m^2$) within 10 min of an insulin priming injection. Various amounts of 20 % glucose solution were infused to maintain euglycemia (clamp), which is equal to the metabolized glucose uptake in the whole body. In most cases, the monitored glucose level and the glucose infusion rate (GIR, mg/kg/min), which were equal to the metabolized glucose uptake, were increased gradually to reach the steady state after 120 min of the clamp. The metabolized glucose uptake (*M value*) is defined as the mean of the GIRs for every 20 min of the 120-min clamp, and the *M/I value* is an index where the *M value* is corrected by the IRI during the 120 min steady state. The *M value* is often expressed as the glucose disposal rate.

15.2.3 Literature About the Adoption of a Euglycemic-Hyperinsulinemic Clamp

Since the euglycemic-hyperinsulinemic clamp was proposed [1], many clinical studies have been reported. In a *PubMed* literature search using the keywords glucose clamp, euglycemic-hyperinsulinemic clamp, and/or hyperglycemic clamp, 1,491 English publications were found, out of which 1,343 (90 %) were regarding the euglycemic-hyperinsulinemic clamp, and 101 (7 %) were from Japan. After the mid-2000s, publications have been decreasing gradually both worldwide and in Japan (Fig. 15.1). To date, there are 20 reports in English where the standard protocol of the clamp was performed using an artificial pancreas (AP) [5–24].

15.3 Artificial Pancreas in Japan

15.3.1 History of the Development of the Artificial Pancreas

Professor E Perry McCullagh, an endocrinologist at the Cleveland Clinic, proposed the concept of the *AP* in 1959, as a substitute for decreased pancreatic beta cell function and insulin secretion in response to blood glucose levels [25]. The AP is

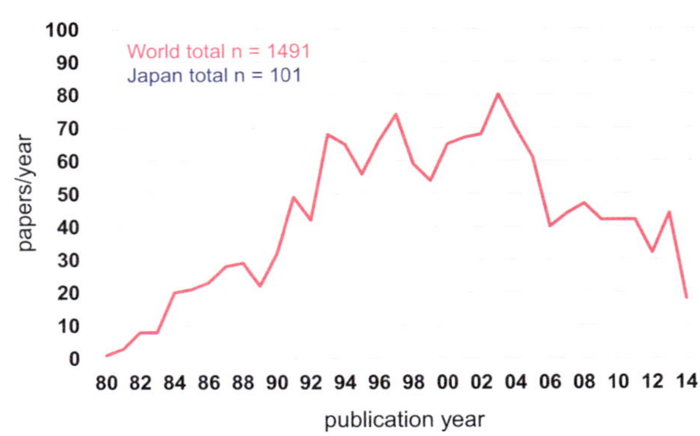

Fig. 15.1 Change in the number of clinical research publications in English regarding the glucose clamp technique, euglycemic-hyperinsulinemic clamp, and/or hyperglycemic clamp, from 1979 to 2014. A PubMed search was conducted using the following parameters: "glucose clamp" or "euglycemic clamp" or "hyperglycemic clamp" in any field, "subjects" or "patients" in the abstract, and English as the language

strictly the *artificial endocrine pancreas* (AEP) because it is unable to perform the pancreas's *exocrine* functions. However, the word "*artificial pancreas, AP*" is adopted in this review because the STG model produced by the Nikkiso Co. Ltd. has a Japanese name "Zinkosuizou," which corresponds to artificial pancreas and is approved by the Pharmaceuticals and Medical Devices Agency in Japan. The bedside-type AP with a closed-loop regulatory system consists of a continuous glucose monitoring system, a computer system equipped with a regulatory algorithm, and an insulin infusion system [25]. Albisser [26, 27] in 1974 in Toronto and Shichiri in 1975 in Osaka [28, 29] were the first to successfully use the AP clinically. This AP consisted of an Autoanalyzer for blood glucose determination, a minicomputer system, and a pump-drive system. After downsizing and improving the equipment, the bedside-type AP was introduced into the clinical and research fields of diabetes. Two models are available, namely, the Biostator (Miles Laboratory Inc., Elkhart, IN, USA) and the STG model (Nikkiso Co. Ltd., Tokyo, Japan). The induction of Biostator into the market started in 1983 and its production ended in 1987. The STG model was introduced to the market in 1987 and is now available in Japan. The various applications of the STG model in the clinic and in the research of diabetes and related diseases have been vigorously examined by the Osaka University and Kumamoto University study groups in Japan. Since 1988, medical insurance in Japan has approved clinical applications of the STG model on a short-term basis, including blood glucose control in diabetic coma, surgery, delivery, hypoglycemia, and the prediction of insulin requirements in special medical institutes and hospitals with specialist Japan Diabetes Association-approved diabetologists. According to the 2002 report by the Artificial Organs Registry in Japan, the STG model has been cumulatively used in 14,418 cases from 1983 to 2002. In 2002, 465 cases reportedly used the STG model, among which 29 (6.2 %) were used for glycemic control, 341 (73.3 %) for laboratory and clinical research (mainly glucose clamp [61.9 %]), and 95 (20.4 %) for animal experiments [25].

15.3.2 The STG-22 Model and the New STG-55 Model

To date, the STG-22 AP model (Fig. 15.2a) produced by Nikkiso Co. Ltd. has been used most widely. Its new model, STG-55 (Fig. 15.2b), was approved by the Pharmaceuticals and Medical Devices Agency in 2009 and was introduced into the clinic in 2010. The STG-55 models are largely improved; they are more convenient and highly precise. First, the equipment is more compact and lightweight (STG-22, 505[W] × 565[D] × 1,600[H] mm, 62 kg; STG-55, 375[W] × 425 [D] × 1,630[H] mm, 36 kg). Second, a largely improved enzyme membrane has been included for continuous blood glucose measurement. Third, the complex circuits for glucose measurement were combined to one-set apron (Fig. 15.3). Fourth, an automatic priming system was introduced for the preparation of the machine. Fifth, the cost of the equipment was largely reduced. Among these improvements, the improved enzyme membrane in STG-55 has great advantages

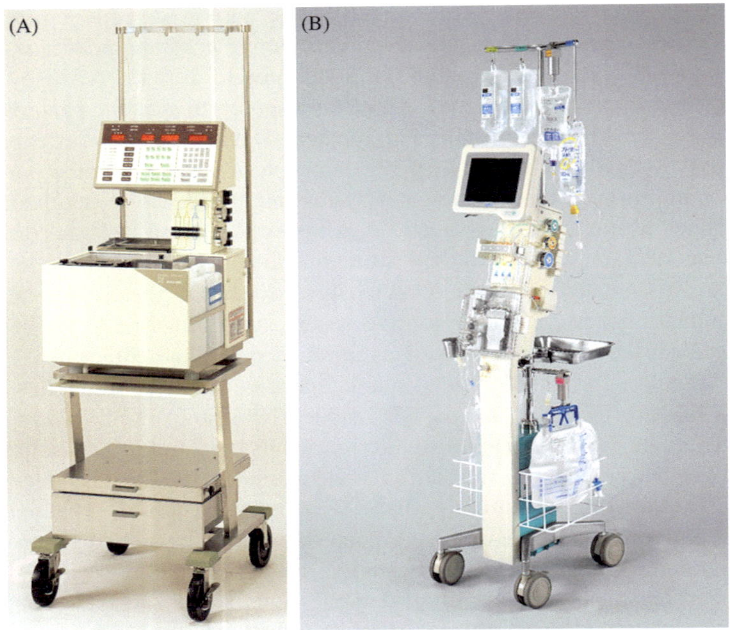

Fig. 15.2 STG-22 (**a**) and STG-55 (**b**) models of the artificial pancreas (Nikkiso Co. Ltd., Tokyo), which are widely used in Japan and have been approved by the Pharmaceuticals and Medical Devices Agency since 1987 (The photographs are provided courtesy of Nikkiso Co. Ltd.)

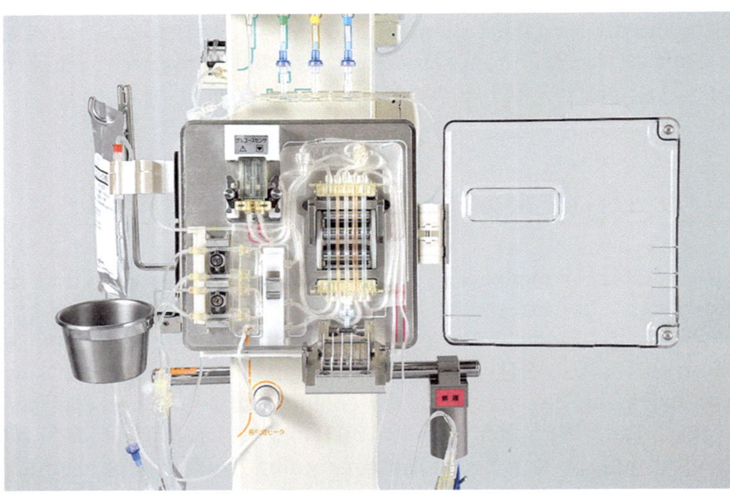

Fig. 15.3 One-set apron circuit for glucose measurement with the glucose and insulin infusion system in model STG-55 of the artificial pancreas (The photograph is provided courtesy of Nikkiso Co. Ltd.)

over the STG-22 model in terms of the improvement in the validity and stability of glucose measurements and the shortened calibration time in the preparation step. As stated below, the parameters of variability for the clamp using STG-55 demonstrate the same degree of validity as with STG-22 in spite of fewer subjects.

15.4 Standard Protocol for a Euglycemic-Hyperinsulinemic Clamp Using the STG Artificial Pancreas

15.4.1 Standard Protocol for a Euglycemic-Hyperinsulinemic Clamp Using an Artificial Pancreas

The euglycemic-hyperinsulinemic clamp was performed, 10–12 h after an overnight fast, according to a previously described standard protocol, using the AP models STG-22 or STG-55 [6, 8–10, 15, 16, 18]. On the morning of the study, a 20-gauge catheter was inserted into a forearm vein in a retrograde manner for constant monitoring of blood glucose levels. In the same arm, a 22-gauge catheter was inserted into the wrist vein for blood sampling. Blood sampling was performed every 30 min during the clamp study to assay the plasma insulin level. Another 22-gauge catheter was inserted into an antecubital vein of the other arm for the administration of human regular insulin (Humulin; Eli Lilly and Company, Indianapolis, IN) and a 10 or 20 % glucose solution. After baseline blood sampling, insulin was first manually infused at a priming infusion dose during the first 9 min of the clamp according to the manipulation manual for STG-22 or STG-55 and afterward automatically at a continuous rate of 1.25 mU/kg/min. The dose of constantly infused insulin corresponded to the dose in DeFronzo's original protocol [1].

Blood glucose levels were determined every 1 min in both STG-22 and STG-55 models during the 120-min clamp study, and euglycemia (90 mg/dL, 5.0 mmol/L) was automatically maintained by infusion of different amounts of a 10 or 20 % glucose solution according to the glycemic control algorithm. The parameters for the algorithm were always set at the same constant values according to the STG-22 or STG-55 manipulation manual; in particular, setting the inputs at 1.25 mU/kg/min for insulin infusion rate was important. This is very crucial in the standard protocol as performing the glucose clamp in the same condition is required for the comparison of insulin sensitivity among subjects and/or within the same subject. If the parameters for the algorithm are set up differently for each subject or each clamp, it is difficult to compare GIR between and within subjects.

Figure 15.4 shows the schematic representative time course for monitored blood glucose, IRI, and GIR according to the aforementioned standard protocol. The real reports for a patient, a printout sheet in STG-22 and a control panel in STG-55, are shown in Fig. 15.5a, b. The various parameters for the standard protocol of a euglycemic-hyperinsulinemic clamp using the artificial pancreas, STG-22 or STG-55, are defined in Table 15.1. The *M* value, an index of insulin sensitivity in

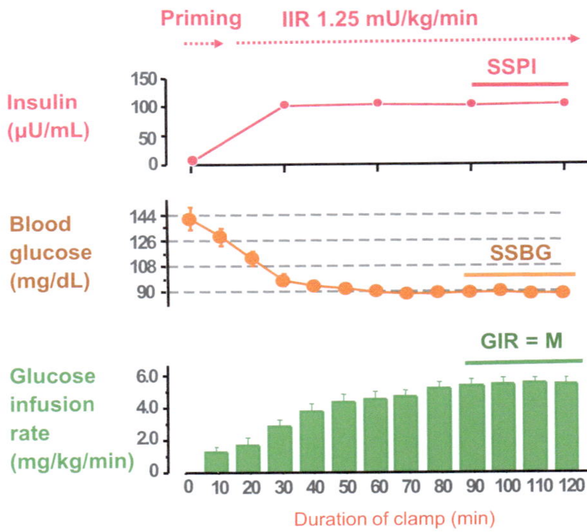

Fig. 15.4 Schematic time course of monitored steady-state blood glucose (SSBG), steady-state plasma insulin (SSPI) levels, and glucose infusion rates (GIR) according to the standard protocol for a euglycemic-hyperinsulinemic clamp using the STG model of the artificial pancreas. The bar represents mean ± SE (standard error). Priming, insulin priming infusion during the first 9 min; *IIR* insulin infusion rate

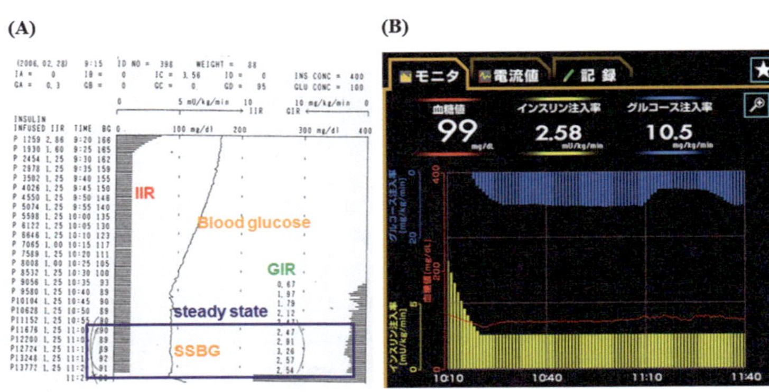

Fig. 15.5 Real printout sheet for a patient in the STG-22 model and control panel in the STG-55 model of the artificial pancreas. *IIR* insulin infusion rate, *GIR* glucose infusion rate, *SSBG* steady-state blood glucose

the original report [1], is represented as the mean of the *GIR*s during the last 30 min of the 120-min clamp. Finally, we use the *M*/*I* value, which is obtained by dividing the mean *GIR* by the steady-state plasma insulin (*SSPI*) levels during the last 30 min of the clamp. This is an index of insulin sensitivity as previously reported. For convenience, the *M*/*I* value is multiplied by 100.

Table 15.1 Definitions of parameters for the standard protocol of a euglycemic-hyperinsulinemic clamp using the artificial pancreas models STG-22 or STG-55

Abbreviation	Units	Term	Definition
SSBG	[mg/dL]	Steady-state blood glucose	Blood glucose level in the steady state*
CV of SSBG	[%]	Coefficient of variance for SSBG	An index of precision of the clamp blood glucose levels
SSPI	[μU/mL]	Steady-state* plasma insulin level	
MCR of insulin	[/kg]	Metabolic clearance rate of insulin	Calculated as IIR × 1,000/(SSPI – (pre-IRI × post-CPR/pre-CPR))
GIR	[mg/kg/min]	Glucose infusion rate	Equal to *M* value or glucose disposal rate (mg/kg/min); mean of each glucose infusion rate in the steady state*
SD of GIR	[mg/kg/min]	Standard deviation of GIR	An index of the stability of the GIR
M/I value	[mg/kg/min (μU/mL)]	M value corrected by SSPI	Calculated as (GIR/SSPI) × 100; M value corrected by the plasma insulin level

The steady state (*) means 90–120 min of the clamp. *IIR* insulin infusion rate, *pre-IRI* immunoreactive insulin level before the clamp, *pre- and post-CPR* serum immunoreactive C-peptide level before and at the end of the clamp

15.4.2 Precision of the Standard Protocol Using the STG Model of the Artificial Pancreas

Since 1993, we have performed the euglycemic-hyperinsulinemic clamp according to the aforementioned standard protocol using the AP model STG-22 in 394 Japanese subjects. Among these subjects, clamp studies could not be performed in only nine subjects (2.3 %) mainly because of difficulties and/or troubles with the blood sampling route in the forearm vein. Finally, GIR/M values were measured from the clamp study in 385 subjects (97.5 %). In order to examine insulin resistance in Japanese subjects with different glucose tolerances, we excluded patients with factors strongly affecting insulin resistance, morbid obesity (BMI [body mass index] greater than 35 kg/m^2), chronic renal insufficiency, and type 1 diabetes. Finally, the data from 337 subjects, including 38 with normal glucose tolerance (NGT), 12 with impaired glucose tolerance (IGT), and 287 with type 2 diabetes (T2DM), were analyzed for the STG-22 model. The clinical characteristics are shown in Table 15.2. These age, BMI, and glycated hemoglobin profiles are concordant with those in Japanese patients who are admitted to hospitals for health checks/education programs.

For all 337 subjects, the coefficient of variance of steady-state blood glucose (SSBG) was found to be 2.49 ± 2.1 %, while in each of the NGT, IGT, or T2DM

Table 15.2 Clinical characteristics, precision of the clamp, and the insulin resistance index for the standard protocol for the euglycemic-hyperinsulinemic clamp using the models STG-22 or STG-55 artificial pancreas

	STG-22			STG-55
	NGT	IGT	T2DM	T2DM
Characteristics of subjects				
N (M/F)	38 (25/13)	12 (3/9)	287 (171/116)	14 (7/7)
Age, years	38.1 ± 20.2 (17–75)	46.3 ± 15.0	53.3 ± 12.8 (15–74))	61.6 ± 13.8 (33–77)
BMI, kg/m^2	23.7 ± 4.2 (17.3–34.7)	29.0 ± 3.2	25.2 ± 3.9 (14.6–34.9)	26.2 ± 3.4 (20.8–32.5)
FPG, mg/dL	89.6 ± 8.8	93.0 ± 11.6	143.7 ± 40.7	121.0 ± 29.6
HbA1c, %	4.87 ± 0.55	5.25 ± 0.43	8.66 ± 1.93	8.71 ± 1.92
IRI, μU/ml	7.0 ± 6.3	11.1 ± 8.3	9.0 ± 7.1	10.4 ± 4.5
Parameters of precision of clamp				
SSBG[a]	92.2 ± 5.1	92.5 ± 1.6	91.0 ± 2.9	92.2 ± 1.7
CV of SSBG[a]	3.56 ± 2.79	3.20 ± 1.85	2.39 ± 2.0	2.27 ± 2.7
SSPI[a]	116.5 ± 45.0	123.6 ± 34.6	112.1 ± 32.4	114.8 ± 23.8
MCR of insulin	12.49 ± 5.49	12.73 ± 5.39	12.41 ± 3.37	11.59 ± 2.65
Insulin resistance index				
M or GIR	9.43 ± 4.69	4.42 ± 1.9	4.52 ± 2.12	3.95 ± 1.52
SD of GIR	0.85 ± 0.62	0.79 ± 0.47	0.73 ± 0.61	0.67 ± 0.49
M/I value	9.33 ± 5.74	4.09 ± 2.07	4.56 ± 2.89	3.74 ± 2.31

All values represent mean ± SD or (range)
All abbreviations and units are the same in Table 16.1. *BMI* body mass index, *FPG* fasting plasma glucose mg/dL, *HbA1c* glycated hemoglobin (%), *IRI* immunoreactive insulin level (μU/ml), *SD* standard deviation
[a]The steady state means 90–120 min of the clamp

groups, it was approximately 3 %, which was within a very narrow range compared to that (around 5–10 %) for the manual program without AP (Tables 15.2 and 15.3). Because of the strict glucose clamp in the steady state, the standard deviation (SD)/standard error for each GIR in the steady state was also small indicating less variability in each subject (Table 15.3). These parameters of the clamp demonstrated the high precision of the standard protocol using STG-22. Although the precision of a euglycemic clamp has not been fully clarified in the available literature, superiority of the standard protocol using STG-22 is expected compared to the manual protocol without artificial pancreas.

On the other hand, the steady-state plasma insulin (SSPI) level varies considerably in spite of a constant insulin infusion rate (IIR, 1.25 mU/kg/min) after the same priming dose in the standard protocol. This is mainly attributed to different metabolic clearance rates of insulin in mainly the liver and the kidneys, which could not be predicted by other data before the clamp study. The mean ± SD, median, and interquartile of the range of SSPI for all 337 subjects were 113 ± 34.6, 105.1, and 37.5 μU/mL, respectively. In terms of the distribution of SSPI (Fig. 15.6), SSPI values of 51.9 % of all subjects were within 80–130 μU/mL. When the formula for

Table 15.3 Insulin resistance index and parameters of precision in a euglycemic-hyperinsulinemic clamp using STG-22 according to the standard protocol in 337 Japanese subjects

	Mean	SD/SE	Median	IQR	Range
SSBG	91.2	3.2/0.2	91.3	2.9	76.0–116.8
CV of SSBG	2.49	2.06/0.13	1.83	1.82	0.45–16.22
SSPI	113.0	34.6/1.9	105.1	37.5	47.0–245.0
MCR of insulin	12.4	3.6/0.2	12.2	4.3	5.2–27.5
GIR (=M)	5.07	2.97/0.16	4.63	2.96	0.82–21.20
SD of GIR	0.74	0.60/0.04	0.56	0.58	0.07–4.36
M/I	5.09	3.64/0.20	4.04	3.74	0.54–22.20

The abbreviations and units are the same as in Table 15.1. *SD/SE* standard deviation and error of each GIR in the steady state, *IQR* interquartile of the range

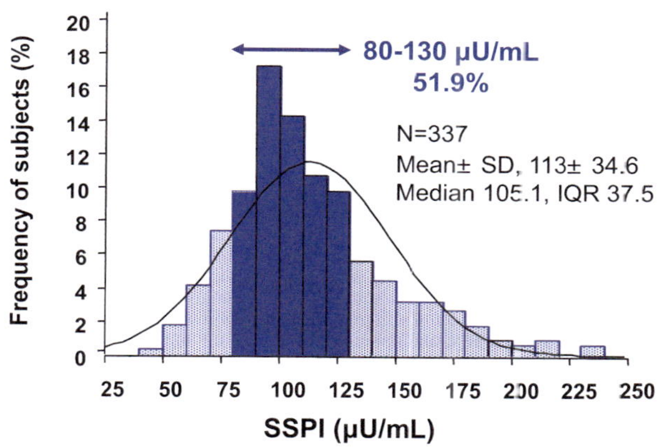

Fig. 15.6 Distribution of steady-state plasma insulin (SSPI) levels according to the standard protocol for a euglycemic-hyperinsulinemic clamp in 337 Japanese subjects with normal glucose tolerance, impaired glucose tolerance with obesity, and type 2 diabetes. *SD* standard deviation, *IQR* interquartile of the range

predicting SSPI from simple clinical parameters was examined by multiple regression analysis, approximately 40 % of SSPI could be explained by the following formula:

$$\text{SSPI} = 18.2 + 0.6 \times (\text{age}) + 2.6 \times (\text{BMI}) + 1.9 \times (\text{IRI}) - 13.7 \times (1/\text{sCre})$$

where age is represented in years, BMI in kg/m^2, fasting IRI in μU/mL, and serum creatinine level (sCre) in mg/dL ($R^2 = 0.398$, $p < 0.0001$).

According to this formula, the SSPI of a 60-year-old patient with a BMI of 25 kg/m^2, fasting IRI of 6 μU/mL, and sCre of 0.6 mg/dL will be 114 μU/mL before the clamp protocol.

15.4.3 Arterialization of the Forearm Vein for Glucose Monitoring: A Controversial Issue

The issue of whether blood flow in the forearm vein should be arterialized by warming for continuous glucose measurement in a euglycemic-hyperinsulinemic clamp or not has been controversial [30–33]. In DeFronzo's original technique [1], continuous sampling for glucose monitoring was performed from the *brachial artery*, which is invasive and risky. An alternative technique for arterial blood sampling as described in the literature is sampling from forearm veins arterialized by warming to various temperatures using a warming box. However, most recent publications do not include a detailed description of the clamp technique, including the arterialization of venous sampling for glucose monitoring.

The mechanism of how arterialization of venous blood sampling affects the result of the euglycemic-hyperinsulinemic clamp has not been elucidated. Andrews et al. demonstrated no significant differences in the SSPI, SSBG, and M values with or without arterialization using a water heat pad at 40–50 °C in 16 healthy and diabetic patients [30]. Wahab et al. also failed to find any significant differences between arterialization using a 55 °C warm air box and non-arterialization in nine healthy subjects in terms of the GIRs and coefficients of variance of SSBG for a euglycemic-hyperinsulinemic clamp with high and low SSPI levels [31]. On the other hand, using almost the same arterialization technique in six healthy subjects, Morris et al. demonstrated that arterialization induced increases in monitored blood glucose levels and oxygen saturation, as well as significant increases in M/I values (from 10.5 ± 3.0 to 11.7 ± 3.2) despite no changes in either SSPI or SSBG [32]. Increased heart rates and decreased blood pressure were also observed. In another report, using only nine healthy subjects, both the monitored blood glucose levels and oxygen saturation (%) increased (0.2–0.5 mM [3.6–9 mg/dL] and 9 %, respectively), although there were no data regarding M or M/I values [33].

In the early days of our study, the forearm used in glucose monitoring was warmed by a heater. However, some patients showed a mild decrease in blood pressure and increased heart rates, probably as a response to warming, via the autonomic nervous system. Possibly, they could not endure the forearm warming during the clamp. Therefore, in most cases, we do not arterialize the forearm vein by warming to avoid risks to the patient.

15.5 Insulin Resistance in Japanese Type 2 Diabetes Patients

It is well established that GIR in the steady state is largely affected by SSPI [3]. In our previous studies [6, 8–10, 15, 16, 18], the mean SSPI levels in the examined groups were greater than 100 μU/mL, the aforementioned target level of SSPI. However, as SSPI differs considerably in each subject, we adopted the M value corrected by SSPI, i.e., the M/I value, as an insulin resistance or sensitivity index in most of our previous reports. As expected, M/I values in IGT patients with obesity

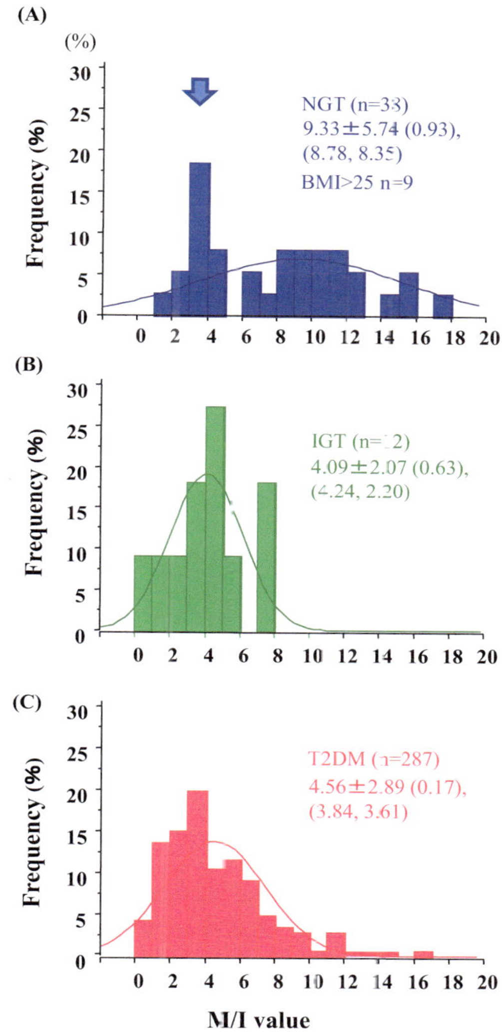

Fig. 15.7 Frequency distributions of M/I values (an insulin resistance index) in subjects with normal glucose tolerance (NGT, **a**), impaired glucose tolerance with obesity (IGT, **b**), and type 2 diabetes (T2DM, **c**). The M/I values were calculated using the standard protocol for a euglycemic-hyperinsulinemic clamp. Some patients with NGT as shown in downward arrow had severe obesity. The values represent n, mean ± SD(SE), and (median, IQR) in each group. *SD* standard deviation, *SE* standard error, *IQR* interquartile of the range, *BMI* body mass index

and T2DM patients were approximately 44 % and 49 % lower, respectively, than those for patients with NGT. There was no significant difference between the M/I values for IGT patients with obesity and T2DM patients (Table 15.2). When the M values among these three groups were compared, almost the same results were seen (Table 15.2). These findings were in accordance with those for Caucasian data. The frequency distributions of M/I values in NGT, IGT, and T2DM patients are shown in Fig. 15.7. The distributions for IGT and T2DM patients are clearly shifted toward the left, i.e., these patients are more insulin resistant than patients with NGT. Furthermore, it is noteworthy that subjects with NGT are widely distributed between an insulin-resistant and an insulin-sensitive state. Some patients with

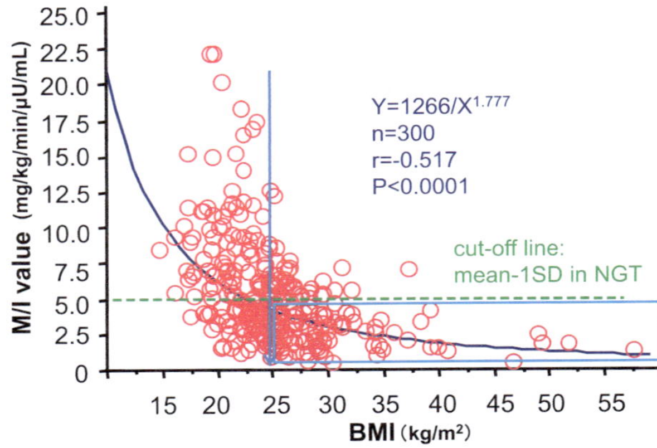

Fig. 15.8 Strong hyperbolic association of the body mass index (BMI) with an insulin resistance index, the M/I value, in type 2 diabetic patients. The percentage of subjects with an M/I value less than 5.0, a tentative cutoff level of mean-1SD in subjects with normal glucose tolerance (NGT), and a BMI greater than 25 kg/m^2 is 79 % among 300 type 2 diabetic patients. *SD* standard deviation

NGT showed severe insulin resistance because of severe obesity and were admitted for weight reduction (as indicated by a downward arrow in Fig. 15.7).

Among 300 Japanese type 2 diabetes patients, there is a strong hyperbolic association of BMI with the insulin resistance index as follows (Fig. 15.8):

$$\mathrm{M/I\ value} = 1266/(\mathrm{BMI})^{1.777}(r = -0.517,\ p < 0.0001)$$

Thus, if a patient who has a lower M/I value of 5.0, which is approximately equal to the mean-1 SD of a healthy subject, is insulin resistant, approximately 60 % of Japanese T2DM patients and approximately 80 % of people with BMIs greater than 25 kg/m^2 are estimated to be insulin resistant.

15.6 Clinical Application of the Standard Protocol Using the STG Model of the Artificial Pancreas

15.6.1 Search for Surrogate Clinical Indexes of Insulin Resistance

15.6.1.1 HOMA-R and Related Indexes

In general, euglycemic-hyperinsulinemic clamps to evaluate insulin resistance in humans are very laborious, invasive to some extent, and time-consuming. Therefore, a simple and precise surrogate index of insulin resistance is needed in a clinical setting in order to evaluate insulin resistance repeatedly and/or in many subjects. To date, several surrogate indexes of insulin resistance have been proposed, and their validity has been examined in comparison with an index for the euglycemic-hyperinsulinemic clamp. Among these indexes, the simplest index is the homeostasis model assessment (HOMA-R) insulin resistance index, which has been proposed by the Oxford group [34–36]. Furthermore, a reciprocal index of logarithmic HOMA-R, the quantitative insulin sensitivity check index (QUICKI), was also reported to be a useful index for insulin resistance [37, 38]. These indexes are calculated using conventional units for convenience as follows:

$$\text{HOMA-R} = \text{FIRI} \times \text{FPG}/405$$
$$\text{QUICKI} = 1/\{\text{Log}(\text{FIRI}) + \text{Log}(\text{FPG})\}$$
$$\text{QUICKI} = 1/\{\text{Log}(\text{HOMA-R}) + 6.00\}$$

where FIRI represents fasting IRI (μU/mL) and FPG is the fasting plasma glucose level (mg/dL).

We also found that in T2DM patients treated with diet therapy alone and sulfonylurea, HOMA-R is closely associated with M/I values obtained according to the standard protocol of the euglycemic-hyperinsulinemic clamp as stated above [9]. Furthermore, such close associations were also found in T2DM patients with and without obesity or with relatively higher fasting plasma glucose up to <200 mg/dL [15, 16]. The QUICKI, a reciprocal index of logarithmic HOMA-R, also showed an association with M/I values [15, 16]. Furthermore, we have also proposed a HOMA-R index combined with serum adiponectin level, HOMA-AD [19], using a collaborative study of three university hospitals using AP in Japan. Adiponectin, an adipocytokine specifically secreted from the adipose tissue, is abundant in serum, and its level is also inversely correlated with insulin resistance [18]. HOMA-AD is calculated from the following formula:

$$\text{HOMA-AD} = \text{FPG} \times \text{Fasting IRI}/\text{AD}$$

where AD is the serum level of adiponectin (mg/dL).

In 117 subjects with T2DM, IGT, or NGT, HOMA-AD showed a stronger association with the M value than HOMA-R or the adiponectin level alone.

15.6.1.2 The Insulin Tolerance Test, K_{ITT}

An insulin tolerance test is a direct method for measuring insulin sensitivity in humans and animals. In 1962, Lundbaek first proposed the concept and method of an insulin tolerance test, K_{ITT} (%/min), as an index for insulin sensitivity [39]. K_{ITT} indicates the slope of the decreasing line of the log-transformed blood glucose level against time (min) after an intravenous bolus injection of insulin (0.1 U/kg). The formula is as follows:

$$\text{Log}(\text{PG}) = a + b \times \text{Time}$$
$$\text{t}_{1/2} = \text{Log}(1/2)/\text{b} = -0.3 \times \text{b}$$
$$K_{ITT} = \left(0.693/\text{t}_{1/2}\right) \times 100 = -230.2 \times b$$

where PG is the plasma glucose level (mg/dL), time is the min after insulin injection, a is the intercept, and b is the slope of the regression line.

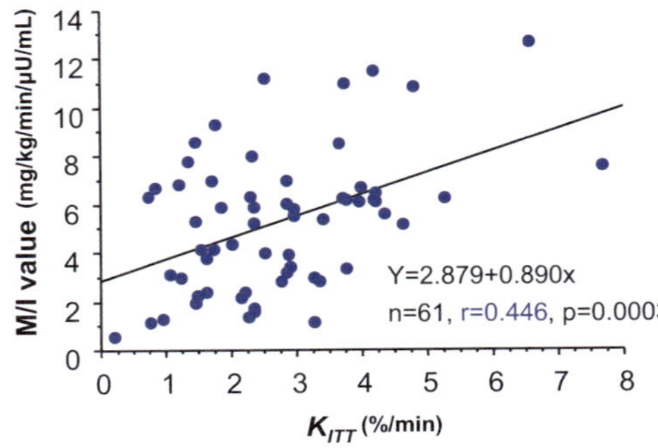

Fig. 15.9 Relatively moderate association of K_{ITT} measured by the insulin tolerance test with an insulin resistance index, the M/I value, which is calculated by the standard protocol of a euglycemic-hyperinsulinemic clamp in 61 type 2 diabetic patients ($r = 0.446$, $p = 0.0003$)

Bonora et al. have reported a strong association of K_{ITT} with an index measured by the euglycemic-hyperinsulinemic clamp. Only 25 healthy, obese, or T2DM patients were analyzed in the study, and the correlation coefficient between the two indexes was 0.811 [40]. To clarify the usefulness of K_{ITT} in a clinical setting, we evaluated K_{ITT} according to the original methods of Lundbaek and Bonora et al. and the M/I value by the standard protocol for a euglycemic-hyperinsulinemic clamp in 61 Japanese T2DM patients. Figure 15.9 shows the relatively moderate association of K_{ITT} with M/I values ($r = 0.446$, $p = 0.0003$), which is not much stronger than the previously reported association with HOMA-R, HOMA-AD, or QUICKI [9, 15, 16].

In addition, we have summarized the correlation coefficients of surrogate indexes as well as the M/I value and possible cutoff level of each surrogate marker for clinical use (Table 15.4). The cutoff level for insulin resistance in each index is equal to the mean-1 SD for 30 healthy subjects. The determination of cutoff levels for the evaluation of insulin resistance has a lot of limitations and issues, since the cutoff levels are widely distributed even in healthy subjects. However, the cutoff levels of each index (Table 15.4) are likely to be reasonable and plausible for clinical diabetologists and physicians. Further studies with a sufficient number of subjects from multicenter, multiethnic populations using the standard protocol for a euglycemic clamp study is needed for a more precise and definitive surrogate index of insulin resistance.

15.6.1.3 New Reports Using the Standard Protocol with the STG Model of the Artificial Pancreas

Tajiri et al. have proposed a new index, estimated glucose infusion rate (EGIR), as a surrogate index for insulin resistance, from a study of 25 healthy subjects and 24 T2DM patients. They used multiple regression models and the standard euglycemic-hyperinsulinemic clamp protocol with the STG-22 model of the AP [22]. EGIR is calculated from waist circumference (WC, cm), serum triglyceride

Table 15.4 The correlation coefficient for surrogate indexes of insulin resistance (IR) with M/I values and possible cutoff levels for insulin resistance for the clinical use of each surrogate marker

	Healthy with NGT ($n = 120$)	Type 2 diabetes mellitus ($n = 121$)	Correlation coefficient, r[a]	Cutoff level for IR[b]	Practical cutoff level[c]
M/I value	10.3 ± 5.1[d]	5.41 ± 2.87	–	<5.20	–
K_{ITT}[e]	–	2.72 ± 1.4[d]	0.446[e]	<2.61[a]	–
HOMA-R	1.22 ± 1.16	2.06 ± 1.60	−0.540	>2.28	>2.5
FIRI	5.16 ± 4.4	5.87 ± 3.9	−0.579	>6.37	>8.0
1/HOMA-R	1.23 ± 0.82	0.76 ± 0.52	0.681	<0.71	<0.4
QUICKI	0.39 ± 0.04	0.36 ± 0.04	0.685	<0.36	<0.34

NGT normal glucose tolerance, *M/I* value, an insulin resistance index, K_{ITT} a measure of the insulin tolerance test, *FIRI* fasting immunoreactive insulin level, *HOMA-R* homeostasis model assessment insulin resistance index, *QUICKI* quantitative insulin sensitivity check index

[a]Correlation coefficient for each index from univariate regression analysis with M/I values

[b]Cutoff level to mean-1 standard deviation estimated from univariate regression analysis of 120 healthy subjects with NGT

[c]Possible cutoff level for each index in view of simplicity and clinical practice

[d]Mean ± standard deviation of M/I values in 30 healthy subjects with NGT and a mean body mass index of 22.02 kg/m^2

[e]Only 61 subjects with type 2 diabetes mellitus were included in this test

levels (TG, mg/dL), and high-density lipoprotein cholesterol levels (HDL-C, mg/dL) as follows:

$$\text{EGIR} = 25.772 - 0.101 \times \text{WC} - 9.444 \times \text{Log(TG)/Log(HDL-C)}$$

The EGIR index reportedly had a strong correlation with the GIR measured using a euglycemic-hyperinsulinemic clamp in healthy and T2DM patients ($r = 0.791$ and $r = 0.702$, respectively).

Kato et al. examined the association between ectopic fat and organ-specific insulin resistance in insulin-target organs in 69 patients with nonalcoholic fatty liver disease using the standard euglycemic-hyperinsulinemic clamp protocol with tracer infusion [24]. In their study, hepatic glucose production was reduced to an average of 0.69 mg/kg/min (69 %) from the basal level of 2.43 mg/kg/min when the average SSPI was 110 μU/mL. They found that liver fat accumulation as measured by proton magnetic resonance spectroscopy was closely associated with insulin resistance in the liver and skeletal muscle and proposed a central role for liver fat accumulation in insulin resistance in the whole body.

15.6.2 Clinical Implications of Insulin Resistance in Various Diseases

The clinical implications of insulin resistance in various pathophysiological states can be clarified by evaluating the insulin resistance index as measured by the standard euglycemic-hyperinsulinemic clamp protocol using the AP models

STG-22 or STG-55. We have previously demonstrated the impact of insulin resistance on early alterations of atherosclerosis in T2DM patients.

The stiffness parameter β and intima-media thickness (IMT) of the common carotid artery (CCA), which are noninvasively measured by high-resolution ultrasound with an echo-tracking system, are well-established surrogate markers of subclinical atherosclerosis in cardiovascular diseases. Both the stiffness parameter β and IMT of the CCA exhibit significant inverse associations with the insulin resistance index, M/I value, in T2DM patients [8, 13]. Since the stiffness parameter β showed a closer association with the M/I value than IMT, we investigated whether a trial intervention to improve insulin resistance by aerobic exercise would improve the stiffness of the CCA [17]. In T2DM patients who performed aerobic exercise for 3 weeks, the stiffness parameter β of the CCA was improved according to the degree of improvement in the insulin resistance, i.e., the M/I value. Furthermore, microalbuminuria failed to show any significant impact on insulin resistance in T2DM patients after adjustment of obesity, but the decrease in the glomerular filtration rate was significantly associated with insulin resistance [6]. Even in T2DM patients with a decreased glomerular filtration rate, the HOMA-R index was closely associated with the M/I value, which indicates its clinical usefulness even in such patients [11]. In T2DM patients, both nephropathy and insulin resistance contributed independently to the plasma homocysteine level, which is a known risk factor for cardiovascular disease [10]. Similarly, the plasma leptin level was also attributed to insulin resistance as well as the state of diabetic nephropathy in T2DM patients [7].

Furthermore, the combination of a euglycemic-hyperinsulinemic clamp with indirect calorimetry or glucose tracer infusion could allow us further detailed analysis of glucose, fat, and protein metabolism in the whole body [18, 20, 24]. In fact, using the standard protocol with the STG model of AP, we demonstrated that plasma adiponectin level was associated with non-oxidative glucose disposal but not with the oxidative glucose disposal rate [18] and that aerobic exercise improved insulin resistance by restoring the reduced non-oxidative glucose disposal rate in T2DM patients [20].

15.7 Conclusion

Insulin resistance, mainly in the muscle in humans, plays a pivotal role in the pathophysiology not only of glucose homeostasis but also of various diseases such as cardiovascular diseases. The evaluation of insulin resistance is needed in the clinical and research fields. Among several methods for the measurement for insulin resistance, a euglycemic-hyperinsulinemic clamp, a glucose clamp technique, is a gold-standard technique in humans. In Japan, the AP (Nikkiso Co. Ltd., Tokyo, Japan), models STG-22 and STG-55, have been widely used since 1987 to perform glucose clamp techniques as well as to control glucose in surgery, brittle diabetes, etc. for a short-term period. The standard protocol using model STG-22 and STG-55, the new model, which is more advanced than model STG-22, is derived from our data and experience with approximately 400 Japanese patients. The protocol is substantiated by many publications in prestigious journals, although it is faithfully based on the original euglycemic clamp method of DeFronzo. The parameters regarding the validation of the clamp are expected to be highly precise and more reproducible than or at least comparable to those in previous reports, where the clamp was performed manually by specific algorithms. Therefore, the standard protocol for the euglycemic-hyperinsulinemic clamp using models STG-22 and STG-55 would make it possible for us to compare and evaluate insulin resistance among patients in various pathophysiological states. In the near future, further studies are needed to investigate the clinical implications of insulin resistance on various diseases using the standard protocol for the euglycemic-hyperinsulinemic clamp using the STG-22 and/or STG-55 models of the AP in a cross-sectional and/or longitudinal multicenter design.

Acknowledgments We sincerely acknowledge the contribution of our colleagues, known as "clampers" in our hospitals, who have been engaged in euglycemic clamp projects using the STG-22 and STG-55 models of the artificial pancreas since 1993, especially Yoshikazu Hiura MD PhD, Kyoko Satoh-Kogawa MD PhD, Hiroyuki Kanda MD PhD, Miyoko Matsuyoshi-Komatsu MD PhD, Shigehiko Fujiwara MD PhD, Takahiro Araki MD PhD, Megumi Teramura-Okada MD PhD, Eiko Lee-Kobayashi MD PhD, Naoya Kawano MD PhD, and Satoshi Imamura MD PhD.

References

1. DeFronzo RA, Tobin JD, Andres R (1979) Glucose clamp technique: a method for quantifying insulin secretion and resistance. Am J Physiol 237(3):E214–E223
2. Kahn CR (1978) Insulin resistance, insulin insensitivity, and insulin unresponsiveness: a necessary distinction. Metabolism 27(12 Suppl 2):1893–1902
3. Campbell PJ, Mandarino LJ, Gerich JE (1988) Quantification of the relative impairment in actions of insulin on hepatic glucose production and peripheral glucose uptake in non-insulin-dependent diabetes mellitus. Metabolism 37(1):15–21
4. DeFronzo RA (1988) Lilly lecture 1987. The triumvirate: beta-cell, muscle, liver. A collusion responsible for NIDDM. Diabetes 37(6):667–687
5. Ishimura E, Nishizawa Y, Emoto M, Maekawa K, Morii H (1996) Effect of insulin on urinary phosphate excretion in type II diabetes mellitus with or without renal insufficiency. Metabolism 45(6):782–786
6. Emoto M, Nishizawa Y, Maekawa K, Kawagishi T, Kogawa K, Hiura Y, Mori K, Tanaka S, Ishimura E, Inaba M, Okuno Y, Morii H (1997) Insulin resistance in non-obese, non-insulin-dependent diabetic patients with diabetic nephropathy. Metabolism 46(9):1013–1018
7. Shoji T, Nishizawa Y, Emoto M, Maekawa K, Hiura Y, Tanaka S, Kawagishi T, Okuno Y, Morii H (1997) Renal function and insulin resistance as determinants of plasma leptin levels in patients with NIDDM. Diabetologia 40(6):676–679. doi:10.1007/s001250050733
8. Emoto M, Nishizawa Y, Kawagishi T, Maekawa K, Hiura Y, Kanda H, Izumotani K, Shoji T, Ishimura E, Inaba M, Okuno Y, Morii H (1998) Stiffness indexes beta of the common carotid and femoral arteries are associated with insulin resistance in NIDDM. Diabetes Care 21 (7):1178–1182

9. Emoto M, Nishizawa Y, Maekawa K, Hiura Y, Kanda H, Kawagishi T, Shoji T, Okuno Y, Morii H (1999) Homeostasis model assessment as a clinical index of insulin resistance in type 2 diabetic patients treated with sulfonylureas. Diabetes Care 22(5):818–822
10. Emoto M, Kanda H, Shoji T, Kawagishi T, Komatsu M, Mori K, Tahara H, Ishimura E, Inaba M, Okuno Y, Nishizawa Y (2001) Impact of insulin resistance and nephropathy on homocysteine in type 2 diabetes. Diabetes Care 24(3):533–538
11. Shoji T, Emoto M, Nishizawa Y (2001) HOMA index to assess insulin resistance in renal failure patients. Nephron 89(3):348–349, doi:46098
12. Kawasaki I, Tahara H, Emoto M, Shoji T, Shioji A, Okuno Y, Inaba M, Nishizawa Y (2002) Impact of Prol2Ala variant in the peroxisome proliferator-activated receptor (PPAR) gamma2 on obesity and insulin resistance in Japanese Type 2 diabetic and healthy subjects. Osaka City Med J 48(1):23–28
13. Fujiwara S, Emoto M, Komatsu M, Motoyama K, Morioka T, Koyama H, Shoji T, Inaba M, Nishizawa Y (2003) Arterial wall thickness is associated with insulin resistance in type 2 diabetic patients. J Atheroscler Thromb 10(4):246–252
14. Motoyama K, Emoto M, Tahara H, Komatsu M, Shoji T, Inaba M, Nishizawa Y (2003) Association of muscle glycogen synthase polymorphism with insulin resistance in type 2 diabetic patients. Metabolism 52(7):895–899
15. Yokoyama H, Emoto M, Fujiwara S, Motoyama K, Morioka T, Komatsu M, Tahara H, Shoji T, Okuno Y, Nishizawa Y (2003) Quantitative insulin sensitivity check index and the reciprocal index of homeostasis model assessment in normal range weight and moderately obese type 2 diabetic patients. Diabetes Care 26(8):2426–2432
16. Yokoyama H, Emoto M, Fujiwara S, Motoyama K, Morioka T, Komatsu M, Tahara H, Koyama H, Shoji T, Inaba M, Nishizawa Y (2004) Quantitative insulin sensitivity check index and the reciprocal index of homeostasis model assessment are useful indexes of insulin resistance in type 2 diabetic patients with wide range of fasting plasma glucose. J Clin Endocrinol Metab 89(3):1481–1484
17. Yokoyama H, Emoto M, Fujiwara S, Motoyama K, Morioka T, Koyama H, Shoji T, Inaba M, Nishizawa Y (2004) Short-term aerobic exercise improves arterial stiffness in type 2 diabetes. Diabetes Res Clin Pract 65(2):85–93. doi:10.1016/j.diabres.2003.12.005
18. Yokoyama H, Emoto M, Mori K, Araki T, Teramura M, Koyama H, Shoji T, Inaba M, Nishizawa Y (2006) Plasma adiponectin level is associated with insulin-stimulated nonoxidative glucose disposal. J Clin Endocrinol Metab 91(1):290–294. doi:10.1210/jc.2004-2549
19. Matsuhisa M, Yamasaki Y, Emoto M, Shimabukuro M, Ueda S, Funahashi T, Matsuzawa Y (2007) A novel index of insulin resistance determined from the homeostasis model assessment index and adiponectin levels in Japanese subjects. Diabetes Res Clin Pract 77(1):151–154. doi:10.1016/j.diabres.2006.10.005
20. Yokoyama H, Mori K, Emoto M, Araki T, Teramura M, Mochizuki K, Tashiro T, Motozuka K, Inoue Y, Nishizawa Y (2008) Non-oxidative glucose disposal is reduced in type 2 diabetes, but can be restored by aerobic exercise. Diabetes Obes Metab 10(5):400–407. doi:10.1111/j.1463-1326.2007.00716.x
21. Mori K, Emoto M, Motoyama K, Lee E, Yamada S, Morioka T, Imanishi Y, Shoji T, Inaba M (2012) Undercarboxylated osteocalcin does not correlate with insulin resistance as assessed by euglycemic hyperinsulinemic clamp technique in patients with type 2 diabetes mellitus. Diabetol Metab Syndr 4(1):53. doi:10.1186/1758-5996-4-53
22. Tajiri Y, Sato S, Kato T, Nakayama H, Yamada K (2011) Surrogate index for insulin sensitivity composed of factors not using glucose and insulin in Japanese patients with diabetes. J Diabetes Invest 2(2):140–147. doi:10.1111/j.2040-1124.2010.00076.x
23. Tajiri Y, Sato S, Yamada K (2011) Metabolic clearance rate is a more robust and physiological parameter for insulin sensitivity than glucose infusion rate in the isoglycemic glucose clamp technique. Diabetes Technol Ther 13(10):1057–1061. doi:10.1089/dia.2011.0042

24. Kato K, Takamura T, Takeshita Y, Ryu Y, Misu H, Ota T, Tokuyama K, Nagasaka S, Matsuhisa M, Matsui O, Kaneko S (2014) Ectopic fat accumulation and distant organ-specific insulin resistance in Japanese people with nonalcoholic fatty liver disease. PLoS One 9(3), e92170. doi:10.1371/journal.pone.0092170
25. Nishida K, Shimoda S, Ichinose K, Araki E, Shichiri M (2009) What is artificial endocrine pancreas? Mechanism and history. World J Gastroenterol 15(33):4105–4110
26. Albisser AM, Leibel BS, Ewart TG, Davidovac Z, Botz CK, Zingg W (1974) An artificial endocrine pancreas. Diabetes 23(5):389–396
27. Albisser AM, Leibel BS, Ewart TG, Davidovac Z, Botz CK, Zingg W, Schipper H, Gander R (1974) Clinical control of diabetes by the artificial pancreas. Diabetes 23(5):397–404
28. Shichiri M, Kawamori R, Yamasaki Y, Inoue M, Shigeta Y, Abe H (1978) Computer algorithm for the artificial pancreatic beta cell. Artif Organs 2(suppl):247–250
29. Kawamori R, Shichiri M, Goriya Y, Yamasaki Y, Shigeta Y, Abe H (1978) Importance of insulin secretion based on the rate of change in blood glucose concentration in glucose tolerance, assessed by the artificial beta cell. Acta Endocrinol (Copenh) 87(2):339–351
30. Andrews J, Klimes I, Vasquez B, Nagulesparan M, Reaven GM (1984) Can mixed venous blood be used to measure insulin action during the hyperinsulinemic clamp? Horm Metab Res 16(Suppl 1):164–166. doi:10.1055/s-2007-1014924
31. Wahab PJ, Rijnsburger AW, Oolbekkink M, Heine RJ (1992) Venous versus arterialized venous blood for assessment of blood glucose levels during glucose clamping: comparison in healthy men. Horm Metab Res 24(12):576–579. doi:10.1055/s-2007-1003393
32. Morris AD, Ueda S, Petrie JR, Connell JM, Elliott HL, Donnelly R (1997) The euglycemic hyperinsulinemic clamp: an evaluation of current methodology. Clin Exp Pharmacol Physiol 24(7):513–518
33. Liu D, Moberg E, Kollind M, Lins PE, Adamson U, Macdonald IA (1992) Arterial, arterialized venous, venous and capillary blood glucose measurements in normal man during hyperinsulinemic euglycemia and hypoglycemia. Diabetologia 35(3):287–290
34. Matthews DR, Hosker JP, Rudenski AS, Naylor BA, Treacher DF, Turner RC (1985) Homeostasis model assessment: insulin resistance and beta-cell function from fasting plasma glucose and insulin concentrations in man. Diabetologia 28(7):412–419
35. Levy JC, Matthews DR, Hermans MP (1998) Correct homeostasis model assessment (HOMA) evaluation uses the computer program. Diabetes Care 21(12):2191–2192
36. Wallace TM, Levy JC, Matthews DR (2004) Use and abuse of HOMA modeling. Diabetes Care 27(6):1487–1495
37. Katz A, Nambi SS, Mather K, Baron AD, Follmann DA, Sullivan G, Quon MJ (2000) Quantitative insulin sensitivity check index: a simple, accurate method for assessing insulin sensitivity in humans. J Clin Endocrinol Metab 85(7):2402–2410. doi:10.1210/jcem.85.7.6661
38. Chen H, Sullivan G, Yue LQ, Katz A, Quon MJ (2003) QUICKI is a useful index of insulin sensitivity in subjects with hypertension. Am J Physiol Endocrinol Metab 284(4):E804–E812
39. Lundbaek K (1962) Intravenous glucose tolerance as a tool in definition and diagnosis of diabetes mellitus. Br Med J 1(5291):1507–1513
40. Bonora E, Moghetti P, Zancanaro C, Cigolini M, Querena M, Cacciatori V, Corgnati A, Muggeo M (1989) Estimates of in vivo insulin action in man: comparison of insulin tolerance tests with euglycemic and hyperglycemic glucose clamp studies. J Clin Endocrinol Metab 68 (2):374–378. doi:10.1210/jcem-68-2-374

Chapter 16
Sarcopenia in Diabetes Mellitus

Ken Sugimoto, Chung-Chi Wang, and Hiromi Rakugi

Abstract Sarcopenia is an age-related loss of skeletal muscle mass and strength. In this chapter, advances in the association of sarcopenia and diabetes mellitus are discussed. Falls in diabetic patients associate with decline of muscle mass or strength in the elderly. Insulin resistance impairs the protein regeneration in skeletal muscle and also induces the protein breakdown and muscle wasting, leading to development of sarcopenia. This insulin resistance suggests the most important linkage between sarcopenia and diabetes. Sarcopenia and obesity appear to have additive effects on insulin resistance and age-related changes in body composition. Loss of skeletal muscle mass affecting glucose disposal and impaired energy homeostasis affecting muscle protein content, together, might lead to a vicious cycle. Insulin resistance and inflammation leads to muscle wasting through the pathways involved in Akt/PKB, FoxOs, PGC-1*α*, and AMPK. The accumulation of AGEs through glucose intolerance enhanced by mitochondrial ROS with promotion of apoptosis leads to the development of muscle wasting. Exercise is known as the most efficient treatment of sarcopenia with diabetes but less information is known for nutritional replenishment or medications. Sarcopenia in diabetes mellitus would have higher physical dysfunction and mortality risks than those in nondiabetic older adults.

Keywords Sarcopenia • Diabetes mellitus • Obesity • Insulin resistance • AGEs

16.1 Introduction

The aging population is increasing worldwide. The older population of those aged 65 years is expected to reach 16.2 % of the total world's population and the "oldest-old" aged 80 years or older will increase from 1.6 to 4.4 % by 2050 [1]. In the elderly, functional decline is typically associated with the increase of body fat and the reduction of lean muscle quality; this contributes to physical disability [2] known as sarcopenia. Sarcopenia is related to frailty, glucose homeostasis

K. Sugimoto (✉) • C.-C. Wang • H. Rakugi
Geriatric Medicine, Osaka University Graduate School of Medicine, 2-2 Yamadaoka, Suita, Osaka 565-0871, Japan
e-mail: sugimoto@geriat.med.osaka-u.ac.jp

M. Inaba (ed.), *Musculoskeletal Disease Associated with Diabetes Mellitus*,
DOI 10.1007/978-4-431-55720-3_16

impairment [3], and geriatric syndromes [4] which affect 20–50 % of adults aged over 60 [5]. Obesity and diabetes appeared to be at higher risks of processing metabolic dysfunction, contributing to the progression of sarcopenia [6] related to alterations of decreased insulin sensitivity [7], unbalanced fuel oxidation [8], and reduced muscle protein content [9].

Diabetes is currently viewed as the most common metabolic dysfunction of this century and referred to high levels of circulating glucose and overall insulin resistance. Epidemiological studies reported that the number of new diabetic patients has increased by 50 % over the last 10 years [10]. The incidence of type 2 diabetes (T2D) in people older than 60 years old was more than 20 % higher than in younger people [11], and around 80 % of people with T2D were obese [12]. Various clinical studies also indicated that obesity and insulin resistance were associated with T2D, which might play important roles in the pathogenesis of physical function decline and sarcopenia [13]. The interplay between obesity and diabetes in an age-related sarcopenia population is now considered as an important concern in geriatrics. Here, we discussed the interactions and mechanisms of sarcopenia in diabetes mellitus and considered the future perspectives of this area.

16.2 Evidence in Clinical Studies for Sarcopenia and Diabetes

16.2.1 Fall in Skeletal Muscle Function Decline with T2D

The primary function of the skeletal muscle is to generate force and to provide locomotion. Fall is one of the geriatric syndromes, which has approximately 30 % of people aged 65 and older fall each year [14] and frequently leads to the risks of injury and disability. It has been reported that increased falls in diabetic patients with hypoglycemia [15] are associated with 1 % muscle size decline per year after age 50 [16]. Further, older adults with T2D have shown an accelerated decline in leg lean mass, muscle strength, and functional capacity in comparison with normoglycemic controls [17]. In addition, in T2D patients in the elderly, leg muscle strength has been presented to be 30 % lower compared with nondiabetic controls in a 3-year-period study [18]. Therefore, T2D may be associated with increasing fall risks through loss of skeletal muscle mass and strength, especially in older adults.

16.2.2 Insulin Resistance and Skeletal Muscle

Insulin, which maintains blood-glucose homeostasis, induces glucose uptake into muscle tissues and mediates lipolysis in adipose tissues. Skeletal muscle plays an important role in glucose metabolism and mediates whole-body insulin-stimulated glucose uptake [19]. In T2D, insulin resistance impairs the balance between protein synthesis and degradation in skeletal muscle cells, which induces muscle wasting [20] and leads to the development of sarcopenia. This insulin resistance suggests the most important linkage between sarcopenia and T2D. T2D and muscle weakness may provide a vicious cycle: loss of skeletal muscle mass affects glucose disposal and energy homeostasis impairment affects muscle protein content.

16.2.3 Sarcopenic Obesity

Recently, obesity incidence has also increased in the older population. Sarcopenia and obesity in elderly subjects appeared to have additive effects on insulin resistance and age-related changing in body composition compared with the obesity condition [21]. Interestingly, insulin resistance is associated with sarcopenia in both non-obese and obese individuals, but only sarcopenic obese individuals have established the associations with insulin resistance and dysglycemia, with or without diabetes [22]. This suggested that sarcopenia could be developed independently from obesity and sarcopenic obese individuals with more unfavorable physical dysfunction than individuals with neither sarcopenia nor obesity. Altogether, sarcopenic obesity could be described as having a larger amount of fat but lower lean muscle mass, excess of energy intake, physical dysfunction, impairment of insulin sensitivity, and glucose homeostasis [23]. The diagnostic criteria for sarcopenic obesity in the early stages could be helpful in the clinical observation for the reduction of health risks in the aged society. The interactions of sarcopenia, diabetes, and obesity have been summarized in Fig. 16.1.

16.3 Evidences in Basic Studies for Sarcopenia and Diabetes

16.3.1 Muscle Fiber-Type Switching

Evaluation of changes in skeletal muscle fiber composition during the early stages of the metabolic syndrome and diabetes is required to provide essential insights as to fiber-type distribution. Age-related sarcopenia is associated with muscle constitution in differing amounts, in individual skeletal muscle [24], and a decrease of size and number of fast type II muscle fiber has been observed [25, 26]. The EDL, or the extensor digitorum longus glycolytic muscle, is predominantly composed of type IIb fibers which has mainly reduced by 25–30 % in the cross-sectional area of the skeletal muscle of humans aged 70 [27]. In addition, insulin resistance is associated with higher proportions of glycolytic fast-twitch type IIb fibers [28]. The muscle transformation studies of the extended periods of bed rest have

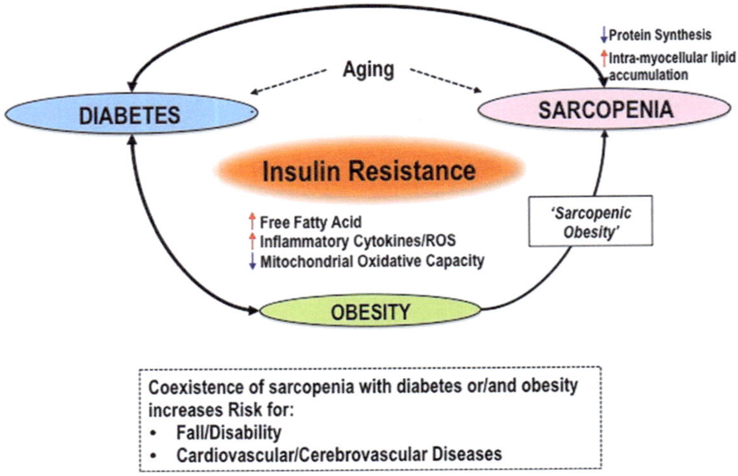

Fig. 16.1 Interaction between sarcopenia and diabetes. Insulin resistance in skeletal muscle is the most important link between sarcopenia and diabetes. Sarcopenia and obesity appear to have additive effects on insulin resistance and age-related changing in body composition. Diabetes, sarcopenia, and obesity may provide a vicious cycle: loss of skeletal muscle mass affects glucose disposal and energy homeostasis impairment affects muscle protein content. Coexistence of sarcopenia with diabetes or/and obesity increases the risk for fall or disability and cardio- and cerebrovascular diseases

observed the slow-to-fast muscle transitions (myosin heavy chain, MyHCI to MyHCII) [29]. This shift in fiber-type composition may lead to the increase of the total EDL content in the aging process of muscle atrophy; however, this increase failed to prevent natural muscle aging and resulted in total skeletal muscle mass reduction in sarcopenia. The decrease in total type II fiber may have negative effects on the production of essentially muscular power in daily life, which is a pathognomonic change in sarcopenia or sarcopenia in diabetes.

16.3.2 Inflammation in Skeletal Muscle

Inflammation, an important mediator in the pathogenesis of insulin resistance, has been observed in both diabetes mellitus and sarcopenia. Since the muscle is the primary tissue which produces and responds to a variety of hormones and cytokines, it has been involved in modulating muscle protein degradation and myogenesis through the prevention of inflammation; further, pro-inflammation is counteracted by insulin resistance [30]. TNF-α is highly expressed in adipose tissues from obese subjects, which develops insulin resistance, induces IL-6 [31], and blocks muscle tissues differentiation leading to sarcopenia [32]. In addition, IL-6 and TNF-α activate TNF-α-related apoptosis-inducing ligand receptors

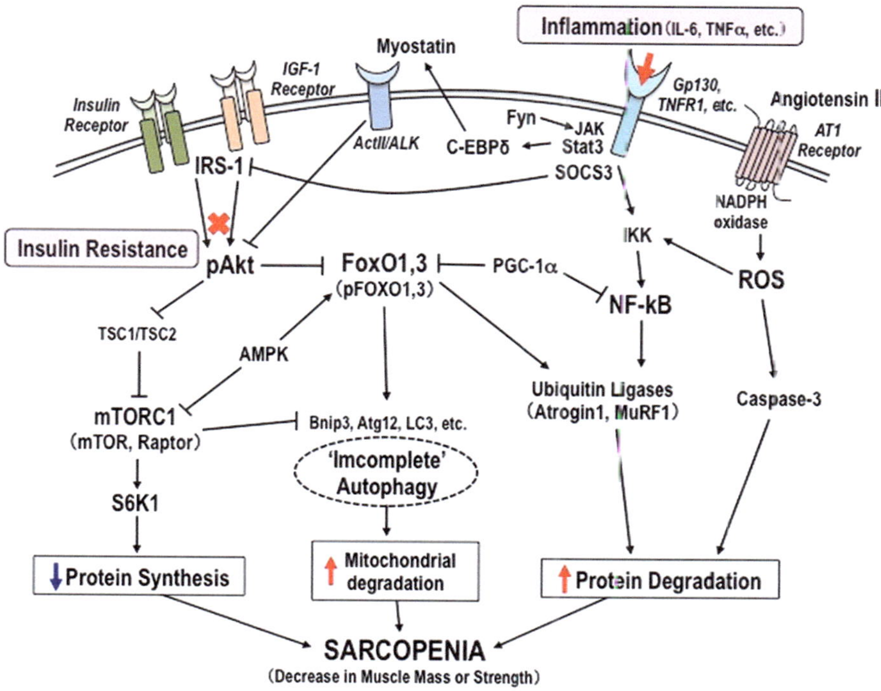

Fig. 16.2 Molecular mechanism of muscle wasting in diabetes. Decline of skeletal muscle mass or strength occurs under a variety of conditions and involves the regulation of muscle protein catabolism and mitochondrial dysfunction: FoxO1 and FoxO3 induce a decrease in muscle mass associated with an upregulation of ubiquitin E3 ligases MAFbx/atrogin-1 and MuRF1 expression. In cancer cachexia and sepsis, FoxOs inhibit the MAFbx/atrogin-1, MuRF1, and Bnip3 mRNA expression, which has been associated with inhibition of muscle fiber atrophy. NF-kB induces muscle breakdown by promoting protein degradations in skeletal muscle by regulation of ubiquitin-proteasome pathway (UPS). AGEs and angiotensin II via the angiotensin type 1 (AT1) receptor activate NADPH oxidase and lead to ROS production, facilitating activation of caspases, which contributes to muscle mass loss. IL-6 and TNF-α activate TNF-α-related apoptosis-inducing ligand receptors (TNFR1) which stimulate inhibitor of κB kinase (IKK) and cause NF-κB activation, thus processing the protein degradations in muscle. Signal transducer and activator of transcription 3 (STAT3) links the activation of signal transducers of the Janus kinase (JAK) protein and increases activity of the transcription factor C-EBPß and C-EBPδ involved in muscle wasting through ActII receptor and myostatin. Suppressor of cytokine signaling (SOCS3) targets IRS-1 in inflammation-induced insulin resistance. IRS-1 is rapidly degraded after IGF-1 stimulation and blocks FoxO1, leading to inhibition of atrophy. IRS-1 phosphorylation links to dephosphorylation of Akt, which mediates insulin resistance. Inactivation of tuberous sclerosis complex 1/2 (TSC1/TSC2) stimulates Akt–mTOR signaling and leads to "incomplete" autophagy in muscle wasting. AMPK inactivates mTOR and decreases the activation of ribosomal protein S6 kinase 1 (S6K1), an activator of protein synthesis, thereby increasing the rates of muscle mass loss. The autophagic regulator proteins, Atg12, LC3-II, and apoptotic genes Bnip3, promote mitochondrial disruption by activation of FoxOs during muscle atrophy

(TNFR1) which stimulate inhibitor of κB kinase [33, 34], causing NF-κB activation resulting in processing protein degradation in the muscle. The effects of insulin antagonizing mediated by IL-6 on skeletal muscle have been described and chronic exposure to IL-6 caused inflammation which impaired insulin-stimulated GLUT4 translocation in skeletal muscle [35]. STAT3, signal transducer and activator of transcription 3, has been characterized in myokines signaling [36] which can link the activation of signal transducers of the Janus kinase (JAK) protein [37] and increased activity of the transcription factor C-EBPß and C-EBPδ involved in muscle wasting [38] through ActII receptor and myostatin [39] (Fig. 16.2).

On the other hand, IL-6 or IL-15 [40, 41], which is secreted from skeletal muscle, suppresses TNF-α effects on the exercise conditions [42]. These cytokines produced from skeletal muscle are called "myokines" and exert autocrine, paracrine, or endocrine effects. The interaction between myokines production and diabetes is still unclear, but myokines can be the candidate biomarkers for metabolic disorders, including diabetes.

16.3.3 Molecule-Related Signaling Pathways in Muscle Wasting

Many reports have shown the molecular mechanisms for muscle wasting using animal models which fed on high-fat or sucrose diet and of diabetes. The molecules signaling pathways related to muscle wasting has been shown in this section.

16.3.3.1 Akt/PKB Signaling

In skeletal muscle, Akt/PKB plays a key role in insulin and PI3K/Akt/mTOR signaling pathway, which is regulating energy metabolism and protein synthesis. Previous studies have shown that SOCS3, suppressor of cytokine signaling, targeted to IRS-1 in inflammation-induced insulin resistance [43]. IRS-1 is rapidly degraded after IGF-1 stimulation and blocking of FoxO1 leads to inhibition of atrophy. The activation of Akt/PKB results in the glucose uptake through the stimulation and translocation of GLUT4, leading to the increased uptake of glucose, thus decreasing the amount of circulating glucose and regulating glucose metabolism upon insulin exposure [44, 45]. However, IRS-1 phosphorylation is linked to dephosphorylation of Akt/PKB [46], which mediates insulin resistance and further inactivates tuberous sclerosis complex 1/2 (TSC1/TSC2) [47] which stimulated Akt–mTOR signaling and autophagy in muscular dystrophy (Fig. 16.2), since signaling through IGF-1/PI3K/Akt activated the mechanistic target of rapamycin (mTOR) pathway [48] and critically mediated the fork head boxO (FoxO) transcription factors [49]. Protein synthesis in skeletal muscle is strongly related to Akt/PKB signaling, through the activation of mTOR [48], to regulate GSK3 (glycogen synthase kinase 3) activity which results in enhanced glycogen synthesis [50]. Furthermore, the defected of insulin actions may produce the increase of protein degradation [51]; this is supposed the Akt/FoxO pathway may contribute to sarcopenia-related muscle protein degradation.

16.3.3.2 FoxOs Transcription Factors

Decline of skeletal muscle mass or strength involves regulation of muscle protein catabolism and mitochondrial dysfunction. FoxOs are important regulators of muscle energy homeostasis and carbohydrate catabolism in the fast state [52]. FoxO1 and FoxO3 induced a decreasing of muscle mass which associated with an upregulation of ubiquitin E3 ligases MAFbx/atrogin-1 and the muscle ring-finger protein 1 (MuRF1) expression [53]. Recently, defect in autophagy-dependent signaling, an important mechanism for maintaining cell self-renew and protein turnover, is also observed in various muscular dystrophies [54]. The autophagic regulator proteins, LC3-II, Atg12, and Bnip3, promote mitochondrial disruption by activation of FoxOs during muscle atrophy [55]. Furthermore, mitochondrial dysfunction has been proposed through FoxOs, switching of muscle type from slow-twitch oxidative type I fiber to fast-twitch glycolytic fiber (MyHCI to MyHCII).

16.3.3.3 PGC-1α and AMPK

In sarcopenia and sarcopenic obese individuals, insulin resistance is involved in developing muscle atrophy in aging and diabetes mellitus [56]. Importantly, high-fat diet-induced insulin resistance observed the reduction of skeletal muscle mitochondrial function and decreased expression of peroxisome proliferator-activated receptor gamma coactivator 1 alpha (PGC-1α) [57]; thus, the hypothesis of mitochondrial dysfunction leading to sarcopenia has been in attention. The downregulation of PGC-1α by high-fat diet implicated the development of skeletal muscle insulin resistance of T2D individuals compared to nondiabetic individuals [58–61]. It was also suggested that PGC-1α plays an important role in fiber-type switching from fast-twitch glycolytic fiber into slow-twitch oxidative type I fiber [62]. These fiber-type switching effects through PGC-1α might be induced by PGC-1α1. However, muscle-specific induction of PGC-1α4, but not PGC-1α1, has shown the increase of muscle mass and strength, resistance to cancer cachexia through activating IGF-1, and suppressing myostatin gene expression [63]. Altogether, PGC-1α and its isoforms may play a crucial role in regulating mitochondrial biogenesis and muscle mass and strength.

AMP-activated protein kinase (AMPK) is a primary regulator of skeletal muscle metabolic homeostasis [64]. AMPK impacts the insulin-mediated effects on muscle protein synthesis through the interfering by the Akt/PKB signaling pathway [65] and promotes glucose uptake and oxidation through migration of GLUT4 to the cellular membrane [66]. Importantly, AMPK activation by AICAR in skeletal muscle [67, 68] improved muscle function and mitochondrial activity in muscle atrophy. In addition, AMPK inactivated mTOR and decreased the activation of ribosomal protein S6 kinase 1, an activator of protein synthesis, thereby increasing the rates of sarcopenic muscle mass loss. On the other hand, AMPK-mediated activation of FoxO3 contributed to the proteolysis with the expression of muscle atrophy F-box (MAFbx/atrogin-1) and MuRF1 [69]. AMPK also was found to promote directly the phosphorylation of PGC-1α and to induce mitochondrial biogenesis [70, 71]. Further investigations will be needed to clarify these conflicting findings on the role of AMPK in the development of sarcopenia.

16.3.4 ROS and Mitochondrial Dysfunction

ROS and oxidative stress have been considered as important pathogenic components of metabolic diseases [72]. Mitochondrial dysfunction produces increased amounts of ROS, resulting in oxidative damage, which includes decreased mitochondrial content and oxidative capacity and increased mitochondrial DNA mutations [73]. Activation of the renin-angiotensin system (RAS) is commonly observed in patients either with diabetes, obesity, or both. ROS production could be enhanced by angiotensin II (Ang II), which stimulated the angiotensin type 1 (AT1, G-protein-coupled) receptor and activated NADPH oxidase. In rodent model, RAS blockade increases survival rate and prevents age-related defects [74]. Thus, it is suggested that Ang II contributes to mitochondrial dysfunction in the aging process. This indicated that diabetes mellitus and age-related sarcopenia may have additive effects for ROS production. Furthermore, NF-kB induces muscle breakdown by promoting protein degradations in skeletal muscle through regulation of ubiquitin-proteasome pathway (UPS) [75]. The maintenance of mitochondrial morphology and regeneration of self-renewal could be due to the mitochondrial fusion and fission interactions. This mitochondrial fission contributes to the quality control of creating new mitochondria and removing of damaged mitochondria during high cellular stress [76]. Disruptions of either event may induce metabolic disorders and leads to developmental defects and diseases [77], suggesting that the maintenance in aging muscle cell mitochondrial morphology may prevent cell dysfunction.

16.3.5 AGE Accumulation and Diabetic Neuropathy

The formation of advanced glycation end products (AGEs) is generated through nonenzymatic glycation of many heterogenous compounds and the complex and diverse possibilities of reaction of glucose with proteins, lipids, and nucleic acids [78]. AGEs are regarded as key molecules to be one source of oxidative stress in aging [79]. It is well known that long-term high-fat diet and endogenously formed AGEs contribute to the progression of diabetic complications [80]. AGEs are produced endogenously via food, and the concentration of circulating AGEs increases in high-fat diet [81]. Interestingly, it has been reported that AGE accumulation was decreased in association with administration of insulin and greater in fast-twitch fibers in non-insulin diabetic animal model [82]. AGE/RAGE in aging stimulates the activation of ERK1/2 and P38 MAPK pathways and increased apoptosis transcription factor such as NF-kB [83]. In recent years, the modified protein methylglyoxal (MG) was observed to involve AGE formation in aged individuals [84, 85]. MG is believed to induce protein glycation leading to the formation of AGEs; some reports indicated that MG or AGEs administration to Sprague-Dawley rats resulted in increased glucose levels and insulin resistance [86, 87]. Moreover, the direct effects of AGEs from Tanaka's group have shown that AGE2 or AGE3 markedly suppressed the expressions of MyoD and myogenin protein on myoblastic differentiation in C2C12 cells and significantly inhibited mRNA expression. This suggested that AGEs have direct negative effects on myogenesis [88].

T2D leads to chronic hyperglycemia and is related to the major age-related microvascular complications such as microangiopathic and macroangiopathic damage and motor neuropathies (diabetic neuropathy) [89]. Enhanced mitochondrial apoptosis has also been observed in muscle denervation and implicated in diabetes and neuropathy in human neuromuscular disorders, which exhibited significant muscle weakness and reduced functional capacity in the ankle and knee [90]. In addition, the AGE-RAGE axis and accumulation of AGEs in the peripheral nerve also play important roles in the pathogenesis of diabetic neuropathy [91], thus impairing the quality of life of diabetic patients. It is not yet established, but increasing studies suggested that accumulation of AGEs through glucose intolerance enhanced by mitochondrial ROS together with promotion of apoptosis leads to an elevated risk of developing sarcopenia.

16.4 Potential Treatments for Sarcopenia with Diabetes

Epidemiological and intervention studies for exercise training have strongly supported its efficacy for prevention, leading to the management of diabetes and sarcopenia. In exercising and amino acid supplementation (AAS) study [92], not only enhanced muscle mass or walking speed but also enhanced muscle strength was observed in sarcopenic women. In addition, high-intensity progressive resistance training was effective in improving glycemic control and physical activity, increasing lean mass among high-risk older adults with T2D [93]. Thus, resistance training and a combination of training and nutritional replenishment, like amino acids, might also be a beneficial intervention in sarcopenia with diabetes.

As for antidiabetic drugs, a class of thiazolidinediones (TZDs) can activate AMPK in insulin-resistant animals [94] and mediate mitochondrial effects on neurodegeneration [95]. In T2D patients, rosiglitazone [96] and pioglitazone [97] both enhanced insulin reactions and reduced plasma nonesterified fatty acids [97], which improved insulin-stimulated muscle glucose disposal. These TZDs may involve a potential role of age-related mitochondrial dysfunction, neurodegeneration diseases [98], and diabetes with sarcopenia. Indeed, a combination of pioglitazone and resistance training leads to a potentiated effect on muscle power compared with resistance training alone in older obese women [99]. Metformin also activates AMPK and enhances insulin sensitivity in skeletal muscle, thereby stimulating glucose uptake [100]; however, there has been no reliable clinical evidence so far. At any rate, insulin resistance and glucose intolerance can contribute to muscle wasting; therefore, the therapies for improving insulin resistance and glucose intolerance are supposed to have a potential to prevent sarcopenia.

16.5 Closing Remarks and Perspectives

We conclude that subjects with sarcopenia in diabetes mellitus would have higher physical dysfunction and mortality risks than those nondiabetic older adults. Sarcopenic obesity could be described as independent of sarcopenia and obesity, both related to insulin resistance and inflammation in diabetes mellitus. We introduce the molecular pathways underlying the pathogenesis of sarcopenia in diabetes in this chapter and, in particular, mitochondrial dysfunction and AGE accumulation might be significant targets common to sarcopenia and diabetes. Further studies will be needed to improve our knowledge on the interaction between diabetes and sarcopenia and to establish beneficial therapeutic interventions combined with exercise for slowing down and reversing the loss of muscle mass and strength in older adults with T2D.

References

1. United Nations (2007) World population prospects, the 2006 revision: highlights. United Nations, New York
2. Smalley KJ, Knerr AN, Kendrick ZV, Colliver JA, Owen OE (1990) Reassessment of body-mass indexes. Am J Clin Nutr 52(3):405–408
3. Dutta C, Hadley EC, Lexell J (1997) Sarcopenia and physical performance in old age: overview. Muscle Nerve 5:S5–S9
4. Kinney JM (2004) Nutritional frailty, sarcopenia and falls in the elderly. Curr Opin Clin Nutr Metab Care 7(1):15–20. doi:10.1097/01.mco.0000109601.04238.46
5. Berger MJ, Doherty TJ (2010) Sarcopenia: prevalence, mechanisms, and functional consequences. Interdiscip Top Gerontol 37:94–114. doi:10.1159/000319997
6. Villareal DT, Banks M, Siener C, Sinacore DR, Klein S (2004) Physical frailty and body composition in obese elderly men and women. Obes Res 12(6):913–920. doi:10.1038/oby.2004.111
7. Goodman MN, Ruderman NB (1979) Insulin sensitivity of rat skeletal muscle: effects of starvation and aging. Am J Physiol 236(5):E519–E523

8. Sial S, Coggan AR, Carroll R, Goodwin J, Klein S (1996) Fat and carbohydrate metabolism during exercise in elderly and young subjects. Am J Physiol-Endocrinol Metab 271(6):E983–E989
9. Dardevet D, Sornet C, Balage M, Grizard J (2000) Stimulation of in vitro rat muscle protein synthesis by leucine decreases with age. J Nutr 130(11):2630–2635
10. Danaei G, Finucane MM, Lu Y, Singh GM, Cowan MJ, Paciorek CJ et al (2011) National, regional, and global trends in fasting plasma glucose and diabetes prevalence since 1980: systematic analysis of health examination surveys and epidemiological studies with 370 - country-years and 2.7 million participants. Lancet 378(9785):31–40. doi:10.1016/s0140-6736(11)60679-x
11. Styskal J, Van Remmen H, Richardson A, Salmon AB (2012) Oxidative stress and diabetes: what can we learn about insulin resistance from antioxidant mutant mouse models? Free Radic Biol Med 52(1):46–58. doi:10.1016/j.freeradbiomed.2011.10.441
12. Laaksonen DE, Niskanen L, Lakka HM, Lakka TA, Uusitupa M (2004) Epidemiology and treatment of the metabolic syndrome. Ann Med 35(5):332–346. doi:10.1080/07853890410031849
13. Stenholm S, Harris TB, Rantanen T, Visser M, Kritchevsky SB, Ferrucci L (2008) Sarcopenic obesity: definition, cause and consequences. Curr Opin Clin Nutr Metab Care 11(6):693–700. doi:10.1097/MCO.0b013e328312c37d
14. Gillespie LD, Gillespie WJ, Robertson MC, Lamb SE, Cumming RG, Rowe BH (2003) Interventions for preventing falls in elderly people. Cochrane Database Syst Rev (4): Cd000340. doi: 10.1002/14651858.cd000340
15. Marzetti E, Leeuwenburgh C (2006) Skeletal muscle apoptosis, sarcopenia and frailty at old age. Exp Gerontol 41(12):1234–1238. doi:10.1016/j.exger.2006.08.011
16. Goodpaster BH, Park SW, Harris TB, Kritchevsky SB, Nevitt M, Schwartz AV et al (2006) The loss of skeletal muscle strength, mass, and quality in older adults: the health, aging and body composition study. J Gerontol Ser A-Biol Sci Med Sci 61(10):1059–1064
17. Leenders M, Verdijk LB, van der Hoeven L, Adam JJ, van Kranenburg J, Nilwik R et al (2013) Patients with type 2 diabetes show a greater decline in muscle mass, muscle strength, and functional capacity with aging. J Am Med Dir Assoc 14(8):585–592. doi:10.1016/j.jamda.2013.02.006
18. Park SW, Goodpaster BH, Strotmeyer ES, Kuller LH, Broudeau R, Kammerer C et al (2007) Accelerated loss of skeletal muscle strength in older adults with type 2 diabetes: the health, aging, and body composition study. Diabetes Care 30(6):1507–1512. doi:10.2337/dc06-2537
19. Corcoran MP, Lamon-Fava S, Fielding RA (2007) Skeletal muscle lipid deposition and insulin resistance: effect of dietary fatty acids and exercise. Am J Clin Nutr 85(3):662–677
20. Russell ST, Rajani S, Dhadda RS, Tisdale MJ (2009) Mechanism of induction of muscle protein loss by hyperglycaemia. Exp Cell Res 315(1):16–25. doi:10.1016/j.yexcr.2008.10.002
21. Lim S, Kim JH, Yoon JW, Kang SM, Choi SH, Park YJ et al (2010) Sarcopenic obesity: prevalence and association with metabolic syndrome in the Korean Longitudinal Study on Health and Aging (KLoSHA). Diabetes Care 33(7):1652–1654. doi:10.2337/dc10-0107
22. Srikanthan P, Hevener AL, Karlamangla AS (2010) Sarcopenia exacerbates obesity-associated insulin resistance and dysglycemia: findings from the National Health and Nutrition Examination Survey III. PLoS One 5(5):e10805. doi:10.1371/journal.pone.0010805
23. de Simone G, Pasanisi F, Ferrara AL, Roman MJ, Lee ET, Contaldo F et al (2013) Relative fat-free mass deficiency and left ventricular adaptation to obesity: the strong heart study. Int J Cardiol 168(2):729–733. doi:10.1016/j.ijcard.2012.09.055
24. Grimby G (1995) Muscle performance and structure in the elderly as studied cross-sectionally and longitudinally. J Gerontol A Biol Sci Med Sci 50(Spec No):17–22
25. Blough ER, Linderman JK (2000) Lack of skeletal muscle hypertrophy in very aged male Fischer 344 x Brown Norway rats. J Appl Physiol (Bethesda, Md: 1985) 88(4):1265–1270
26. Holloszy JO, Chen M, Cartee GD, Young JC (1991) Skeletal muscle atrophy in old rats: differential changes in the three fiber types. Mech Ageing Dev 60(2):199–213

27. Porter MM, Vandervoort AA, Lexell J (1995) Aging of human muscle: structure, function and adaptability. Scand J Med Sci Sports 5(3):129–142
28. Lillioja S, Young AA, Culter CL, Ivy JL, Abbott WG, Zawadzki JK et al (1987) Skeletal muscle capillary density and fiber type are possible determinants of in vivo insulin resistance in man. J Clin Invest 80(2):415–424. doi:10.1172/jci113088
29. Ohlendieck K (2011) Skeletal muscle proteomics: current approaches, technical challenges and emerging techniques. Skelet Muscle 1(1):6. doi:10.1186/2044-5040-1-6
30. Pedersen BK (2010) Muscle-to-fat interaction: a two-way street? J Physiol 588(Pt 1):21. doi:10.1113/jphysiol.2009.184747
31. Briaud I, Lingohr MK, Dickson LM, Wrede CE, Rhodes CJ (2003) Differential activation mechanisms of Erk-1/2 and p70(S6K) by glucose in pancreatic beta-cells. Diabetes 52 (4):974–983
32. Plomgaard P, Bouzakri K, Krogh-Madsen R, Mittendorfer B, Zierath JR, Pedersen BK (2005) Tumor necrosis factor-alpha induces skeletal muscle insulin resistance in healthy human subjects via inhibition of Akt substrate 160 phosphorylation. Diabetes 54(10):2939–2945
33. Mikkelsen HB (2010) Interstitial cells of Cajal, macrophages and mast cells in the gut musculature: morphology, distribution, spatial and possible functional interactions. J Cell Mol Med 14(4):818–832. doi:10.1111/j.1582-4934.2010.01025.x
34. Yeh WC, Shahinian A, Speiser D, Kraunus J, Billia F, Wakeham A et al (1997) Early lethality, functional NF-kappaB activation, and increased sensitivity to TNF-induced cell death in TRAF2-deficient mice. Immunity 7(5):715–725
35. Benito M (2011) Tissue specificity on insulin action and resistance: past to recent mechanisms. Acta Physiol 201(3):297–312. doi:10.1111/j.1748-1716.2010.02201.x
36. Yu H, Jove R (2004) The STATs of cancer – new molecular targets come of age. Nat Rev Cancer 4(2):97–105. doi:10.1038/nrc1275
37. Boulton TG, Zhong Z, Wen Z, Darnell JE Jr, Stahl N, Yancopoulos GD (1995) STAT3 activation by cytokines utilizing gp130 and related transducers involves a secondary modification requiring an H7-sensitive kinase. Proc Natl Acad Sci U S A 92(15):6915–6919
38. Penner G, Gang G, Sun X, Wray C, Hasselgren PO (2002) C/EBP DNA-binding activity is upregulated by a glucocorticoid-dependent mechanism in septic muscle. Am J Physiol Regul Integr Comp Physiol 282(2):R439–R444. doi:10.1152/ajpregu.00512.2001
39. Toledo M, Busquets S, Ametller E, Lopez-Soriano FJ, Argiles JM (2011) Sirtuin 1 in skeletal muscle of cachectic tumour-bearing rats: a role in impaired regeneration? J Cachex Sarcopenia Muscle 2(1):57–62. doi:10.1007/s13539-011-0018-6
40. Kern PA, Ranganathan S, Li C, Wood L, Ranganathan G (2001) Adipose tissue tumor necrosis factor and interleukin-6 expression in human obesity and insulin resistance. Am J Physiol Endocrinol Metab 280(5):E745–E751
41. Marzetti E, Carter CS, Wohlgemuth SE, Lees HA, Giovannini S, Anderson B et al (2009) Changes in IL-15 expression and death-receptor apoptotic signaling in rat gastrocnemius muscle with aging and life-long calorie restriction. Mech Ageing Dev 130(4):272–280
42. Pedersen BK, Steensberg A, Keller P, Keller C, Fischer C, Hiscock N et al (2003) Muscle-derived interleukin-6: lipolytic, anti-inflammatory and immune regulatory effects. Pflugers Arch: Eur J Physiol 446(1):9–16. doi:10.1007/s00424-002-0981-z
43. Rui L, Yuan M, Frantz D, Shoelson S, White MF (2002) SOCS-1 and SOCS-3 block insulin signaling by ubiquitin-mediated degradation of IRS1 and IRS2. J Biol Chem 277 (44):42394–42398. doi:10.1074/jbc.C200444200
44. Huang L, Gong L, Jiang X, Xing D (2014) Photoactivation of GLUT4 translocation promotes glucose uptake via PI3-K/Akt2 signaling in 3T3-L1 adipocytes. J Innov Opt Health Sci 7 (3):1–10. doi: 10.1142/s1793545813500673
45. Hajduch E, Alessi DR, Hemmings BA, Hundal HS (1998) Constitutive activation of protein kinase B alpha by membrane targeting promotes glucose and system A amino acid transport, protein synthesis, and inactivation of glycogen synthase kinase 3 in L6 muscle cells. Diabetes 47(7):1006–1013

46. Andreozzi F, Procopio C, Greco A, Mannino GC, Miele C, Raciti GA et al (2011) Increased levels of the Akt-specific phosphatase PH domain leucine-rich repeat protein phosphatase (PHLPP)-1 in obese participants are associated with insulin resistance. Diabetologia 54 (7):1879–1887. doi:10.1007/s00125-011-2116-6
47. Inoki K, Li Y, Zhu T, Wu J, Guan KL (2002) TSC2 is phosphorylated and inhibited by Akt and suppresses mTOR signalling. Nat Cell Biol 4(9):648–657. doi:10.1038/ncb839
48. Nader GA (2007) Muscle growth learns new tricks from an old dog. Nat Med 13 (9):1016–1018. doi:10.1038/nm0907-1016
49. Sandri M (2008) Signaling in muscle atrophy and hypertrophy. Physiology (Bethesda) 23:160–170. doi:10.1152/physiol.00041.2007
50. van der Velden JL, Langen RC, Kelders MC, Willems J, Wouters EF, Janssen-Heininger YM et al (2007) Myogenic differentiation during regrowth of atrophied skeletal muscle is associated with inactivation of GSK-3beta. Am J Physiol Cell Physiol 292(5):C1636–C1644. doi:10.1152/ajpcell.00504.2006
51. Welch AA (2014) The 5th international symposium of the nutrition society nutritional influences on age-related skeletal muscle loss. Proc Nutr Soc 73(1):16–33. doi:10.1017/s0029665113003698
52. Furuyama T, Kitayama K, Yamashita H, Mori N (2003) Forkhead transcription factor FOXO1 (FKHR)-dependent induction of PDK4 gene expression in skeletal muscle during energy deprivation. Biochem J 375(Pt 2):365–371. doi:10.1042/bj20030022
53. Kamei Y, Miura S, Suzuki M, Kai Y, Mizukami J, Taniguchi T et al (2004) Skeletal muscle FOXO1 (FKHR) transgenic mice have less skeletal muscle mass, down-regulated type I (slow twitch/red muscle) fiber genes, and impaired glycemic control. J Biol Chem 279 (39):41114–41123. doi:10.1074/jbc.M400674200
54. Irwin ML, Yasui Y, Ulrich CM, Bowen D, Rudolph RE, Schwartz RS et al (2003) Effect of exercise on total and intra-abdominal body fat in postmenopausal women: a randomized controlled trial. JAMA 289(3):323–330
55. McLoughlin TJ, Smith SM, DeLong AD, Wang H, Unterman TG, Esser KA (2009) FoxO1 induces apoptosis in skeletal myotubes in a DNA-binding-dependent manner. Am J Physiol Cell Physiol 297(3):C548–C555. doi:10.1152/ajpcell.00502.2008
56. Cleasby ME, Jarmin S, Eilers W, Elashry M, Andersen DK, Dickson G et al (2014) Local overexpression of the myostatin propeptide increases glucose transporter expression and enhances skeletal muscle glucose disposal. Am J Physiol-Endocrinol Metab 306(7):E814–E823. doi:10.1152/ajpendo.00586.2013
57. Henagan TM, Lenard NR, Gettys TW, Stewart LK (2014) Dietary quercetin supplementation in mice increases skeletal muscle PGC1 alpha expression, improves mitochondrial function and attenuates insulin resistance in a time-specific manner. Plos One 9(2):1–11. doi: 10.1371/journal.pone.0089365
58. Mootha VK, Lindgren CM, Eriksson KF, Subramanian A, Sihag S, Lehar J et al (2003) PGC-1alpha-responsive genes involved in oxidative phosphorylation are coordinately downregulated in human diabetes. Nat Genet 34(3):267–273. doi:10.1038/ng1180
59. Patti ME, Butte AJ, Crunkhorn S, Cusi K, Berria R, Kashyap S et al (2003) Coordinated reduction of genes of oxidative metabolism in humans with insulin resistance and diabetes: potential role of PGC1 and NRF1. Proc Natl Acad Sci U S A 100(14):8466–8471. doi:10.1073/pnas.1032913100
60. Crunkhorn S, Dearie F, Mantzoros C, Gami H, da Silva WS, Espinoza D et al (2007) Peroxisome proliferator activator receptor gamma coactivator-1 expression is reduced in obesity: potential pathogenic role of saturated fatty acids and p38 mitogen-activated protein kinase activation. J Biol Chem 282(21):15439–15450. doi:10.1074/jbc.M611214200
61. Sparks LM, Xie H, Koza RA, Mynatt R, Hulver MW, Bray GA et al (2005) A high-fat diet coordinately downregulates genes required for mitochondrial oxidative phosphorylation in skeletal muscle. Diabetes 54(7):1926–1933

62. Lin J, Wu H, Tarr PT, Zhang CY, Wu Z, Boss O et al (2002) Transcriptional co-activator PGC-1 alpha drives the formation of slow-twitch muscle fibres. Nature 418(6899):797–801. doi:10.1038/nature00904
63. Ruas JL, White JP, Rao RR, Kleiner S, Brannan KT, Harrison BC et al (2012) A PGC-1alpha isoform induced by resistance training regulates skeletal muscle hypertrophy. Cell 151 (6):1319–1331. doi:10.1016/j.cell.2012.10.050
64. Steinberg GR, Kemp BE (2009) AMPK in health and disease. Physiol Rev 89(3):1025–1078. doi:10.1152/physrev.00011.2008
65. Ohanna M, Sobering AK, Lapointe T, Lorenzo L, Praud C, Petroulakis E et al (2005) Atrophy of S6K1(-/-) skeletal muscle cells reveals distinct mTOR effectors for cell cycle and size control. Nat Cell Biol 7(3):286–294. doi:10.1038/ncb1231
66. Pehmoller C, Treebak JT, Birk JB, Chen S, Mackintosh C, Hardie DG et al (2009) Genetic disruption of AMPK signaling abolishes both contraction- and insulin-stimulated TBC1D1 phosphorylation and 14-3-3 binding in mouse skeletal muscle. Am J Physiol Endocrinol Metab 297(3):E665–E675. doi:10.1152/ajpendo.00115.2009
67. Sanchez AM, Csibi A, Raibon A, Cornille K, Gay S, Bernardi H et al (2012) AMPK promotes skeletal muscle autophagy through activation of forkhead FoxO3a and interaction with Ulk1. J Cell Biochem 113(2):695–710. doi:10.1002/jcb.23399
68. Tong JF, Yan X, Zhu MJ, Du M (2009) AMP-activated protein kinase enhances the expression of muscle-specific ubiquitin ligases despite its activation of IGF-1/Akt signaling in C2C12 myotubes. J Cell Biochem 108(2):458–468. doi:10.1002/jcb.22272
69. Nakashima K, Yakabe Y (2007) AMPK activation stimulates myofibrillar protein degradation and expression of atrophy-related ubiquitin ligases by increasing FOXO transcription factors in C2C12 myotubes. Biosci Biotechnol Biochem 71(7):1650–1656
70. Birkenfeld AL, Lee HY, Guebre-Egziabher F, Alves TC, Jurczak MJ, Jornayvaz FR et al (2011) Deletion of the mammalian INDY homolog mimics aspects of dietary restriction and protects against adiposity and insulin resistance in mice. Cell Metab 14(2):184–195. doi:10.1016/j.cmet.2011.06.009
71. Jager S, Handschin C, St-Pierre J, Spiegelman BM (2007) AMP-activated protein kinase (AMPK) action in skeletal muscle via direct phosphorylation of PGC-1alpha. Proc Natl Acad Sci U S A 104(29):12017–12022. doi:10.1073/pnas.0705070104
72. Whaley-Connell A, McCullough PA, Sowers JR (2011) The role of oxidative stress in the metabolic syndrome. Rev Cardiovasc Med 12(1):21–29. doi:10.3909/ricm0555
73. Rooyackers OE, Adey DB, Ades PA, Nair KS (1996) Effect of age on in vivo rates of mitochondrial protein synthesis in human skeletal muscle. Proc Natl Acad Sci U S A 93 (26):15364–15369
74. de Cavanagh EMV, Inserra F, Ferder L (2011) Angiotensin II blockade: a strategy to slow ageing by protecting mitochondria? Cardiovasc Res 89(1):31–40. doi:10.1093/cvr/cvq285
75. Cai D, Frantz JD, Tawa NE Jr, Melendez PA, Oh BC, Lidov HG et al (2004) IKKbeta/NF-kappaB activation causes severe muscle wasting in mice. Cell 119(2):285–298. doi:10.1016/j.cell.2004.09.027
76. Nicolson GL, Ash ME (2014) Lipid replacement therapy: a natural medicine approach to replacing damaged lipids in cellular membranes and organelles and restoring function. Biochim Biophys Acta Biomemb 1838(6):1657–1679. doi:10.1016/j.bbamem.2013.11.010
77. Zuchner S, Mersiyanova IV, Muglia M, Bissar-Tadmouri N, Rochelle J, Dadali EL et al (2004) Mutations in the mitochondrial GTPase mitofusin 2 cause charcot-marie-tooth neuropathy type 2A. Nat Genet 36(5):449–451. doi:10.1038/ng1341
78. Thorpe SR, Baynes JW (2003) Maillard reaction products in tissue proteins: new products and new perspectives. Amino Acids 25(3–4):275–281. doi:10.1007/s00726-003-0017-9
79. Yan SD, Schmidt AM, Anderson GM, Zhang J, Brett J, Zou YS et al (1994) Enhanced cellular oxidant stress by the interaction of advanced glycation end products with their receptors/binding proteins. J Biol Chem 269(13):9889–9897

80. Teshima Y, Takahashi N, Nishio S, Saito S, Kondo H, Fukui A et al (2014) Production of reactive oxygen species in the diabetic heart – roles of mitochondria and NADPH oxidase. Circ J 78(2):300–306. doi:10.1253/circj.CJ-13-1187
81. Van Puyvelde K, Mets T, Njemini R, Beyer I, Bautmans I (2014) Effect of advanced glycation end product intake on inflammation and aging: a systematic review. Nutr Rev 72 (10):638–650. doi:10.1111/nure.12141
82. Snow LM, Thompson LV (2009) Influence of insulin and muscle fiber type in nepsilon-(carboxymethyl)-lysine accumulation in soleus muscle of rats with streptozotocin-induced diabetes mellitus. Pathobiology J Immunopathol Mol Cell Biol 76(5):227–234. doi:10.1159/000228898
83. Alves M, Calegari VC, Cunha DA, Saad MJ, Velloso LA, Rocha EM (2005) Increased expression of advanced glycation end-products and their receptor, and activation of nuclear factor kappa-B in lacrimal glands of diabetic rats. Diabetologia 48(12):2675–2681. doi:10.1007/s00125-005-0010-9
84. Thornalley PJ (2005) Dicarbonyl intermediates in the maillard reaction. Ann N Y Acad Sci 1043:111–117. doi:10.1196/annals.1333.014
85. Stadtman ER (2006) Protein oxidation and aging. Free Radic Res 40(12):1250–1258. doi:10.1080/10715760600918142
86. Dhar A, Desai KM, Wu L (2010) Alagebrium attenuates acute methylglyoxal-induced glucose intolerance in Sprague-Dawley rats. Br J Pharmacol 159(1):166–175. doi:10.1111/j.1476-5381.2009.00469.x
87. Falone S, D'Alessandro A, Mirabilio A, Petruccelli G, Cacchio M, Di Ilio C et al (2012) Long term running biphasically improves methylglyoxal-related metabolism, redox homeostasis and neurotrophic support within adult mouse brain cortex. PLoS One 7(2):e31401. doi:10.1371/journal.pone.0031401
88. Tanaka K, Kanazawa I, Yamaguchi T, Yano S, Kaji H, Sugimoto T (2014) Active vitamin D possesses beneficial effects on the interaction between muscle and bone. Biochem Biophys Res Commun 450(1):482–487. doi:10.1016/j.bbrc.2014.05.145
89. Brownlee M (1995) The pathological implications of protein glycation. Clin Invest Med Clin Exp 18(4):275–281
90. Andersen H (2012) Motor dysfunction in diabetes. Diabetes Metab Res Rev 28:89–92. doi:10.1002/dmrr.2257
91. El-Mesallamy HO, Hamdy NM, Ezzat OA, Reda AM (2011) Levels of soluble advanced glycation end product-receptors and other soluble serum markers as indicators of diabetic neuropathy in the foot. J Invest Med 59(8):1233–1238. doi:10.231/JIM.0b013e318231db64
92. Kim HK, Suzuki T, Saito K, Yoshida H, Kobayashi H, Kato H et al (2012) Effects of exercise and amino acid supplementation on body composition and physical function in community-dwelling elderly Japanese sarcopenic women: a randomized controlled trial. J Am Geriatr Soc 60(1):16–23. doi:10.1111/j.1532-5415.2011.03776.x
93. Castaneda C, Layne JE, Munoz-Orians L, Gordon PL, Walsmith J, Foldvari M et al (2002) A randomized controlled trial of resistance exercise training to improve glycemic control in older adults with type 2 diabetes. Diabetes Care 25(12):2335–2341
94. Lessard SJ, Chen ZP, Watt MJ, Hashem M, Reid JJ, Febbraio MA et al (2006) Chronic rosiglitazone treatment restores AMPKalpha2 activity in insulin-resistant rat skeletal muscle. Am J Physiol Endocrinol Metab 290(2):E251–E257. doi:10.1152/ajpendo.00096.2005
95. Feinstein DL, Spagnolo A, Akar C, Weinberg G, Murphy P, Gavrilyuk V et al (2005) Receptor-independent actions of PPAR thiazolidinedione agonists: is mitochondrial function the key? Biochem Pharmacol 70(2):177–188. doi:10.1016/j.bcp.2005.03.033
96. Miyazaki Y, He H, Mandarino LJ, DeFronzo RA (2003) Rosiglitazone improves downstream insulin receptor signaling in type 2 diabetic patients. Diabetes 52(8):1943–1950
97. Bajaj M, Baig R, Suraamornkul S, Hardies LJ, Coletta DK, Cline GW et al (2010) Effects of pioglitazone on intramyocellular fat metabolism in patients with type 2 diabetes mellitus. J Clin Endocrinol Metab 95(4):1916–1923. doi:10.1210/jc.2009-0911

98. Colca JR, Feinstein DL (2012) Altering mitochondrial dysfunction as an approach to treating Alzheimer's disease. Adv Pharmacol 64:155–176. doi:10.1016/b978-0-12-394816-8.00005-2, San Diego, Calif
99. Marsh AP, Shea MK, Vance Locke RM, Miller ME, Isom S, Miller GD et al (2013) Resistance training and pioglitazone lead to improvements in muscle power during voluntary weight loss in older adults. J Gerontol A Biol Sci Med Sci 68(7):828–836. doi:10.1093/gerona/gls258
100. Owen MR, Doran E, Halestrap AP (2000) Evidence that metformin exerts its anti-diabetic effects through inhibition of complex 1 of the mitochondrial respiratory chain. Biochem J 348 (Pt 3):607–614

Chapter 17
Body Temperature Regulation During Exercise Training

Kazunobu Okazaki

Abstract Physical work and exercise in the heat cause early exhaustion and heat-related illnesses compared with cooler conditions, and the incidence of the disorders is associated with intensity of activity and ambient conditions. Thermoregulatory function is critical during working in the heat, which is affected by individual somatotype, fitness level, and physiological status. Exercise-induced decrease in plasma volume (PV) and elevation in plasma osmolality attenuate heat dissipative responses, skin blood flow, and sweating responses to an increased core temperature during exercise in a hot environment; furthermore, these responses are exacerbated with thermal dehydration. Aerobic exercise training as well as thermal acclimation improves thermoregulatory responses which is associated with exercise-induced increase in PV. Thermoregulatory responses are reduced with biological aging, which would be also improved after exercise training accompanied with an improved maximal oxygen consumption rate, although the improvement is limited in elderly persons relative to young counterparts. Post-exercise protein and carbohydrate intake during training period accelerates exercise training-induced PV expansion and therefore thermoregulatory adaptations both in young and elderly persons (170 wards).

Keywords Thermoregulation • Sweat rate • Skin blood flow • Plasma volume • Aging

17.1 Introduction

When we perform physical work or sporting activities for a prolonged time in the heat or under the blazing sun, we are more likely to be exhausted and develop heat-related illnesses than in cooler conditions. Thermoregulation is the most important physiological function when we are exposed to such a severe hot environment.

K. Okazaki (✉)
Research Center for Urban Health and Sports, Osaka City University, 3-3-138 Sugimoto, Sumiyoshi, Osaka 558-8585, Japan

Department of Environmental Physiology for Exercise, Osaka City University Graduate School of Medicine, 3-3-138 Sugimoto, Sumiyoshi, Osaka 558-8585, Japan
e-mail: okazaki@sports.osaka-cu.ac.jp

M. Inaba (ed.), *Musculoskeletal Disease Associated with Diabetes Mellitus*,
DOI 10.1007/978-4-431-55720-3_17

Especially, the incidence of heat-related illnesses is greater if physical work or exercise is performed at higher intensities and in conditions with higher ambient temperatures (T_a) and relative humidity (RH) [1]. On the other hand, the incidence is greater in persons who are dehydrated, are not heat acclimated, or are healthy but had little daily activity [1]. In addition, the incidence is greater in individuals with impaired thermoregulatory responses such as obesity, diabetes mellitus, and cardiovascular diseases [1, 2] and also in individuals with diminished thermoregulatory responses such as skin grafts, spinal cord injuries, and multiple sclerosis [3–5]. Moreover, such a severe environment is serious for elderly people, even for those who are healthy [1, 2]. Actually, the morbidity and mortality of heat-related illnesses have rapidly increased for these two decades in Japan [6] because of rapid aging of the population and global warming. In this chapter, in the first, thermoregulation during work and exercise in the heat and effects of humoral and other considerable factors on thermoregulation are described physiologically, and then based on these mechanisms, the effects of exercise training to improve thermoregulatory responses are described.

17.2 Thermoregulation During Work and Exercise in the Heat

Body core temperature is determined by the heat equilibrium between heat gain and loss [1]. In general, body core temperature is increased during whole-body continuous work and exercise. That is because energy produced in contracting muscles is used for muscle contraction by about 20 %, and the other 80 % is converted to heat energy and therefore increases muscle temperature. Obviously, the higher the intensity of exercise, the greater the heat production during exercise. For example, when a person with 65 kg of body weight works at an intensity of 135 W (equivalent to intensity of running at 160 m/min) for 30 min, the heat energy produced in contracting muscles is estimated as 233 kcal, and if the heat is not dissipated from body surface at all, core temperature would increase from 37 °C to about 41 °C. However, empirically, core temperature increases rapidly within several minutes after the start of exercise but eventually reaches a steady state when heat dissipation mechanisms are activated sufficiently to balance the heat production.

Thermoregulatory effectors in the skin are the cutaneous vasculature and the sweat glands, and increase in skin blood flow (SkBF, cutaneous vasodilation) and sweating are two major heat dissipation mechanisms in human [1]. The heat produced in contracting muscles is transferred to the skin surface with the circulation; thus, the increased SkBF elevates skin surface temperature. The heat at skin surface is transferred to the surrounding air according to the temperature gradient between the skin and the air (non-evaporative heat dissipation). Therefore, non-evaporative heat dissipation is effective in a cool environment, but it becomes negligible or even negative at a warm environment with T_a higher than skin temperatures (~30 °C) and acts as a source of heat gain. On the other hand, sweating enhances heat dissipation from the skin surface to the air with evaporation of sweat (evaporative heat dissipation). Evaporative heat dissipation is determined by the water vapor gradient between the skin surface and surrounding air; therefore, it is effective regardless of T_a and is the main and critical heat dissipation mechanism at T_a above ~30 °C, whereas it is limited in a humid environment. Consequently, body core temperature increases rapidly when heat gain exceeds heat dissipation such as during heavy work and exercise in a hot and humid environment, and therefore we become extrasusceptible to heat-related illnesses in these situations.

SkBF and sweating are under the regulatory control related to body core and skin temperatures (thermal factors) and also other factors (nonthermal factors) [1]. Core and skin temperatures are monitored continuously by the central and peripheral thermoreceptors, respectively, through an afferent path to the thermoregulatory center in the preoptic/anterior hypothalamus [1]. SkBF and sweating are increased through reflex efferent paths of the sympathetic nerve system [1] when the thermoregulatory center determines core and skin temperatures higher than the set point. In humans, neural control of skin blood flow and sweating is accomplished via two distinct skin sympathetic nerves. Skin blood flow is controlled by a sympathetic adrenergic vasoconstrictor system and a separate sympathetic cholinergic vasodilator system, and sweating is controlled by sympathetic cholinergic nerves [1]. The thermal reflex is modulated by nonthermal factors, such as central commands, mechano- and metaboreflexes, arterial and cardiopulmonary baroreflexes, blood volume and osmolality, mental stimulus, and so on [1]. These nonthermal factors affect SkBF and sweating responses differently during exercise [1]. Basically, SkBF at the same core and skin temperatures is restricted during exercise compared to resting conditions, and the restriction is greater at higher intensities of exercise. On the other hand, sweating at the same core and skin temperatures is likely to be enhanced during exercise compared to resting conditions.

17.3 Effects of Humoral Factors on Thermoregulation

Most importantly, during work or exercise in a hot environment, the risk of heat-related illnesses is much higher when levels of dehydration worsen [7]. Rothstein et al. [8] first suggested the effects of dehydration on thermoregulation in human by reporting that rectal temperature at breaks between exercises increased by ~0.3 °C per 1 % loss of body weight by sweating in soldiers marching in the desert. That is because hypovolemia and hyperosmolality induced by dehydration restrict the response of SkBF and sweating to increased body temperatures as nonthermal factors.

17.3.1 Body Fluid Change During Exercise in a Hot Environment

Body fluid volume and osmolality are changed dramatically during exercise even in a cool environment. Indeed, plasma volume (PV) is decreased with an increased relative intensity of exercise by about 300–500 mL (8–15 %) at maximal exercise. The PV change during exercise is associated with an increased capillary fluid filtration from the intra- to the extravascular spaces because of an increased blood pressure and peripheral vasodilation and with an increased free-water shift from plasma to intracellular fluid through the interstitium based on osmotic gradient with accumulated metabolites such as lactic acid in intracellular fluid of contracting muscles [9]. The volume shifted to the contracting muscles is estimated to be ~1 L at maximal exercise and about half of the volume is from PV [10]. In addition, plasma osmolality (P_{osm}) is increased from ~285 mosmol/kgH_2O at rest to over 300 mosmol/kgH_2O at maximal exercise due to an accumulation of metabolites. These humoral changes are observed within several minutes after the start of exercise, therefore those are not caused by dehydration with sweating but associated with exercise per se.

In addition to the above, the decrease in PV (hypohydration) and the increase in P_{osm} (hyperosmolality) during exercise are exacerbated when exercise is performed in a hot environment because of an enhanced SkBF and sweating for thermoregulation. Increased SkBF causes a decreased venous return to the heart due to excessive pooling of blood in dilated peripheral skin vasculatures. For example, blood pooling in a person with 75 kg body weight is ~400–500 mL at 18 °C of skin temperature but increases to ~700–900 mL at 44 °C of skin temperature [11]. Sweat rate during exercise in a hot environment exceeds ~2 L in 1 h and reaches ~5–6 L after 2–3 h of intense exercise; therefore, PV is decreased more than ~500 mL with a profuse sweating because generally ~10 % volume of sweat is lost from plasma fluid. Moreover, P_{osm} is increased according to sweat rate because sweat is hypotonic. For example, 2 L sweating (1.2 % of 60 kg body weight) increases P_{osm} by ~2–3 mosmol/kgH_2O. These humoral changes increase load to the circulation and act as limiting factors for thermoregulation.

17.3.2 Effects of Hypovolemia on Thermoregulation

Nadel et al. [12] first reported that isotonic hypovolemia achieved by diuretics administration (change in PV, −700 mL; body weight, −2.7 %) before exercise significantly increased the esophageal temperature (T_{es}) threshold for the onset of cutaneous vasodilation by 0.4 °C and decreased the maximal SkBF by 50 % during exercise at 55 % of maximal oxygen consumption rate (VO_{2max}) in a hot environment (T_a, 35 °C). In addition, Mack et al. [13] reported that acute reduction in venous return to the heart achieved by −40 mmHg of lower body negative pressure

(LBNP) reduced SkBF and increased T_{es} during exercise at an intensity corresponding to heart rate of 125 beats/min in a warm environment (T_a, 28 °C). In contrast, maneuvers to acutely increase venous return to the heart and cardiac filling pressure during exercise, isotonic saline infusion [11], change of body position from upright to supine [14, 15], head-out water immersion [16], and continuous negative pressure breathing [17] all enhanced SkBF during exercise. These observations suggest that dehydration-induced hypovolemia suppresses the response to increase SkBF to an increased core temperature during exercise via cardiopulmonary baroreflex.

Several previous studies have also suggested that hypovolemia suppresses the response to increase sweat rate during exercise. Fortney et al. [18] reported that diuretics-induced isotonic hypovolemia by 9 % before exercise significantly reduced the sensitivity to increase sweat rate on chest and forearm in response to increased T_{es} although T_{es} threshold for the onset of sweating remained unchanged during exercise at 65–70 % VO_{2max} in a warm environment (T_a, 30 °C; RH, 40 %). Mack et al. [13] reported that −40 mmHg of LBNP during exercise noted above reduced the response to increase in sweat rate as well as SkBF, and another group [19] reported a reduced skin sympathetic nervous activity by LBNP in passively heated subjects. In contrast, Kamijo et al. [20] suggested that diuretics-induced isotonic hypovolemia by 10 % before exercise reduced the response to increase SkBF similarly as reported by Nadel et al. [12], while it did not change the response to increase sweat rate at all during exercise at 60 % VO_{2max} in a warm environment (T_a, 30 °C; RH, 45 %). Thus, the effects of hypovolemia on sweat rate are still controversial.

17.3.3 Effects of Hyperosmolality on Thermoregulation

The response to increase SkBF and sweat rate during exercise is suppressed by plasma hyperosmolality. Fortney et al. [21] reported that increase in P_{osm} by 10 mosmol/kgH_2O achieved by hypertonic saline infusion before exercise caused an upward shift of T_{es} thresholds for cutaneous vasodilation and sweating by 0.2 °C and also decreased the sensitivity to increase SkBF in response to increased T_{es} during exercise at 70 % VO_{2max} in a warm environment (T_a, 30 °C; RH, 40 %). Additionally, Takamata et al. [22] suggested that T_{es} thresholds for cutaneous vasodilation and sweating during passive heating (lower legs immersion in 42 °C water) at rest shifted upward by 0.044 °C and 0.034 °C per 1 mosmol/kgH_2O increase, respectively, by showing a linear upward shift of the T_{es} thresholds with several levels of increase in P_{osm} by hypertonic saline infusion before heating. More importantly, they also suggested that upward-shifted T_{es} thresholds during exercise were caused by an increased P_{osm} with exercise per se, by showing that the upward shift of T_{es} thresholds at a given increase in P_{osm} during exercise was identical to that during passive heating at rest [22]. Mitono et al. [23] supported this evidence by showing that the upward-shifted T_{es} threshold for cutaneous vasodilation during exercise was attenuated when the increase in P_{osm} during exercise was attenuated by hypotonic saline infusion prior to exercise. It has been supposed that plasma hyperosmolality suppresses the response of the thermoregulatory center via osmoreceptors.

As described above, dehydration suppresses heat dissipative mechanisms during exercise in the heat, which is a mechanism to prevent cardiovascular failure caused by reduced venous return to the heart due to excessive pooling of blood in dilated peripheral skin vasculatures and decrease in PV with sweating. Indeed, it has been reported that stimulation of oropharyngeal reflexes by drinking such a small amount of water so as not to change PV and P_{osm} in dehydrated subjects rapidly reduces thirst sensation and plasma vasopressin secretion [24, 25] and simultaneously releases the dehydration-induced suppression of SkBF [20] and SR responses [25], which are followed by a fall in mean arterial pressure [20].

17.4 Effects of Exercise Training on Thermoregulation

It has been well known that aerobic exercise training improves thermoregulatory responses and reduces physiological strain and therefore enhances cardiovascular and exercise capacities during exercise in the heat. These adaptations are remarkable when exercise training is performed under the heat [1]. As shown in Fig. 17.1, the responses to increase SkBF and sweat rate to an increased T_{es} during exercise (T_a, 25 °C) increased after a 10-day training in a temperate condition (T_a, 20 °C) and further after a subsequent 10-day training in a hot condition (T_a, 35 °C) [26]. The increased SkBF and sweating responses are characterized by the lowered shift of T_{es} thresholds for cutaneous vasodilation and sweating [27, 28] and the enhanced sensitivity to increase SkBF and sweat rate in response to an increased T_{es} [27, 28]. The mechanisms of the increase in thermoregulatory responses with exercise training are suggested to be similar to those with acclimation to repeated heat

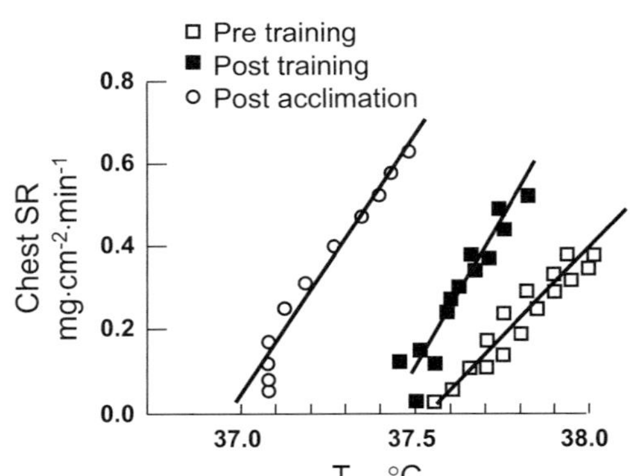

Fig. 17.1 Chest sweat rate (chest SR) plotted against esophageal temperature (T_{es}) for one subject exercising at an ambient temperature (T_a) of 25 °C. The responses to increase chest SR to an increased T_{es} during exercise increased after a 10-day training in a temperate condition (T_a, 20 °C) and further after a subsequent 10-day training in a hot condition (T_a, 35 °C) [26]

exposures, including adaptations of the thermoregulatory center and thermoregulatory effectors [1, 12] as well as an increase in VO_{2max} [29] and PV [27, 30, 31].

17.4.1 Effects of PV Expansion on Thermoregulation

The exercise-induced PV expansion is suggested to be primarily associated with an increase in total volume of extracellular fluid [32] and secondary with an increase in plasma protein, mainly albumin content, resulting in drawing fluids into the intravascular space from the interstitium [32–34]. As for the mechanisms about the former, a facilitated Na^+ and water reabsorption [32, 35] and also an increased voluntary fluid intake with an enhanced thirst sensation [36] due to an activated renin-angiotensin-aldosterone system and vasopressin release during and after exercise or dehydration are suggested [37]. As for the mechanisms about the latter, an enhanced plasma protein synthesis in the liver [38, 39] and an increased protein translocation from the interstitium to the intravascular space [40] with a decreased transcapillary protein escape ratio [41] are suggested.

Expanded PV after exercise training associates with an attenuated increase in P_{osm} due to reduced lactic acid concentration in blood (enhanced lactate threshold) during exercise at the same absolute intensity and therefore shifts the core temperature threshold for cutaneous vasodilation and sweating downward. Moreover, expanded PV increases venous return to the heart and cardiac filling pressure and therefore enhances cardiac stroke volume and the response to increase SkBF and sweat rate to an increased core temperature during exercise [11, 16, 17]. Indeed, Ichinose et al. [27] suggested that an increase in cardiac stroke volume and also the sensitivity to increase SkBF in response to an increased T_{es} during exercise in a warm environment (T_a, 30 °C) were closely associated with an increased PV after 10-day endurance training (60 % VO_{2max} for 1 h/day) in the same condition. More directly, Goto et al. [42] examined the effects of post-exercise protein and carbohydrate (CHO) mixture (Pro-CHO; 3.6 kcal and 0.36 g protein/kg) intake during 5-day exercise training (70 % VO_{2max} for 30 min/day) in a warm environment (T_a, 30 °C) on PV and thermoregulatory responses. They suggested that plasma albumin content (Alb_{cont}) and therefore PV in the Pro-CHO group increased by ~10 % and ~8 %, respectively, which were significantly higher than ~4 % in the placebo intake group (CNT; 0.9 kcal and 0 g protein/kg body weight). They attributed that the increase in Alb_{cont} was caused by an enhanced hepatic albumin synthesis after exercise because of an enhanced bioavailability of the substance [38, 39] and anabolic effects of insulin on hepatocytes [43]. Most importantly, they found that the sensitivity to increase SkBF and sweat rate in response to an increased T_{es} in the Pro-CHO group increased by 44 % and 56 %, respectively, after training, which were significantly higher than those in the CNT group increased by 10 % and 19 %, respectively (Fig. 17.2). Moreover, the increases in heart rate and T_{es} during exercise were attenuated after training in both groups but more prominent in the

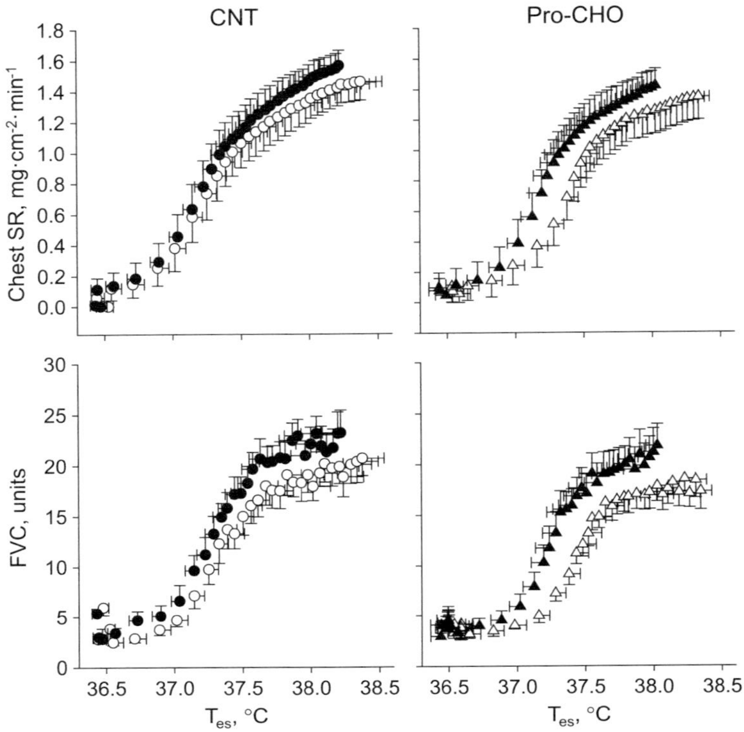

Fig. 17.2 Chest sweat rate (chest SR) (**a**, **b**) and forearm vascular conductance (FVC) (**c**, **d**) responses to increased esophageal temperature (T_{es}) during exercise in a warm environment (T_a, 30 °C) (*open symbols*) and after (*closed symbols*) 5-day training in the same condition. CNT, placebo intake group; Pro-CHO, protein and carbohydrate intake group. Means and SE bars are presented for nine subjects [42]

Pro-CHO group than in the CNT group, indicating decreased cardiovascular and thermal strains after training with PV expansion (Fig. 17.3).

In addition, Ikegawa et al. [30] confirmed the observations by Goto et al. [42] by showing an increased PV with a downward-shifted T_{es} threshold for cutaneous vasodilation and sweating after the same training protocol and further the downward-shifted T_{es} threshold were totally or at least in part abolished after the increased PV was normalized by administration of diuretics after training. Furthermore, Ichinose et al. [27] suggested that the sensitivity of the upward shift of T_{es} threshold for cutaneous vasodilation at a given increase in P_{osm} by hypertonic saline infusion was reduced after 10-day exercise training (60 % VO_{2max} for 60 min/day) in a warm environment (T_a, 30 °C) although that for sweating remained unchanged. They further suggested that the reduction in each subject was significantly correlated with the increase in PV after training, suggesting that the stretch of cardiopulmonary baroreceptors due to PV expansion was associated with the reduction. These results clearly demonstrate that the enhanced thermoregulatory responses

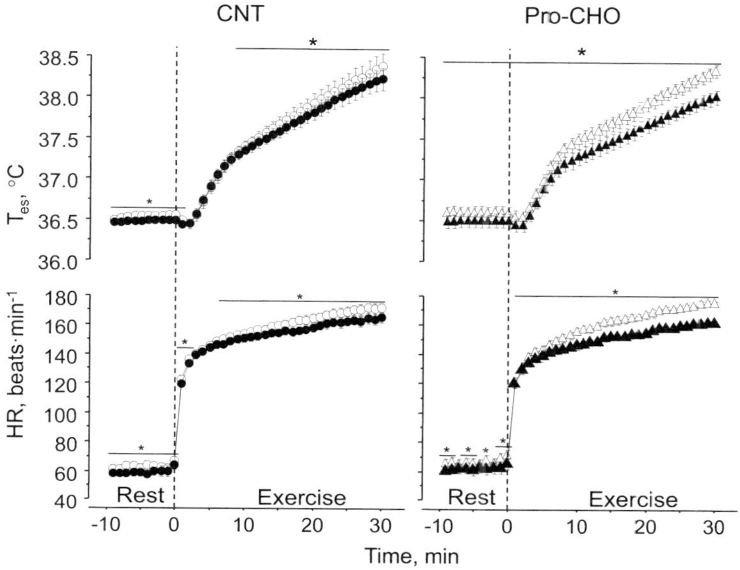

Fig. 17.3 Esophageal temperature (T_{es}) and heart rate (*HR*) responses during exercise in a warm environment (T_a, 30 °C) before (*open symbols*) and after (*closed symbols*) 5-day training. CNT, placebo intake group; Pro-CHO, protein and carbohydrate intake group. Means and SE bars are presented for nine subjects. *significant differences vs. before training, $P < 0.05$ [42]

and cardiovascular capacities after exercise training are closely associated with PV expansion in addition to the neural adaptation of the thermoregulatory center and thermoregulatory effectors [1, 12].

17.4.2 *Effects of Other Adaptations with Training on Thermoregulation*

In addition, Na^+ concentration of sweat decreased after exercise training or heat acclimation due to an enhanced Na^+ reabsorption at the sweat gland duct with an enhanced sensitivity to aldosterone [44]. Hypotonic sweat is advantageous for maintaining PV during exercise because hypotonic sweat loss causes a greater increase in osmolality of extracellular fluid that facilitates water movement from intracellular fluid to extracellular fluid space according to osmotic gradient between the spaces [44] and therefore attenuates the reduction in venous return to the heart. As a result, the decrease in thermoregulatory responses with a given loss of sweat is attenuated with low sweat Na^+ concentration [45]. Moreover, the upward shift of T_{es} thresholds for cutaneous vasodilation and sweating at a given increase in P_{osm} was reduced in heat-acclimated subjects in whom an increase in P_{osm} at a given loss of sweat was enhanced due to low sweat Na^+ concentration [45].

17.5 Effects of Biological Aging on Thermoregulation

The susceptibility to heat-related illnesses in the elderly [6] is caused by deteriorated thermoregulatory responses with aging [46]. Actually, previous studies have indicated that healthy elderly individuals have an impaired thermal perception [47] and impaired autonomic [48, 49] and behavioral [50, 51] thermoregulatory responses. Decreased VO_{2max} and cardiovascular capacity are associated with the deteriorated thermoregulatory responses in the elderly [49]. However, it has been suggested that elderly subjects with matched VO_{2max} to younger subjects show a lowered SkBF response to total body or local passive heating as well as during exercise in a hot environment than younger subjects [52, 53]. Kenney et al. [53] suggested that the limited SkBF response to hyperthermia during exercise in a hot condition was caused not by an enhanced vasoconstrictor system but mainly by a decreased sensitivity of active vasodilator system to increased T_{es}, by using bretylium tosylate to block local release of norepinephrine on the forearm skin. In addition, total body and local sweat rate in response to passive heating or exercise are lower in the elderly than in young adults [54].

Moreover, decreased PV and increased P_{osm} at baseline condition [55], diminished thirst sensation [55] and responses in antidiuretic hormone and aldosterone after thermal dehydration [37], decreased renal concentrating ability [56], and lower reabsorptive ability of sweat gland ducts [56] with advancing age are suggested to be associated with the decreased thermoregulatory responses in the elderly. Splanchnic and renal vasoconstriction during exercise, which enhance the redistribution of cardiac output to the skin vasculatures and associate with an increased cutaneous vasodilation in the youth, were also decreased in the elderly [57]. Furthermore, it is not uncommon for the elderly to be taking a variety of prescription drugs that may affect thermoregulatory responses and body fluid regulation [1]. These diminished body fluid regulations and thermoregulatory functions with aging can be improved with exercise training and heat acclimation, although generally the gain is lower or limited relative to their younger counterparts.

17.5.1 Effects of Exercise Training on Thermoregulation in the Elderly

Several longitudinal studies have suggested that thermoregulatory responses during exercise in a hot environment are enhanced with aerobic training performed under cool, thermoneutral, or hot conditions in initially sedentary elderly subjects [29, 57, 58] as well as in young subjects [26–28]. Thomas et al. [29] reported that a 16-week aerobic training lowered the mean body temperature threshold for cutaneous vasodilation during exercise in a hot environment (T_a, 36 °C) both in young and elderly subjects, whose VO_{2max} increased by ≥ 5 %. They also suggested that the enhanced cutaneous vasodilation is caused by an enhanced sensitivity of active vasodilator system [29]. Additionally, Okazaki et al. [58] confirmed and extended these results by showing that T_{es} thresholds for cutaneous vasodilation and sweating during exercise in a warm environment (T_a, 30 °C) were lowered after an 18-week aerobic and resistance training under cool and thermoneutral conditions, with improved VO_{2max}, by 20 % and 10 %, respectively, in initially sedentary elderly subjects. In both studies, on the other hand, the sensitivities to increase SkBF and sweat rate in response to an increased mean body temperature or T_{es} remained unchanged after training in elderly subjects. Okazaki et al. [58] attributed the results to an attenuated PV expansion after training in elderly subjects, by showing a linear correlation between changes in the sensitivities and those in PV after training. As above, in young subjects, PV expansion is considered to be a major mechanism involved in the training-induced enhancement of thermoregulatory responses by increasing cardiac stroke volume and/or by suppressing baroreflex-induced attenuation of skin vasodilation by increasing venous return to the heart [11]. Additionally, Ho et al. [57] showed that splanchnic and renal vasoconstriction during exercise were enhanced in young subjects but not in elderly subjects after aerobic training. Thus, the beneficial effects of training on thermoregulation in elderly people involve an increased VO_{2max} but are generally attenuated compared with younger counterparts [57, 58].

The blunted increase in PV with aerobic training in elderly people is likely to be associated with a reduced fluid intake after thermal dehydration [37, 55] or water deprivation [59] with aging; however, an attenuated increase in Alb_{cont} with exercise [34, 58, 60] appears to be a primary limiting factor. As above, one mechanism of the increased Alb_{cont} after aerobic training is likely to be an enhanced hepatic albumin synthesis response to exercise in the younger group [38, 39]; the smaller increase in Alb_{cont} after training in the elderly group could be caused, in part, by the blunted response of the albumin synthesis to exercise [61, 62] due to reduced gene expression with aging. However, it is also plausible that this is caused by protein intake insufficient for albumin synthesis in elderly people since they are likely habituated to low energy and protein diets due to minimal daily physical activity, and therefore it would be improved if substrates for plasma albumin synthesis are given immediately after exercise where albumin synthesis is reportedly enhanced [39, 62]. In this regard, one study showed that recoveries in Alb_{cont} and PV after acute high-intensity interval exercise were generally attenuated in elderly versus young subjects when they consumed a non-energy placebo just after exercise, whereas Alb_{cont} and PV recovered more when they consumed a protein and CHO mixture than when they consumed the placebo in elderly and young subjects [34].

Based on these results, Okazaki et al. [63] examined the effects of post-exercise protein and CHO intake during 8 weeks of aerobic training under cool and thermoneutral conditions on PV and thermoregulatory responses during exercise in elderly subjects. They suggested that Alb_{cont} and PV increased by 6 %, and these increases were accompanied by enhanced sensitivities for SkBF and sweat rate to an increased T_{es} by 18 % and 80 %, respectively, in subjects with protein and CHO

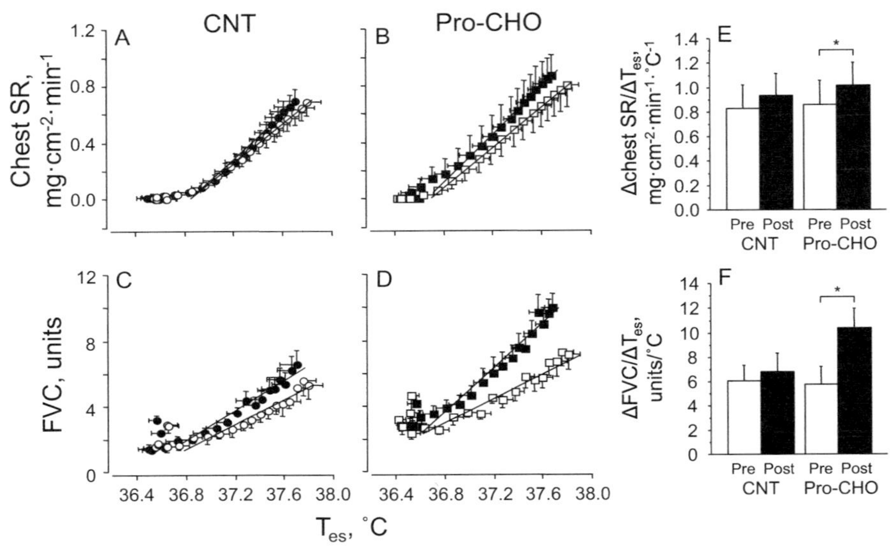

Fig. 17.4 Chest sweat rate (chest SR) (**a**, **b**) and forearm skin vascular conductance (FVC) (**c**, **d**) responses to increased esophageal temperature (T_{es}), and the sensitivity of the increase in chest SR (Δcheat SR/ΔT_{es}; E) and FVC (ΔFVC/ΔT_{es}; F) at a given increase in T_{es} during exercise in a warm environment (T_a, 30 °C) before (*open symbols*) and after (*closed symbols*) 8-week aerobic training in elderly men. CNT, placebo intake group; Pro-CHO, protein and carbohydrate intake group. Means and SE bars are presented for seven subjects. * significant differences, $P < 0.05$ [63]

intake, whereas those remained unchanged in subjects taking the placebo [63]. Additionally, the enhanced sensitivity was observed with increased stroke volume during exercise by 10 % [63]. Thus, the blunted increase in cardiovascular and thermoregulatory capacity in elderly individuals compared with younger counterparts was normalized by increasing PV with exercise in conjunction with post-exercise protein and CHO intake (Fig. 17.4).

Recent studies have shown that aerobic training improves cutaneous vasodilation by local mechanisms in aged skin [64]. Black et al. [65] blocked NO production with cutaneous microdialysis of L-NAME (a NO synthase inhibitor) during acetylcholine infusions and demonstrated that increased vascular responsiveness following 12 and 24 weeks of aerobic training in initially sedentary elderly subjects was achieved through the increased action of NO in the skin. Similar results were reported in a longitudinal study [66] although a cross-sectional study reported no effect [67].

The enhancement of sweating function in summer occurred later and its reduction in winter occurred earlier, despite a smaller range of seasonal variation in an elderly group compared with a younger group [68]. To prevent heat disorders in elderly individuals, we strongly recommend that they engage in exercise training prior to the summer seasons and regular exercise in general to improve thermoregulatory capacity with VO_{2max} and to adopt protein and CHO intake after exercise to achieve adequate training adaptations.

17.6 Oral Rehydration During Exercise

Finally, to prevent extra thermal and cardiovascular strains during exercise in the heat and heat-related illnesses, dehydration prior to and during exercise should be prevented or fairly restituted. Oral rehydration with CHO-electrolytes solutions (NaCl, 0.1–0.2 %; CHO, 4–8 %) based on thirst sensation is recommended but body weight reduction during exercise should not exceed 2 % [7]. Persons who work or exercise with high intensities in the heat and the elderly should start fluid ingestion prior to and in the early period of work before they feel thirst [7].

References

1. Taylor NAS, Kondo N, Kenney WL (2008) The physiology of acute heat exposure, with implications for human performance in the heat. In: Taylor NAS, Groeller H (eds) Physiological bases of human performance during work and exercise. Elsevier, Philadelphia, pp 341–358
2. Kenny GP, Yardley J, Brown C, Sigal RJ, Jay O (2010) Heat stress in older individuals and patients with common chronic diseases. CMAJ 182(10):1053–1060
3. Crandall CG, Davis SL (2010) Cutaneous vascular and sudomotor responses in human skin grafts. J Appl Physiol 109(5):1524–1530
4. Davis SL, Wilson TE, White AT, Frohman EM (2010) Thermoregulation in multiple sclerosis. J Appl Physiol 109(5):1531–1537
5. Price MJ, Campbell IG (1999) Thermoregulatory responses of spinal cord injured and able-bodied athletes to prolonged upper body exercise and recovery. Spinal Cord 37(11):772–779
6. Nakai S, Shin-ya H, Yoshida T, Yorimoto A, Inoue Y, Morimoto T (2007) Proposal of new guidelines for prevention of heat disorders during sports and daily activities based on age, clothing and heat acclimatization. Jpn J Phys Fitness Sports Med 56:437–444
7. Sawka MN, Burke LM, Eichner ER, Maughan RJ, Montain SJ, Stachenfeld NS (2007) American College of Sports Medicine position stand. Exercise and fluid replacement. Med Sci Sports Exerc 39(2):377–390
8. Rothstein A, Towbin EJ (1947) Blood circulation and temperature of men dehydrating in the heat. In: Adolph EF (ed) Physiology of man in the desert. Interscience, New York, pp 172–196
9. Nose H, Takamata A, Mack GW, Oda Y, Okuno T, Kang DH, Morimoto T (1991) Water and electrolyte balance in the vascular space during graded exercise in humans. J Appl Physiol 70 (6):2757–2762
10. Lundvall J, Mellander S, Westling H, White T (1972) Fluid transfer between blood and tissues during exercise. Acta Physiol Scand 85(2):258–269
11. Nose H, Mack GW, Shi XR, Morimoto K, Nadel ER (1990) Effect of saline infusion during exercise on thermal and circulatory regulations. J Appl Physiol 69(2):609–616
12. Nadel ER, Fortney SM, Wenger CB (1980) Effect of hydration state of circulatory and thermal regulations. J Appl Physiol 49(4):715–721
13. Mack G, Nishiyasu T, Shi X (1995) Baroreceptor modulation of cutaneous vasodilator and sudomotor responses to thermal stress in humans. J Physiol 483(Pt 2):537–547

14. Johnson JM, Rowell LB, Brengelmann GL (1974) Modification of the skin blood flow-body temperature relationship by upright exercise. J Appl Physiol 37(6):880–886
15. Gonzalez-Alonso J, Mora-Rodriguez R, Coyle EF (1999) Supine exercise restores arterial blood pressure and skin blood flow despite dehydration and hyperthermia. Am J Physiol 277 (2 Pt 2):H576–H583
16. Nielsen B, Rowell LB, Bonde-Petersen F (1984) Cardiovascular responses to heat stress and blood volume displacements during exercise in man. Eur J Appl Physiol Occup Physiol 52 (4):370–374
17. Nagashima K, Nose H, Takamata A, Morimoto T (1998) Effect of continuous negative-pressure breathing on skin blood flow during exercise in a hot environment. J Appl Physiol 84(6):1845–1851
18. Fortney SM, Nadel ER, Wenger CB, Bove JR (1981) Effect of blood volume on sweating rate and body fluids in exercising humans. J Appl Physiol 51(6):1594–1600
19. Dodt C, Gunnarsson T, Elam M, Karlsson T, Wallin BG (1995) Central blood volume influences sympathetic sudomotor nerve traffic in warm humans. Acta Physiol Scand 155 (1):41–51
20. Kamijo Y, Okumoto T, Takeno Y, Okazaki K, Inaki M, Masuki S, Nose H (2005) Transient cutaneous vasodilatation and hypotension after drinking in dehydrated and exercising men. J Physiol 568(Pt 2):689–698
21. Fortney SM, Wenger CB, Bove JR, Nadel ER (1984) Effect of hyperosmolality on control of blood flow and sweating. J Appl Physiol 57(6):1688–1695
22. Takamata A, Nagashima K, Nose H, Morimoto T (1998) Role of plasma osmolality in the delayed onset of thermal cutaneous vasodilation during exercise in humans. Am J Physiol 275 (1 Pt 2):R286–R290
23. Mitono H, Endoh H, Okazaki K, Ichinose T, Masuki S, Takamata A, Nose H (2005) Acute hypo-osmolality attenuates the suppression of cutaneous vasodilation with increased exercise intensity. J Appl Physiol 99(3):902–908
24. Geelen G, Keil LC, Kravik SE, Wade CE, Thrasher TN, Barnes PR, Pyka G, Nesvig C, Greenleaf JE (1984) Inhibition of plasma vasopressin after drinking in dehydrated humans. Am J Physiol 247(6 Pt 2):R968–R971
25. Takamata A, Mack GW, Gillen CM, Jozsi AC, Nadel ER (1995) Osmoregulatory modulation of thermal sweating in humans: reflex effects of drinking. Am J Physiol 268(2 Pt 2):R414–R422
26. Roberts MF, Wenger CB, Stolwijk JA, Nadel ER (1977) Skin blood flow and sweating changes following exercise training and heat acclimation. J Appl Physiol 43(1):133–137
27. Ichinose T, Okazaki K, Masuki S, Mitono H, Chen M, Endoh H, Nose H (2005) Ten-day endurance training attenuates the hyperosmotic suppression of cutaneous vasodilation during exercise but not sweating. J Appl Physiol 99(1):237–243
28. Takeno Y, Kamijo YI, Nose H (2001) Thermoregulatory and aerobic changes after endurance training in a hypobaric hypoxic and warm environment. J Appl Physiol 91(4):1520–1528
29. Thomas CM, Pierzga JM, Kenney WL (1999) Aerobic training and cutaneous vasodilation in young and older men. J Appl Physiol 86(5):1676–1686
30. Ikegawa S, Kamijo Y, Okazaki K, Masuki S, Okada Y, Nose H (2011) Effects of hypohydration on thermoregulation during exercise before and after 5-day aerobic training in a warm environment in young men. J Appl Physiol 110(4):972–980
31. Okazaki K, Goto M, Nose H (2009) Protein and carbohydrate supplementation increases aerobic and thermoregulatory capacities. J Physiol 587(Pt 23):5585–5590
32. Convertino VA, Brock PJ, Keil LC, Bernauer EM, Greenleaf JE (1980) Exercise training-induced hypervolemia: role of plasma albumin, renin, and vasopressin. J Appl Physiol 48 (4):665–669
33. Gillen CM, Lee R, Mack GW, Tomaselli CM, Nishiyasu T, Nadel ER (1991) Plasma volume expansion in humans after a single intense exercise protocol. J Appl Physiol 71(5):1914–1920

34. Okazaki K, Hayase H, Ichinose T, Mitono H, Doi T, Nose H (2009) Protein and carbohydrate supplementation after exercise increases plasma volume and albumin content in older and young men. J Appl Physiol 107(3):770–779
35. Nagashima K, Wu J, Kavouras SA, Mack GW (2001) Increased renal tubular sodium reabsorption during exercise-induced hypervolemia in humans. J Appl Physiol 91 (3):1229–1236
36. Greenleaf JE, Brock PJ, Keil LC, Morse JT (1983) Drinking and water balance during exercise and heat acclimation. J Appl Physiol: Respir Environ Exerc Physiol 54(2):414–419
37. Takamata A, Ito T, Yaegashi K, Takamiya H, Maegawa Y, Itoh T, Greenleaf JE, Morimoto T (1999) Effect of an exercise-heat acclimation program on body fluid regulatory responses to dehydration in older men. Am J Physiol 277(4 Pt 2):R1041–R1050
38. Nagashima K, Cline GW, Mack GW, Shulman GI, Nadel ER (2000) Intense exercise stimulates albumin synthesis in the upright posture. J Appl Physiol 88(1):41–46
39. Yang RC, Mack GW, Wolfe RR, Nadel ER (1998) Albumin synthesis after intense intermittent exercise in human subjects. J Appl Physiol 84(2):584–592
40. Mack GW, Yang R, Hargens AR, Nagashima K, Haskell A (1998) Influence of hydrostatic pressure gradients on regulation of plasma volume after exercise. J Appl Physiol 85 (2):667–675
41. Haskell A, Gillen CM, Mack GW, Nadel ER (1998) Albumin infusion in humans does not model exercise induced hypervolemia after 24 hours. Acta Physiol Scand 164(3):277–284
42. Goto M, Okazaki K, Kamijo Y, Ikegawa S, Masuki S, Miyagawa K, Nose H (2010) Protein and carbohydrate supplementation during 5-day aerobic training enhanced plasma volume expansion and thermoregulatory adaptation in young men. J Appl Physiol 109(4):1247–1255
43. Ahlman B, Charlton M, Fu A, Berg C, O'Brien P, Nair KS (2001) Insulin's effect on synthesis rates of liver proteins. A swine model comparing various precursors of protein synthesis. Diabetes 50(5):947–954
44. Nose H, Mack GW, Shi XR, Nadel ER (1988) Shift in body fluid compartments after dehydration in humans. J Appl Physiol 65(1):318–324
45. Takamata A, Yoshida T, Nishida N, Morimoto T (2001) Relationship of osmotic inhibition in thermoregulatory responses and sweat sodium concentration in humans. Am J Physiol Regul Integr Comp Physiol 280(3):R623–R629
46. Blatteis CM (2012) Age-dependent changes in temperature regulation – a mini review. Gerontology 58(4):289–295
47. Guergova S, Dufour A (2011) Thermal sensitivity in the elderly: a review. Ageing Res Rev 10 (1):80–92
48. Holowatz LA, Kenney WL (2010) Peripheral mechanisms of thermoregulatory control of skin blood flow in aged humans. J Appl Physiol 109(5):1538–1544
49. Kenney WL (1997) Thermoregulation at rest and during exercise in healthy older adults. Exerc Sport Sci Rev 25:41–76
50. Kenney WL, Chiu P (2001) Influence of age on thirst and fluid intake. Med Sci Sports Exerc 33 (9):1524–1532
51. Van Someren EJ, Raymann RJ, Scherder EJ, Daanen HA, Swaab DF (2002) Circadian and age-related modulation of thermoreception and temperature regulation: mechanisms and functional implications. Ageing Res Rev 1(4):721–778
52. Kenney WL, Tankersley CG, Newswanger DL, Hyde DE, Puhl SM, Turner NL (1990) Age and hypohydration independently influence the peripheral vascular response to heat stress. J Appl Physiol 68(5):1902–1908
53. Kenney WL, Morgan AL, Farquhar WB, Brooks EM, Pierzga JM, Derr JA (1997) Decreased active vasodilator sensitivity in aged skin. Am J Physiol 272(4 Pt 2):H1609–H1614
54. Inoue Y, Shibasaki M, Ueda H, Ishizashi H (1999) Mechanisms underlying the age-related decrement in the human sweating response. Eur J Appl Physiol Occup Physiol 79(2):121–126

55. Mack GW, Weseman CA, Langhans GW, Scherzer H, Gillen CM, Nadel ER (1994) Body fluid balance in dehydrated healthy older men: thirst and renal osmoregulation. J Appl Physiol 76 (4):1615–1623
56. Geelen G, Corman B (1992) Relationship between vasopressin and renal concentrating ability in aging rats. Am J Physiol 262(5 Pt 2):R826–R833
57. Ho CW, Beard JL, Farrell PA, Minson CT, Kenney WL (1997) Age, fitness, and regional blood flow during exercise in the heat. J Appl Physiol 82(4):1126–1135
58. Okazaki K, Kamijo Y, Takeno Y, Okumoto T, Masuki S, Nose H (2002) Effects of exercise training on thermoregulatory responses and blood volume in older men. J Appl Physiol 93 (5):1630–1637
59. Phillips PA, Rolls BJ, Ledingham JG, Forsling ML, Morton JJ, Crowe MJ, Wollner L (1984) Reduced thirst after water deprivation in healthy elderly men. N Engl J Med 311(12):753–759
60. Zappe DH, Bell GW, Swartzentruber H, Wideman RF, Kenney WL (1996) Age and regulation of fluid and electrolyte balance during repeated exercise sessions. Am J Physiol 270(1 Pt 2): R71–R79
61. Gersovitz M, Munro HN, Udall J, Young VR (1980) Albumin synthesis in young and elderly subjects using a new stable isotope methodology: response to level of protein intake. Metabolism 29(11):1075–1086
62. Sheffield-Moore M, Yeckel CW, Volpi E, Wolf SE, Morio B, Chinkes DL, Paddon-Jones D, Wolfe RR (2004) Postexercise protein metabolism in older and younger men following moderate-intensity aerobic exercise. Am J Physiol Endocrinol Metab 287(3):E513–E522
63. Okazaki K, Ichinose T, Mitono H, Chen M, Masuki S, Endoh H, Hayase H, Doi T, Nose H (2009) Impact of protein and carbohydrate supplementation on plasma volume expansion and thermoregulatory adaptation by aerobic training in older men. J Appl Physiol 107(3):725–733
64. Simmons GH, Wong BJ, Holowatz LA, Kenney WL (2011) Changes in the control of skin blood flow with exercise training: where do cutaneous vascular adaptations fit in? Exp Physiol 96(9):822–828
65. Black MA, Green DJ, Cable NT (2008) Exercise prevents age-related decline in nitric-oxide-mediated vasodilator function in cutaneous microvessels. J Physiol 586(14):3511–3524
66. Hodges GJ, Sharp L, Stephenson C, Patwala AY, George KP, Goldspink DF, Tim Cable N (2010) The effect of 48 weeks of aerobic exercise training on cutaneous vasodilator function in post-menopausal females. Eur J Appl Physiol 108(6):1259–1267
67. Tew GA, Saxton JM, Klonizakis M, Moss J, Ruddock AD, Hodges GJ (2011) Aging and aerobic fitness affect the contribution of noradrenergic sympathetic nerves to the rapid cutaneous vasodilator response to local heating. J Appl Physiol 110(5):1264–1270
68. Inoue Y, Nakao M, Okudaira S, Ueda H, Araki T (1995) Seasonal variation in sweating responses of older and younger men. Eur J Appl Physiol Occup Physiol 70(1):6–12

Chapter 18
Clinical Application of Exercise Therapy in Diabetes

Masayuki Hosoi, Yosuke Yakushiji, and Shiro Tanaka

Abstract This chapter describes the practical prescription for exercise therapy for diabetes mellitus. After careful medical check, a prescription for exercise must be ordered from the following viewpoints: the purpose of exercise, the mode of exercise, the frequency and duration of exercise, the intensity of exercise, the place for exercise, and the patients to be prohibited or restricted from exercise.

Keywords Diabetes mellitus • Aerobic • Resistance • Exercise • Physical activities

18.1 Clinical Benefits of Exercise in Diabetes Therapy

Exercise, together with diet and pharmacologic therapies, is important as part of the overall approach to improving glycemic control. In patients with type 2 diabetes, the improvement of the cardiorespiratory function, blood sugar control, improvement of the lipid metabolism, and improvement of the insulin sensitivity are found by exercising. Besides, osteoporosis prophylaxis, dementia prevention, and cancer onset protective efficacy are expected, too.

In type 1 diabetes mellitus, we reduce the cardiovascular risk factor and improve quality of life. The significance called the mental health maintenance is important.

The many clinical benefits of exercise in diabetic patients are as follows:

- An immediate effect of exercise is to increase the utilization of glucose and fatty acids and lower blood glucose.
- A long-term glycemic control as a result of the improvement of insulin resistance.

(continued)

M. Hosoi, M.D. (✉) • Y. Yakushiji, M.D.
Department of Diabetic Medicine, Osaka City General Hospital, 2-13-22, Miyakojima-hondori, Miyakojima-ku, Osaka, Japan
e-mail: my-hosoi@yb3.so-net.ne.jp

S. Tanaka, M.D.
Department of Sport and Health Science, Osaka Sangyo University, Osaka, Japan

M. Inaba (ed.), *Musculoskeletal Disease Associated with Diabetes Mellitus*,
DOI 10.1007/978-4-431-55720-3_18

- The improved balance between energy intake and expenditure is effective for the reduction of body weight.
- Exercise can promote loss of adipose tissue with preservation of lean body mass.
- Exercise can promote a beneficial redistribution of body fat.
- Osteoporosis caused by aging and insufficient exercise can be prevented.
- Exercise can improve dyslipidemia.
- Exercise can lower blood pressure.
- Cardiorespiratory function is improved.
- Mental health maintenance and the prevention of dementia.
- The prevention of cancer.
- Exercise capacity can be increased.
- Exercise can improve QOL, accompanied by the feeling of exhilaration and increased energy.

18.2 Medical Check and Adaptation for Exercise

When patients start doing exercise, an evaluation (medical check) should be done beforehand concerning medical questions such as the age of the patients, an exercise custom, the physical situation, the physical strength, and the degree of the diabetic complications such as neuropathy, retinopathy, nephropathy, brain cardiovascular disease, and orthopedic disease.

It is important to take a history of patients' medication. If they take the beta-blocker remedy, not having a pulse rise or arrhythmia by exercising may mislead the medical check. Also it is important to watch out for the presence of orthostatic hypotension, a sensory nerve disorder, and the pulse beat of the dorsalis pedis artery.

It is desirable to perform the stress test to detect ischemia in higher-risk patients. Criteria for consideration of graded exercise stress testing are as follows:

- Patients with insufficient blood glucose control
- Elderly patients
- Patients treated with insulin
- Type 1 diabetes patients (duration of a disease is 15 years or more)
- Type 2 diabetes patients (duration of a disease is 10 years or more)
- Patients with mild or severe hypertension
- Patients with severe obesity

The treadmill test, CT coronary angiography, and myocardium scintigraphy are useful. Particularly, the search of the silent myocardial ischemia lesion becomes the problem. Careful evaluation must be needed because of the sensitivity and specificity of each stress testing.

18.3 Universal Risks of Exercise in Patients with Diabetes

In the same way as medical therapy, there are a main effect and a side effect in the exercise therapy. A condition worsens and causes new complications when we take the wrong adaptation.

There are some significant risks associated with exercise in diabetic patients, including symptomatic hypoglycemia which can occur in up to 24 h after exercise, exacerbation of known cardiac disease, worsening of symptoms secondary to degenerative joint disease, and possible damage to joints in the setting of neuropathy [1].

18.3.1 Hypoglycemia

Twenty to sixty minutes after exercise, endogenous insulin secretion decreases and increases the glucogenesis with the liver, but hypoglycemia occurs in the healthy subject because this insulin secretion inhibition does not occur in patients with use of insulin and oral hypoglycemic agents.

Also, the insulin sensitivity with the muscle is improved by exercise, and the blood sugar level decreases for glycogenesis increase.

As for this effect, we might produce hypoglycemia as tardive hypoglycemia after exercise on the second day of the exercise to continue after exercise for a few days for several hours.

It is desirable to take an absorption of 80–160 kcal of good carbohydrates when blood glucose level before the exercise is 100 mg/dl or less.

Especially, insulin adjustment is necessary in type 1 diabetic patients.

Insulin regimen for exercise:

- Multiple injections:

  Decrease short-acting insulin dose by 30–50 % before exercise.
  Adjust post-exercise doses based on glucose monitoring and experience with post-exercise hypoglycemia.

- Insulin pump therapy:

  Decrease basal infusion rate.
  Decrease or omit pre-meal boluses before exercise.
  Adjust post-exercise basal rate and boluses based on glucose level.

18.3.2 Hyperglycemia and Ketotic Aggravation

Because there is the rise of insulin antagonism hormones such as glucagon in remarkable hyperglycemia and ketotic state on exercise, metabolism states such as a rise in the further blood glucose level or the ketotic progress aggravate it. Exercise for this purpose is contraindicated. The exercise is contraindicated in patients with urine ketones positive and a fasting blood sugar level of 250 mg/dl or more.

18.3.3 Aggravation of the Diabetic Nephropathy

On the contrary, proteinuria increases and, by exercising, may cause the exacerbation of edema and concurrence of heart failure. It is first, and principle exercise is possible for stage 2.

When proteinuria increases by exercising in stage 3, we lower the exercise intensity and need to limit the aerobic exercise.

We assume it a walk and housework of the degree not to reduce physical active mass for the fourth stage 5.

In patients with advanced complications, it is necessary to prevent them from reducing physical active mass in their everyday lives as much as possible.

18.3.4 Aggravation of the Diabetic Retinopathy

The normal exercise is good for the simple retinopathy, but requires attention not to cause excessive elevated blood pressure. The exercise with the Valsalva maneuver (the movement that demands holding out of one's breath) prevents it from being carried out. When maculopathy and proliferative retinopathy, particularly recent vitreous hemorrhage, are detected, the exercise is contraindicated.

18.3.5 Aggravation of the Diabetic Neuropathy

When there is a sensory nerve disorder, we are unconscious, and an injury by the exercise may be caused; thus foot care is necessary. When there are autonomic nervous system disorders, it shows low blood pressure after high blood pressure and exercise during the exercise and needs attention because lack of self-consciousness-related hypoglycemia is found. With the advanced thing of autonomic nervous system disorders, the sudden death is not rare, too, and as for the exercise except in the everyday life, prohibition is a principle.

18.3.6 Aggravation of Macro-angiopathy (Cardiovascular System)

The presence or absence of myocardial infarction and angina is the complication that is the most serious including anamnestic presence. Particularly, in patients with diabetes, we may have silent myocardial ischemia and need attention for the screening.

Attention is necessary for low blood pressure and for blood pressure, a pulse change by the resistance exercise in particular after high blood pressure, and exercise during the exercise.

18.3.7 Aggravation (Foot Lesion) of the Skeletal System Disorder

We may have a foot ulcer and gangrene by exercise in patients having sensory nerve disorder and peripheral arterial disease (PAD) in particular and are to watch out. An unnoticeable foot deformity (Charcot joint) could be caused by even minutes bone fractures with a sensory nerve disorder (Fig. 18.1).

Exercise should be prohibited or restricted in the following cases:

- When metabolic control is extremely poor (fasting plasma glucose level over 250 mg/dl or urinary ketone bodies positive or above).
- When new hemorrhaging in the ocular fundus caused by proliferative retinopathy occurs. Vigorous exercise can cause retinal hemorrhage or vitreous bleeding in patients with proliferative retinopathy.
- When renal failure (serum creatinine in men over 2.5 mg/dl and in women over 2.0 mg/dl) proteinuria tends to increase with exercise in patients with nephropathy.
- When there is a presence of ischemic heart disease and cardiopulmonary disorders.
- When there is a presence of diabetic gangrene and bone or joint disease. Patients with sensory neuropathy should refrain from high-impact exercise to reduce the risk of soft tissue and joint injury.
- When there is a presence of acute infectious disease.
- When there is presence of severe autonomic neuropathy. The presence of autonomic neuropathy often decreases aerobic capacity and causes postural hypotension.

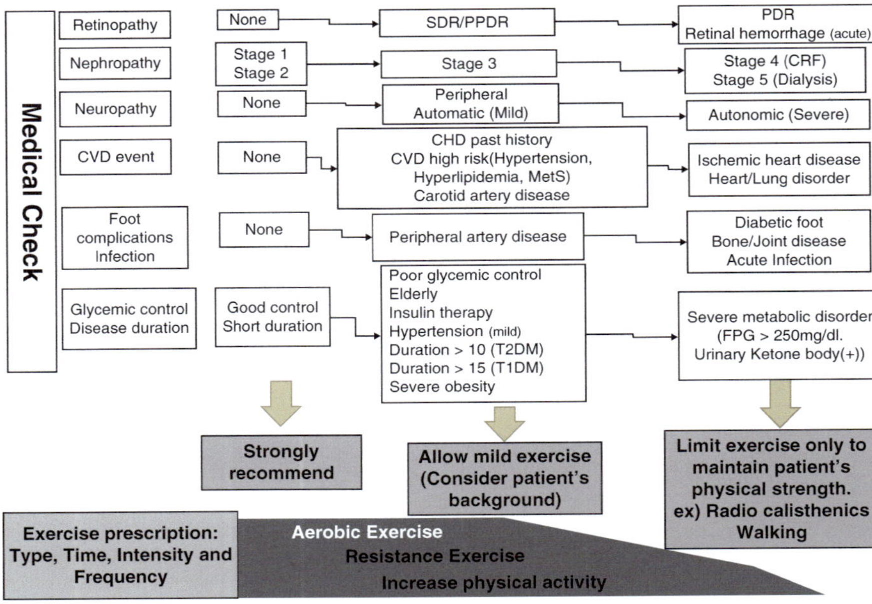

Fig. 18.1 Exercise therapy application criteria for patients with diabetes; after careful medical check, exercise prescription on the type, time, intensity, and frequency must be ordered according to the degree or extension of diabetic complications

18.4 Practical Prescription for Exercise Therapy

After careful medical check, a prescription for exercise must be ordered. You should prescribe the following orders (5W1H):

Why (purpose of exercise)
What (mode of exercise)
When (frequency and duration of exercise)
Where (place for exercise)
Who (patients to be prohibited or restricted from exercise)
How (intensity of exercise)

18.4.1 Mode of Exercise

There are two typical types of exercise, aerobic and resistance. The former consists of exercise whose intensity is proportional to the consumption of oxygen and which, if performed regularly, increases insulin sensitivity. Exercises involving the whole body, such as brisk walking and jogging, belong to this category. Resistance exercise, on the other hand, if performed is anaerobic exercise against a force or resistance. If practiced effectively, this form of exercise can be expected to increase the mass and strength of the muscles.

Recently, physical activities are focused in addition to the above two exercises.

18.4.1.1 Increase of the Physical Activities (Life Activities)

In "the physical activity indicator for the making of health," Ministry of Health, Labor and Welfare advice "Plus 10, let's move bodies for ten minutes more than now." It is said that 3 % of the risks of a disease and the care decrease by moving the body for 10 min.

Therefore at first, in every age group, we aim for the increase of the physical active mass.

Other than the case in which complications such as bleeding of ocular fundus or the highly advanced nephrotic state, we encourage patients to reduce the time spent sitting down, and to do more actively.

A walk, radio exercises, and light housework are recommended.

18.4.1.2 Aerobic Exercise

Aerobic exercise (walking, jogging, cycling, swimming exercise using the major muscle of the whole body) in moderate strength is ideal. However, careful exercise or physical limitation is necessary depending on the degree in patients with nonproliferative retinopathy and/or nephropathy stage 3 or more.

18.4.1.3 Resistance Exercise

We recommend the muscle training (repetition of eight kinds of training, 10–15 times for one set) more than twice a week.

The exercise using a dumbbell and lifting it, self-respect (squat for knee expansion and contraction in standing position), and the tube training is effective.

We can increase muscular strength and quantity of the muscle. We can also expect maintenance, increase of the basal metabolic rate, and the prevention of the arthropathy.

However, it is important that we do not keep on holding our breath (Valsalva breathing, exercise with the straining), which may increase blood pressure.

Resistance exercise doesn't have enough evidence about the contraindications of the exercise therapy.

Past studies reported that resistance exercise is hard to induce ischemic heart disease as compared with aerobic exercise. For example, high-intensity resistance exercise does not cause anginal changes such as an ST change or arrhythmia in patients with coronary artery disease that can occur in electrocardiogram change by moderate aerobic exercise (ADA).

Thus, in patients with cardiovascular complications, resistance exercise may be safer than aerobic exercise if they neither elevate blood pressure nor raise heart rate.

A resistance exercise together with aerobic exercise is more effective.

18.4.1.4 Stretch Exercise

In the case of a stretch exercise, particularly with an old age syndrome, a surveillance bottom is desirable.

18.4.2 Intensity of Exercise

Diabetic patients must select the type of exercise most suitable for themselves.

We recommend moderate aerobic exercise so as to pant lightly. Exercise requiring approximately 50 % of the maximum oxygen consumption is recommended. The degree can be judged by taking the heart rate during exercise. The pulse during exercise is kept between 100 and 120 bpm for subjects under 50 years old, and below 100 for those over 50 years old. The precise target heart rate is set to be as follows: the target heart rate (40–60 % of VO2max.) = {(220-age) – heart rate at rest} × 40–60 % + heart rate at rest.

However, if an index of the heart rate cannot be set, the patient's subjective feeling of their condition must be used as criterion. With a rating of perceived exertion, it is optimal exercise for patients to feel that "the degree is comfortable" or " is moderately strong-minded."

If the patient says, "It's hard," this should generally be taken to indicate that the exercise is excessive.

There is a method to express the exercise intensity as a standard of turn overrate using METs (metabolic equivalent unit, 1METs = turnover rate of 3.5 ml of oxygen consumption per weight, 1 kg per 1 min). Enforcement with or more than 23 exercises (at 1 exercise = 1METs × 1 h time, 4 exercises of those carries out activities 3METS or more) is desirable in a week.

18.4.3 Frequency of Exercise

It is desirable that the patients should include exercise sessions in their daily schedule. The minimum number of sessions should be no less than three times a week. Exercising 3–5 days or more is ideal in a week so that the chronic effect of the exercise decreases within 3 days and disappears in 1 week.

18.4.4 Duration of Exercise

Diabetic patients should spend 15–30 min twice a day for walking. The amount of walking should be approximately 10,000 steps in a day, and the amount of energy expended should be between 160 and 240 kcal.

Even minimal movement is said to be effective even when we carry out activities 150 min or more in total in a week.

18.4.5 Progression of Exercise

It is important that we increase moments in everyday life progressively. We perform setting-up exercises (warm-up) for approximately 3 min and rearranging exercises (cooling down) for approximately 3 min before and after exercise.

18.5 Art of the Exercise to Continue

- We attach a record.
- We take a rest without being unreasonable.
- We keep company such as a family member, a friend, and a pet dog.
- We give reward to ourself.
- Even if a fickle Buddhist priest says no on the third, the Buddhist priest repeats ten times on the third which makes 1 month – it's a positive thinking.

It is important to explain to patients as follows:

> Ii is first to increase physical activities even a little than the present. Depending on complications, a kind, degree of the exercise may include a limit [2].

References

1. Colberg SR (2013) Exercise and diabetes a clinician's guide to prescribing physical activity. American Diabetes Association, Alexandria, Virginia, USA
2. Hosoi M (2015) Exercise therapy for diabetic patients. In: Yamaguchi T, Kitahara M (eds) Today's therapy 2015. Igakushoin, Tokyo, pp 694–696

Chapter 19
Clinical Application of Exercise Therapy in Diabetes with Chronic Kidney Disease

Hisayo Yokoyama

Abstract A small number of patients with chronic kidney disease (CKD), particularly those on maintenance hemodialysis, are in the habit of exercise, and this sedentary lifestyle and poor physical fitness is associated with a high prevalence of fall-associated fracture and an increased mortality risk. However, exercise training has various therapeutic benefits in these patients. It delays the progression of microalbuminuria or CKD, increases physical fitness and strength, improves mental health, enhances dialysis efficacy, results in a better glycemic control, and reduces both cardiovascular and mortality risks.

If possible, undergoing a cardiopulmonary exercise test (CPX) before participating in an exercise program may lead to a safer and more effective training of these patients. Aerobic exercise training should be started with a low level of exercise load, and its intensity should be gradually increased along with the assessment of the patient's perceived exertion during the sessions. Not only ensuring the safety and enough consideration toward the diabetic complications but also the involvement of exercise professionals and attractive programs are included as the key elements of the sustainability of exercise in these patients.

Keywords Intradialytic exercise • Exercise test • Perceived exertion

H. Yokoyama (✉)
Research Center for Urban Health and Sports, Osaka City University, 3-3-138, Sugimoto, Sumiyoshi-ku, Osaka 558-8585, Japan
e-mail: yokoyama@sports.osaka-cu.ac.jp

M. Inaba (ed.), *Musculoskeletal Disease Associated with Diabetes Mellitus*,
DOI 10.1007/978-4-431-55720-3_19

19.1 Physical Frailty Among Patients with Chronic Kidney Disease (CKD)

19.1.1 Physical Inactivity Among Patients with CKD

19.1.1.1 A Small Number of the Patients with CKD Are Habitual of Exercise

Regular exercise is an established non-pharmacological therapeutic strategy for patients with diabetes with or without chronic kidney disease (CKD) and is expected to bring about favorable effects on their physical functions and reduce the cardiovascular and mortality risk factors. In 2005, the National Kidney Foundation recommended in the Kidney Disease Outcomes Quality Initiative (K/DOQI) cardiovascular guidelines that patients with CKD should perform at least 30 min of physical activity of moderate intensity every day, if possible [1]. However, this population, particularly, those on dialysis, has a significantly lower rate of being habitual to exercise as compared with their healthy sedentary counterparts. According to the cross-sectional data of 20,920 participants in the Dialysis Outcomes and Practice Patterns Study (DOPPS), 52.4 % of the patients on maintenance hemodialysis never exercised or exercised less than once a week, and this sedentary lifestyle was remarkable when the facility the patients belonged did not provide specific exercise programs [2]. In addition to the aforementioned findings, obtained using self-reported physical activity levels, investigations by activity monitors have quantitatively revealed the physical inactivity of patients on hemodialysis. Johansen et al. [3] and recently Kim et al. [4] reported in their studies using a three-dimensional accelerometer that the daily physical activity and the estimated daily energy expenditure were reduced in dialysis patients with values corresponding to 60–70 % of those in normal controls.

Several prospective observational studies, including a large cohort of dialysis patients, revealed that sedentary behavior was associated with an increased risk of mortality among not only the general population but also these patients [5–7].

19.1.1.2 Why Are They Sedentary?

Most patients on hemodialysis are forced to spend 3–4 h on bed rest during one dialysis session, which amounts to 9–12 h a week. Actually, the parameters pertaining to the physical activity level, such as the number of daily steps and activity-related energy expenditure, are lower on dialysis days as compared with non-dialysis days [8]. In addition, particularly, patients with diabetes may face difficulties in getting out of bed due to various complications such as blindness, stroke sequelae, and leg amputation. However, physical inactivity among these patients on dialysis is not only a result of this lengthy bed rest period. Delgado et al. conducted a survey on 100 dialysis patients to identify the barriers, which prevent them from participating in exercise [9]. In their report, almost all patients believed that a sedentary lifestyle was a health risk and that exercising was beneficial. Nevertheless, a majority of them had at least one barrier toward physical activity. Shortness of breath, lack of motivation, and having multiple medical problems were the most common barriers, in addition to fatigue or insufficient time to exercise on dialysis days.

Although the patients also answered they would exercise if counseled to do so, the counseling behavior by nephrologists does not seem enough. Few nephrologists make an assessment of their patients' physical activity levels and advise them to increase exercise in spite of the published K/DOQI guidelines [10]. This lack of guidance by the nephrologists is associated with their concerns about risks associated with exercise participation and a lack of confidence in the ability to discuss the topics pertaining to physical activity. Consequently, patients with CKD have little opportunity to increase their physical activity.

19.1.2 Low Exercise Capacity and Motor Ability in the Population

19.1.2.1 Low Peak Oxygen Consumption (Peak VO_2) and Impaired Motor Ability

There are several studies regarding limited aerobic fitness in patients with CKD. It has been reported that patients with stage 3–5 CKD have a lower peak VO_2 as compared with their healthy counterparts, with an average of 50–80 % of reference values [11]. Furthermore, Leehey et al. in an exercise intervention study showed that obese diabetic patients with stage 2–4 CKD had an extremely low peak VO_2, averaging 45 % of healthy levels [12]. Their low exercise capacity corresponded to the Class III determined in New York Heart Function Assessment (NYHA) classification and probably limited their daily activities to slow walking.

In addition to a low aerobic capacity, muscle atrophy (sarcopenia) and reduced muscle strength are common complications among patients with CKD, particularly in the dialysis patients [13]. The cross-sectional areas of thigh muscle are smaller in dialysis patients than in dialysis-independent patients with CKD and are associated with aging and low serum albumin concentration [14]. Quadriceps muscle strength in dialysis patients is also less than 70 % of that in their anthropometrically matched healthy counterparts, and serum albumin concentration is the only significant predictor of the loss of muscle strength [15]. Thus, muscle weakness, a well-recognized feature in dialysis patients, is most likely derived from protein-energy malnutrition.

19.1.2.2 Clinical Consequences of Low Exercise Capacity

In elderly people, physical performance and functional independence in daily life are mainly determined by muscle strength. The same is true for dialysis patients, and muscle weakness contributes to impairment in mobility such as walking at a slow speed. Dialysis patients also have higher chances of falling. Cook et al. have shown by cross-sectional interviews with seniors (65 years and older) on dialysis that 27 % of them had fallen in the past 12 months and that 4 % of them had reported a fall-associated fracture or head injury [16]. They also revealed that the rate of falling in elderly dialysis patients was higher than in the elderly population without CKD [17]. Trauma or fracture by falling inevitably causes hospitalization and functional decline and often results in being bedridden or other life-threatening conditions.

On the other hand, exercise capacity evaluated by peak VO_2 is an important predictor of survival in dialysis patients as well as in the population without CKD [18]. This is because peak VO_2 reflects other factors (e.g., cardiovascular function or complicated medical conditions), which have been previously established as the predictors of survival for the patients. Sietsema et al. analyzed 175 dialysis cohorts over a median follow-up of 39 months and found that a low peak VO_2 was a significant contributor to mortality along with age and chronic heart failure [19]. Recently, a much simpler test measuring the distance walked in 6 min has become widely used as the index of functional capacity. This test is closely associated with peak VO_2, and it has been reported as a useful predictor of survival in dialysis patients, in whom a 100-m increment increased approximately 5 % of the survival rate [20].

In addition, it is a major problem that these impaired physical performances adversely affect the mental health and health-related quality of life (QOL) in patients with CKD, particularly in those on dialysis [21–23], which finally results in dependency on family members and caregivers.

19.1.2.3 Why Are They Unfit?

Besides physical inactivity, various specific factors in CKD seem to contribute to low physical fitness, although the exact mechanism has not been fully resolved. To date, anemia, a very common complication in patients with CKD, has been considered to be very important in the reduction of exercise capacity in these patients. A number of studies have reported an improvement in peak VO_2 by intense treatment of anemia in patients with dialysis-dependent and dialysis-independent CKD. However, in many of these studies, exercise capacity failed to improve as much as was expected post the extent of the achieved amount of correction in hemoglobin concentration. Furthermore, some reports found that exercise performance fell with the progression of chronic renal failure despite the maintenance of hemoglobin concentration [24]. Therefore, the impact of anemia in the impairment of exercise capacity is still controversial. Other potential causes include uremic toxins [25], which have been suggested as a mechanism for impaired physical fitness in CKD, independent of physical inactivity; however, the exact mechanisms remain unknown. Cardiovascular factors such as endothelial dysfunction and high cardiac sympathetic nerve activity, which are common features in CKD, may also contribute to low exercise capacity in this population.

There was an intriguing report which evaluated whether dialysis itself affected exercise capacity. Moore et al. performed peak exercise testing in dialysis patients immediately before and during dialysis and demonstrated that peak VO_2 and cardiovascular responses such as cardiac output or stroke volume on testing were not different between the two conditions [26]. These results suggest that dialysis itself has no effect on the acute response to exercise, i.e., the hemodynamic changes on dialysis or water retention could not explain the low physical fitness of dialysis patients.

19.2 Various Aspects of the Efficacy of Exercise in Patients with CKD

19.2.1 Delaying the Initiation of Dialysis

Can exercise slow the progression of renal dysfunction in predialytic patients with CKD? There are only a few interventional studies with small cohorts on this issue. A non-randomized aerobic exercise trial [27] and a randomized-controlled resistance training trial [28] have shown an increase in glomerular filtration rate (GFR) in patients with CKD after 12-week interventions. In the predialytic state, a low-protein diet is prescribed in almost all cases to delay the progression of CKD, which leads to muscle atrophy and frailty. As a specific effect on this population, exercise can reduce catabolism by low-protein diet and uremia. No previous study has supported the adverse effect of exercise on the progression of CKD.

19.2.2 Increasing Physical Fitness and Strength

The effect of exercise on maximum aerobic capacity has been a major concern in many clinical trials with aerobic exercise protocols in dialysis patients. In a systematic review by Cheema et al., 17 of 19 uncontrolled, non-randomized controlled, and randomized controlled trials (RCTs) succeeded in increasing peak VO_2 by 17–23 % mainly due to aerobic training for a period of 10 weeks to 4 years in patients maintained on hemodialysis [29]. In another review article, Johansen demonstrated that trials with aerobic exercise training for 8 weeks to 6 months enhanced peak VO_2 by 17 %, regardless of the use of erythropoietin to control renal anemia [30]. Smart et al. reported in a more recent systematic review on 365 patients from 8 studies that aerobic training increased peak VO_2 from 70 to 88 % of age-predicted value, corresponding to +5.22 ml/kg/min of peak VO_2 [31]. The improvements in peak VO_2 reported in these studies, although significant, were relatively minor, and the patients could not reach the predicted age-adjusted peak VO_2 even after the intervention.

Muscle strength is the most important contributor to physical performance and independence in daily life. Particularly in the last 5 years, several RCTs on dialysis patients concerning the effect of exercise on muscle strength could be found. These studies reported the positive effect of intradialytic resistance training, with or without cycle ergometer, on the muscle strength of lower extremities [32–35]. Furthermore, the ACTINUT study, an RCT against protein-energy wasting and muscle atrophy, is currently ongoing [36]. In addition, a biopsy study also showed the regeneration of degenerated muscle fibers, increase in capillary density, and favorable changes in the structure and number of mitochondria following exercise training in hemodialysis patients [37]. The improvement in functional abilities evaluated by gait speed, stair-climbing, 10-m walking, or timed up and go test was also found to be associated with increased muscle strength.

19.2.3 Positive Psychiatric Effects

Like many other chronic diseases, CKD probably affects the psychological state of the patients. Based on the high incidence of depression and anxiety among this population, a concept called "psychonephrology" was proposed to refer to this problem, particularly, in patients on maintenance hemodialysis and those who have had a kidney transplant [38]. There are only a few reports that have demonstrated the favorable effects of aerobic exercise on mental health and health-related QOL. Most of these used the Short Form-36 questionnaire, which is frequently used to evaluate QOL in patients on dialysis as well as in the general population [39–41]. For many elderly patients on dialysis, clinical outcomes such as mental status and QOL may become more important than mortality. From this perspective, it is desirable that they increase opportunities to participate in exercise more actively in the clinical settings of dialysis, although further studies on the effects of exercise on mental health in this population are necessary.

19.2.4 Enhancing Dialysis Efficacy

Reduced hemodialysis efficiency with insufficient removal of toxins leads to the accumulation of uremic toxins and systemic damages in a concentration-dependent manner. To address this issue, the methodologies involved in hemodialysis

(HD) such as high-flux HD and online hemodiafiltration (HDF) have been developed, in addition to increasing the dialysis time and frequency. However, the benefits of these therapies are restricted by inter-compartmental resistance, i.e., toxins distributed in intracellular and interstitial compartments are restricted from being removed by cellular membranes or capillary endothelium. Intradialytic exercise increases cardiac output and blood flow to low-perfusion skeletal muscle regions and could possibly increase the exchange between these compartments and the systemic circulation, therefore, enhancing the removal of uremic toxins. Several previous studies have reported the improvement of dialysis efficiency, assessed by Kt/V, clearance of urea and creatinine, and removal of potassium and phosphate, by intradialytic exercise [42, 43]. A prospective-randomized study, comparing toxin removal in online HDF and intradialytic exercise in high-flux HD, is also ongoing [44].

19.2.5 Improving Glycemic Control

Exercise is an established therapeutic strategy for type 2 diabetes, and several meta-analyses have reported that aerobic exercise, resistance exercise, and a combination of the two improved glycemic control in this population with HbA1c levels reduced by 0.6–0.8 % [45–47]. An elevated HbA1c level is an independent contributor to mortality in diabetic patients with and without CKD and in those on maintenance hemodialysis [48–50]. Therefore, improved glycemic control is a very important aspect of health management in patients with diabetes and CKD.

Insulin resistance is a common finding in diabetes with CKD due to impaired insulin signaling in skeletal muscle cells along with muscle atrophy and metabolic acidosis [51]. These features are often masked by the prolonged half-life of insulin secondary to decrease in both the degeneration of insulin and its renal clearance. DeFronzo et al. demonstrated that peripheral insulin-mediated glucose uptake was decreased in patients on dialysis [10]. For these reasons, exercise may be more suitable than therapies with insulin or insulin secretagogues, for glycemic management in patients with CKD. A recent interventional study revealed that the effects of strength training on glucose tolerance by changing in muscle fiber-type composition in type 2 diabetes on dialysis [52].

19.2.6 Reducing Cardiovascular Risks

Patients with CKD not on dialysis are at the highest risk of cardiovascular diseases (CVD), and they are more likely to die of CVD than to progress to dialysis [53]. These patients have a high prevalence of traditional risk factors for CVD, such as diabetes, hypertension, and dyslipidemia. Various conditions closely related to CKD itself, including endothelial dysfunction, high sympathetic activity, oxidative stress, and inflammation, may also increase the risk for cardiovascular diseases in this population. Of course physical inactivity itself contributes to the development of CVD; therefore, exercise or physical activity could ameliorate CKD-associated cardiovascular dysfunction [54, 55]. However, there is no available evidence that exercise intervention can reduce the incidence of CVD in patients with CKD.

Many studies have suggested a counterintuitive relationship between obesity, hypertension, or hypercholesterolemia and CVD risk in dialysis patients. The lack of these CVD risk factors, which are generally expected to be ameliorated by exercise, rather involve malnutrition associated with a higher risk of mortality in dialysis patients, and this phenomenon is known as "reverse epidemiology" [56]. Nevertheless, a sedentary lifestyle is still a risk factor for impaired cardiovascular health and high mortality rate in this population [30].

19.2.7 Reducing Mortality Risks

As mentioned in Sect. 19.1.1.1, several observational studies, including the latest one with a large cohort of dialysis patients, have shown that physical inactivity, assessed by self-report or interview, was associated with an increased risk of mortality among these patients [5–7]. On the other hand, there are only a few studies regarding the effect of exercise intervention on life expectancy in patients on maintenance dialysis. We could only find one study reporting mortality risk reduction by cardiac rehabilitation in dialysis patients who have undergone coronary artery bypass grafting (CABG). Huang et al. have shown that over a 42-month follow-up period, cardiac rehabilitation was associated with a longer cumulative survival time with an increase of up to 76 days in post-CABG dialysis patients [57]. Further longitudinal studies are needed to elucidate whether exercise increases life span in these patients.

19.3 Exercise Practice for Patients with CKD

19.3.1 Cardiopulmonary Exercise Test (CPX)

Exercise testing has mainly been used for screening and identification of myocardial ischemia for a long time. However, there are no available guidelines specifically for conducting CPX in patients with CKD or end-stage renal disease. If "asymptomatic" patients intend to perform low-intensity physical activity such as walking, routine CPX before the participation is not necessarily recommended, because it does not seem to have any significant benefits on serious clinical outcomes even among patients with diabetes who are at a high risk for silent ischemia [58].

In addition, requiring routine CPX before exercise may rather be obstructive to participating in exercises for the patients. Consequently, it is unlikely that pre-exercise CPX is essential for all patients with CKD or end-stage renal disease.

Even so, in a joint statement in 2010, the American College of Sports Medicine (ACSM) and the American Diabetes Association (ADA) proposed recommendations for exercise testing in patients with diabetes. They stated that exercise testing was advisable in patients with type 2 diabetes who had previously been sedentary and now planned to undertake physical activity of an intensity more than brisk walking [59]. The American Heart Association (AHA) guidelines also recommend that individuals at a greater risk for CVD, such as the patients with diabetes or known CVD, should be considered for exercise testing before participating in vigorous exercise programs [60]. According to these statements, it is preferable that patients with CKD, who are also at a high risk for CVD, undergo CPX not only for screening but also for the evaluation of prognosis and effect of therapy, including exercise interventions, if all necessary equipment for the testing is available. According to the AHA guidelines for exercise testing in older people, the testing must include an adequate warm-up period at low resistance and progress with a modest and almost imperceptible increment in exercise load [60]. Such modulation is also ideal for exercise testing in patients with CKD.

A previous survey reported that one to two myocardial infarctions and sustained ventricular tachycardia per 10,000 tests are expected [61]. Therefore, exercise testing is considered an extremely safe procedure. However, a defibrillator and other appropriate medications should be immediately available, and physicians supervising the test must be trained in cardiopulmonary resuscitation.

19.3.2 Exercise Prescription for Dialysis Patients

The aforementioned K/DOQI guidelines recommend that dialysis patients should participate in cardiovascular (aerobic) exercise at a moderate intensity for 30 min most, if not all, days per week [1]. Moderate intensity generally means exercising to reach a target heart rate of 60–70 % of the maximal heart rate (220-age). However, exercise prescriptions based on heart rate may not be suitable for dialysis patients, because their fluid status and medications such as β-adrenergic blocking agents can affect their heart rate response to exercise. If the dialysis patients have undergone CPX, the physicians can prescribe the exercise load at an aerobic threshold as an appropriate intensity. Another way to determine exercise intensity for dialysis patients is to use the highly reproducible Borg's rating of perceived exertion (RPE) scale, which ranges from 6 (no exertion at all) to 20 (maximal exertion) and is widely used to assess perceived patients' exertion during an exercise test in clinical settings. Because a rating of "13 (somewhat hard)" corresponds approximately to an aerobic threshold, around "13" on the scale can be adopted as the target exercise intensity. It is also important to provide several minutes of warm-up at very low levels before the true exercise period followed by an adequate cooling-down period.

In addition to aerobic exercise, resistance training is also recommended with the aim of strengthening the muscles of the lower extremities. This program has to be individualized and gradually stepped up from bodyweight exercise, using the patient's own weight against gravity as resistance to weight training of the hand and ankle weights or Thera-Bands. Furthermore, combining this with flexibility exercises may enhance the efficacy of resistance training and activity level during walking by improving the range of motion and stride.

19.3.3 Special Concerns About Exercise for Diabetes with CKD

In the ACSM/ADA joint position statement of 2010, it was suggested that exercise for diabetes with nephropathy should be started with a low intensity and volume because of reduced aerobic capacity and muscle function in this population [59]. These are essential to avoid the patients from feeling that the exercise program is difficult and losing motivation and to prevent them from unexpected injuries. The statement also mentioned exercise with Valsalva maneuver, which may not only cause retinal hemorrhage in patients with active retinopathy but also cause an excessive elevation of blood pressure (BP) [59]. Although, in many cases, an increase in urinary albumin excretion by BP elevation during exercise is transient, the patients should keep away from further otiose hypertension caused by vigorous exercise. Tight BP control along with the treatment and low-intensity exercise are more beneficial in delaying the progression of microalbuminuria [62].

If a patient is relatively fit and is able to exercise for longer than 1 h even at low intensity, frequent monitoring of blood glucose may minimize the risk of exercise-induced hypoglycemia. The patient may need to decrease insulin dosage by one or two units and take additional carbohydrate snacks before each exercise session. For better glucose control, both the patient and physician must regularly discuss the timing of drug and insulin administration and food intake prior to exercise.

19.3.4 When Should Dialysis Patients Exercise?

19.3.4.1 Exercise During Dialysis

Patients on hemodialysis can participate in facility-based exercise programs during their dialysis sessions. Investigators have shown favorable efficacy of intradialytic exercise training on exercise capacity, muscle strength, functional ability, and mental health [63]. In many cases, exercise professionals supervise intradialytic exercise; therefore, the patients can be advised on how to perform appropriate

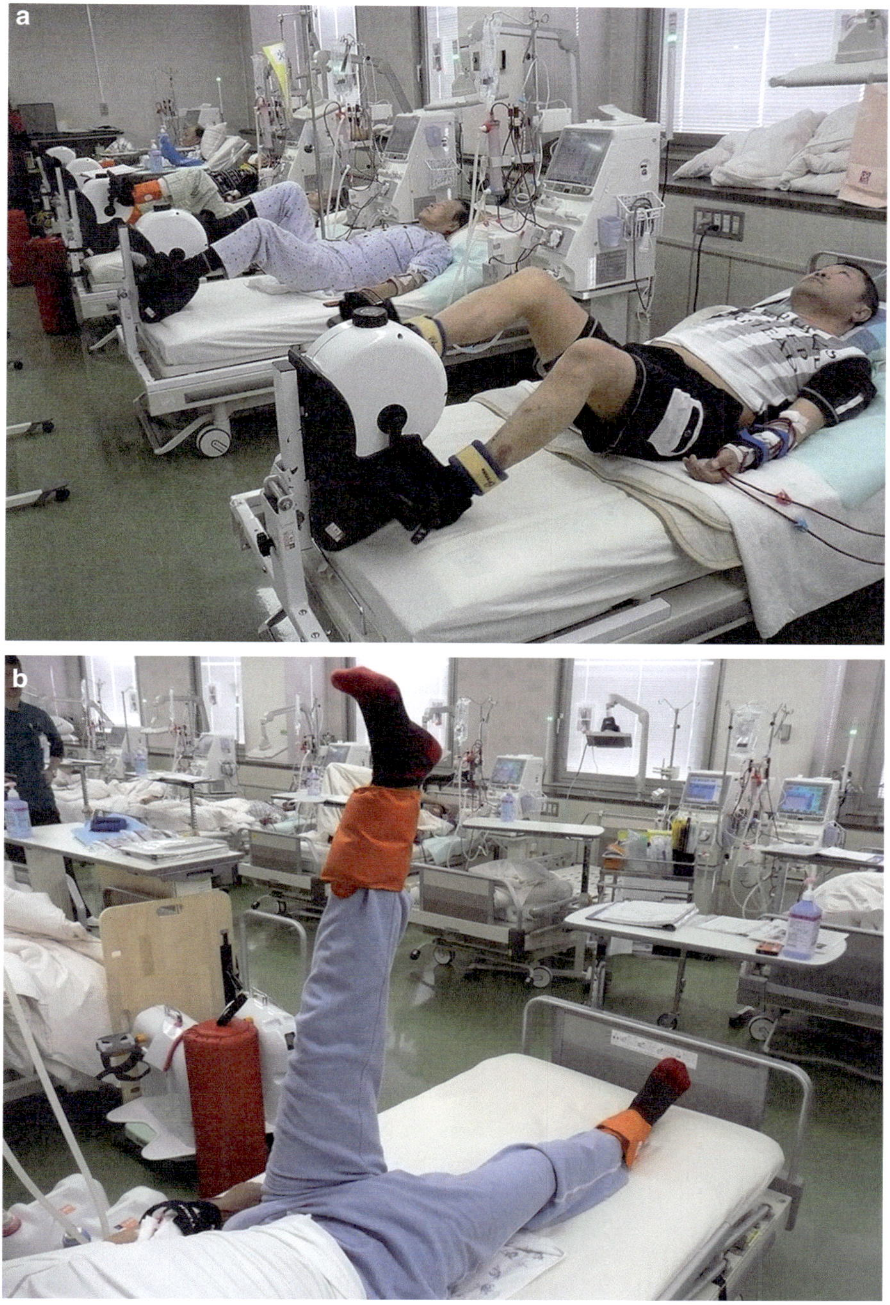

Fig. 19.1 Intradialytic exercise program (i.e., exercise during dialysis sessions). **a** Aerobic exercise using a recumbent cycle ergometer. **b** Strength training using ankle weights

exercises based on individual exercise prescriptions. In addition, intradialytic exercise is expected to enable the patients to save time, improve adherence to exercise, and avoid boredom during the dialysis treatment. Indeed, exercise programs during dialysis sessions often have lower dropout rates than outpatient exercise programs on non-dialysis days [64].

We also have incorporated an intradialytic exercise program into our partnered artificial dialysis facilities. Many patients begin the training program early in the dialysis treatment, which is composed of aerobic exercise using a recumbent cycle ergometer, strength training using silicone rubber bands or ankle weights, and flexibility exercises (Fig. 19.1a, b). The athletic trainers supervise each session and encourage the participants to perform exercise with adequate intensity and procedure. The program has been very successful, particularly, in improving peak VO_2 and physical function.

Exercise professionals often need to be involved in intradialytic exercise programs because dialysis staff may not have the skills or the inclination to attend the exercising patients. Furthermore, exercise performed during dialysis is usually limited to leg exercise because of vascular access complications; therefore, the patient needs to have another opportunity to exercise the upper extremities.

19.3.4.2 Home-Based Exercise on Non-dialysis Days

Home-based exercise training is an alternative for hemodialysis patients. This type of training enables them to exercise at their own convenience without being concerned about fatigue during dialysis, therefore resulting in a low dropout rate. Koh et al. in a randomized 6-month interventional study reported that home-based exercise training equally improved exercise capacity as intradialytic exercise in hemodialysis patients, if they could conduct home-based exercise with appropriate volume or intensity as advised [65]. However, because such programs cannot be supervised at all, it is difficult to ensure patient compliance with exercise. Whether the patients conduct exercise or not may be influenced by their motivation and mood. Therefore, in home-based exercise, practicing time and intensity are often insufficient, and there are a few studies, which report the effects of home-based exercise on cardiorespiratory function to be less than intradialysis exercise [64].

19.3.4.3 In-facility Exercise Programs on Non-dialysis Days

Although some dialysis facilities provide outpatient exercise programs, availability is still too low for the majority of dialysis patients to benefit from them. The survey in DOPPS (2005–2006) reported that only 10–20 % of facilities offered exercise programs to patients not on dialysis in most DOPPS countries [2]. Furthermore, patients' adherence to such programs is not satisfactory. They often stop participating because of lack of spare time on non-dialysis days, transportation difficulties, high morbidity, and lack of motivation [63, 64]. Nevertheless, such supervised exercise training on non-dialysis days enables them to perform more aggressive, high-intensity exercise and further sports activities involving the movement of upper extremities, which is difficult during the dialysis treatment because of vascular access. Therefore, this method of exercise program has the greatest effect on improving cardiorespiratory capacity in maintenance hemodialysis patients as compared with intradialytic or home-based exercise [64].

19.3.5 The Aspects of Sustainability of Exercise Programs

Because it is widely known that the benefits of exercise are lost within a few weeks of non-training (detraining), it is important to incorporate exercise programs into routine care in the population on dialysis. Bennett et al. tried to identify contributing factors for sustaining hemodialysis exercise programs by examining 28 original studies and 14 review articles [66]. Other than the aforementioned elements necessary for improving patients' adherence to exercise, such as exercise professionals' involvement and conducting exercise programs during dialysis sessions, they identified other factors as follows: commitment to exercise by dialysis and medical staff, adequate space and equipment, interesting and stimulating programs or interventions, and addressing cost implications. Although it is not easy to meet all these requirements, the staffs in dialysis facilities need to make some effort toward creating an atmosphere in which the patients feel like participating continuously in physical activity or exercise.

In regard to the patients on continuous ambulatory peritoneal dialysis (CAPD), exercise capacity estimated by peak VO_2 and aerobic threshold remain unchanged regardless of whether the dialysis solution was retained in the peritoneal cavity or drained. However, exercise time was significantly shortened when the solution was retained directly due to the carrying of extra weight [67]. Therefore, exercising under conditions in which the solution is drained may be sustainable for this population.

In addition, difficulty in sustaining physical activity in patients with CKD has been attributed to anemia. A meta-analysis by Johansen et al. demonstrated that the treatment of anemia using erythropoiesis-stimulating agents significantly increased peak VO_2 by 24 % in hemodialysis patients, although many studies included were not controlled trials [68]. The improvement in anemia probably contributes to the sustainability of exercise, because the patients are freed from shortness of breath and fatigue, which are both major barriers to continuously participating in exercise programs, and could overcome discomfort or pain during exercise.

19.3.6 *Safety of Exercise for Patients with CKD*

There is a very small amount of data from controlled studies to discuss or quantify the risks of exercise-induced adverse events in patients with CKD. However, to date, no published study on exercise training in hemodialysis patients has reported deaths or cardiovascular events. Therefore, it does not seem that exercise in dialysis patients necessarily carries additional risks.

According to a scientific statement from AHA, although the incidence of fatal and nonfatal cardiovascular events during exercise varies with the prevalence of cardiac disease in a study population, the rate is extremely low even among patients with chronic heart failure undertaking cardiac rehabilitation programs [69]. In contrast, the relative risk of cardiac arrest during vigorous exercise as compared with risk at other times is notably greater in patients who are unaccustomed to exercise [70]. Regular exercise participation, performed at low to moderate intensity, reduces the long-term risk of cardiac events both during exercise and at rest.

The exercise guide for nephrologists developed by the Life Options Rehabilitation Advisory Council suggested that to minimize the risks of exercise, nephrologists must be sure to provide adequate dialysis, manage ongoing medical concerns, control hypertension, and respond to symptoms suggestive of cardiac disease [71].

19.4 Summary

Patients with CKD, particularly, those on dialysis, have been exposed to the environment where they had a few opportunities to participate in physical activity due to conventional therapeutic policy. However, now it is evident that a sedentary lifestyle and low physical fitness result in a poor prognosis for this population. To engage all the patients in regular exercise, it is important that both patients and nephrologists discuss exercise positively and that the medical staff encourage the patients to exercise with a customized training program according to individual physical strength, medical concerns, and convenience.

References

1. K/DOQI Workgroup (2005) K/DOQI clinical practice guidelines for cardiovascular disease in dialysis patients. Am J Kidney Dis 45:S1–S153
2. Tentori F, Elder SJ, Thumma J, Pisoni RL, Bommer J, Fissell RB et al (2010) Physical exercise among participants in the Dialysis Outcomes and Practice Patterns Study (DOPPS): correlates and associated outcomes. Nephrol Dial Transplant 25:3050–3062
3. Johansen KL, Chertow GM, Ng AV, Mulligan K, Carey S, Schoenfeld PY et al (2000) Physical activity levels in patients on hemodialysis and healthy sedentary controls. Kidney Int 57:2564–2570

4. Kim JC, Shapiro BB, Zhang M, Li Y, Porszasz J, Bross R et al (2014) Daily physical activity and physical function in adult maintenance hemodialysis patients. J Cachex Sarcopenia Muscle 5:209–220
5. O'Hare AM, Tawney K, Bacchetti P, Johansen KL (2003) Decreased survival among sedentary patients undergoing dialysis: results from the dialysis morbidity and mortality study wave 2. Am J Kidney Dis 41:447–454
6. Stack AG, Molony DA, Rives T, Tyson J, Murthy BV (2005) Association of physical activity with mortality in the US dialysis population. Am J Kidney Dis 45:690–701
7. Lopes AA, Lantz B, Morgenstern H, Wang M, Bieber BA, Gillespie BW et al (2014) Associations of self-reported physical activity types and levels with quality of life, depression symptoms, and mortality in hemodialysis patients: the DOPPS. Clin J Am Soc Nephrol 9:1702–1712
8. Avesani CM, Trolonge S, Deleaval P, Baria F, Mafra D, Faxen-Irving G et al (2012) Physical activity and energy expenditure in hemodialysis patients: an international survey. Nephrol Dial Transplant 27:2430–2434
9. Delgado C, Johansen KL (2012) Barriers to exercise participation among dialysis patients. Nephrol Dial Transplant 27:1152–1157
10. Delgado C, Johansen KL (2010) Deficient counseling on physical activity among nephrologists. Nephron Clin Pract 116:c330–c336
11. Johansen KL, Painter P (2012) Exercise in individuals with CKD. Am J Kidney Dis 59:126–134
12. Leehey DJ, Moinuddin I, Bast JP, Qureshi S, Jelinek CS, Cooper C et al (2009) Aerobic exercise in obese diabetic patients with chronic kidney disease: a randomized and controlled pilot study. Cardiovasc Diabetol 8:62
13. Johansen KL, Shubert T, Doyle J, Soher B, Sakkas GK, Kent-Braun JA (2003) Muscle atrophy in patients receiving hemodialysis: effects on muscle strength, muscle quality, and physical function. Kidney Int 63:291–297
14. McIntyre CW, Selby NM, Sigrist M, Pearce LE, Mercer TH, Naish PF (2006) Patients receiving maintenance dialysis have more severe functionally significant skeletal muscle wasting than patients with dialysis-independent chronic kidney disease. Nephrol Dial Transplant 21:2210–2216
15. Spindler A, Paz S, Berman A, Lucero E, Contino N, Penalba A et al (1997) Muscular strength and bone mineral density in hemodialysis patients. Nephrol Dial Transplant 12:128–132
16. Cook WL, Jassal SV (2005) Prevalence of falls among seniors maintained on hemodialysis. Int Urol Nephrol 37:649–652
17. Cook WL, Tomlinson G, Donaldson M, Markowitz SN, Naglie G, Sobolev B et al (2006) Falls and fall-related injuries in older dialysis patients. Clin J Am Soc Nephrol 1:1197–1204
18. Myers J, Prakash M, Froelicher V, Do D, Partington S, Atwood JE (2002) Exercise capacity and mortality among men referred for exercise testing. N Engl J Med 346:793–801
19. Sietsema KE, Amato A, Adler SG, Brass EP (2004) Exercise capacity as a predictor of survival among ambulatory patients with end-stage renal disease. Kidney Int 65:719–724
20. Kohl Lde M, Signori LU, Ribeiro RA, Silva AM, Moreira PR, Dipp T et al (2012) Prognostic value of the six-minute walk test in end-stage renal disease life expectancy: a prospective cohort study. Clinics 67:581–586
21. Laegreid IK, Aasarod K, Bye A, Leivestad T, Jordhoy M (2014) The impact of nutritional status, physical function, comorbidity and early versus late start in dialysis on quality of life in older dialysis patients. Ren Fail 36:9–16
22. Oliveira CM, Costa SP, Costa LC, Pinheiro SM, Lacerda GA, Kubrusly M (2012) Depression in dialysis patients and its association with nutritional markers and quality of life. J Nephrol 25:954–961
23. Da Silva-Gane M, Wellsted D, Greenshields H, Norton S, Chandna SM, Farrington K (2012) Quality of life and survival in patients with advanced kidney failure managed conservatively or by dialysis. Clin J Am Soc Nephrol 7:2002–2009

24. Leikis MJ, McKenna MJ, Petersen AC, Kent AB, Murphy KT, Leppik JA et al (2006) Exercise performance falls over time in patients with chronic kidney disease despite maintenance of hemoglobin concentration. Clin J Am Soc Nephrol 1:488–495
25. Moore GE, Parsons DB, Stray-Gundersen J, Painter PL, Brinker KR, Mitchell JH (1993) Uremic myopathy limits aerobic capacity in hemodialysis patients. Am J Kidney Dis 22:277–287
26. Moore GE, Brinker KR, Stray-Gundersen J, Mitchell JH (1993) Determinants of VO2 peak in patients with end-stage renal disease: on and off dialysis. Med Sci Sports Exerc 25:18–23
27. Toyama K, Sugiyama S, Oka H, Sumida H, Ogawa H (2010) Exercise therapy correlates with improving renal function through modifying lipid metabolism in patients with cardiovascular disease and chronic kidney disease. J Cardiol 56:142–146
28. Castaneda C, Gordon PL, Uhlin KL, Levey AS, Kehayias JJ, Dwyer JT et al (2001) Resistance training to counteract the catabolism of a low-protein diet in patients with chronic renal insufficiency. A randomized, controlled trial. Ann Intern Med 135:965–976
29. Cheema BS, Singh MA (2005) Exercise training in patients receiving maintenance hemodialysis: a systematic review of clinical trials. Am J Nephrol 25:352–364
30. Johansen KL (2007) Exercise in the end-stage renal disease population. J Am Soc Nephrol 18:1845–1854
31. Smart N, Steele M (2011) Exercise training in hemodialysis patients: a systematic review and meta-analysis. Nephrology 16:626–632
32. Cheema B, Abas H, Smith B, O'Sullivan A, Chan M, Patwardhan A et al (2007) Randomized controlled trial of intradialytic resistance training to target muscle wasting in ESRD: the Progressive Exercise for Anabolism in Kidney Disease (PEAK) study. Am J Kidney Dis 50:574–584
33. Dong J, Sundell MB, Pupim LB, Wu P, Shintani A, Ikizler TA (2011) The effect of resistance exercise to augment long-term benefits of intradialytic oral nutritional supplementation in chronic hemodialysis patients. J Ren Nutr 21:149–159
34. Song WJ, Sohng KY (2012) Effects of progressive resistance training on body composition, physical fitness and quality of life of patients on hemodialysis. J Korean Acad Nurs 42:947–956
35. Paglialonga F, Lopopolo A, Scarfia RV, Consolo S, Galli MA, Salera S et al (2014) Intradialytic cycling in children and young adults on chronic hemodialysis. Pediatr Nephrol 29:431–438
36. Magnard J, Deschamps T, Cornu C, Paris A, Hristea D (2013) Effects of a six-month intradialytic physical ACTIvity program and adequate NUTritional support on protein-energy wasting, physical functioning and quality of life in chronic hemodialysis patients: ACTINUT study protocol for a randomized controlled trial. BMC Nephrol 14:259
37. Kouidi E, Albani M, Natsis K, Megalopoulos A, Gigis P, Guiba-Tziampiri O et al (1998) The effects of exercise training on muscle atrophy in hemodialysis patients. Nephrol Dial Transplant 13:685–699
38. Levy NB (2008) What is psychonephrology? J Nephrol 21(Suppl 13):S51–S53
39. Levendoglu F, Altintepe L, Okudan N, Ugurlu H, Gokbel H, Tonbul Z et al (2004) A twelve week exercise program improves the psychological status, quality of life and work capacity in hemodialysis patients. J Nephrol 17:826–832
40. Matsumoto Y, Furuta A, Furuta S, Miyajima M, Sugino T, Nagata K et al (2007) The impact of pre-dialytic endurance training on nutritional status and quality of life in stable hemodialysis patients (Sawada study). Ren Fail 29:587–593
41. Carney RM, Templeton B, Hong BA, Harter HR, Hagberg JM, Schechtman KB et al (1987) Exercise training reduces depression and increases the performance of pleasant activities in hemodialysis patients. Nephron 47:194–198
42. Farese S, Budmiger R, Aregger F, Bergmann I, Frey FJ, Uehlinger DE (2008) Effect of transcutaneous electrical muscle stimulation and passive cycling movements on blood pressure and removal of urea and phosphate during hemodialysis. Am J Kidney Dis 52:745–752

43. Giannaki CD, Stefanidis I, Karatzaferi C, Liakos N, Roka V, Ntente I et al (2011) The effect of prolonged intradialytic exercise in hemodialysis efficiency indices. ASAIO J 57:213–218
44. Maheshwari V, Samavedham L, Rangaiah GP, Loy Y, Ling LH, Sethi S et al (2012) Comparison of toxin removal outcomes in online hemodiafiltration and intradialytic exercise in high-flux hemodialysis: a prospective randomized open-label clinical study protocol. BMC Nephrol 13:156
45. Boule NG, Kenny GP, Haddad E, Wells GA, Sigal RJ (2003) Meta-analysis of the effect of structured exercise training on cardiorespiratory fitness in Type 2 diabetes mellitus. Diabetologia 46:1071–1081
46. Snowling NJ, Hopkins WG (2006) Effects of different modes of exercise training on glucose control and risk factors for complications in type 2 diabetic patients: a meta-analysis. Diabetes Care 29:2518–2527
47. Umpierre D, Ribeiro PA, Kramer CK, Leitao CB, Zucatti AT, Azevedo MJ et al (2011) Physical activity advice only or structured exercise training and association with HbA1c levels in type 2 diabetes: a systematic review and meta-analysis. J Am Med Assoc 305:1790–1799
48. Morioka T, Emoto M, Tabata T, Shoji T, Tahara H, Kishimoto H et al (2001) Glycemic control is a predictor of survival for diabetic patients on hemodialysis. Diabetes Care 24:909–913
49. Oomichi T, Emoto M, Tabata T, Morioka T, Tsujimoto Y, Tahara H et al (2006) Impact of glycemic control on survival of diabetic patients on chronic regular hemodialysis: a 7-year observational study. Diabetes Care 29:1496–1500
50. Kalantar-Zadeh K, Kopple JD, Regidor DL, Jing J, Shinaberger CS, Aronovitz J et al (2007) A1C and survival in maintenance hemodialysis patients. Diabetes Care 30:1049–1055
51. Bailey JL (2013) Insulin resistance and muscle metabolism in chronic kidney disease. ISRN Endocrinol 2013:329606
52. Molsted S, Harrison AP, Eidemak I, Dela F, Andersen JL (2013) Improved glucose tolerance after high-load strength training in patients undergoing dialysis. Nephron Clin Pract 123:134–141
53. Schiffrin EL, Lipman ML, Mann JF (2007) Chronic kidney disease: effects on the cardiovascular system. Circulation 116:85–97
54. Mustata S, Chan C, Lai V, Miller JA (2004) Impact of an exercise program on arterial stiffness and insulin resistance in hemodialysis patients. J Am Soc Nephrol 15:2713–2718
55. Kouidi E, Karagiannis V, Grekas D, Iakovides A, Kaprinis G, Tourkantonis A et al (2010) Depression, heart rate variability, and exercise training in dialysis patients. Eur J Cardiovasc Prev Rehabil 17:160–167
56. Levin NW, Handelman GJ, Coresh J, Port FK, Kaysen GA (2007) Reverse epidemiology: a confusing, confounding, and inaccurate term. Semin Dial 20:586–592
57. Huang Y, Zhang R, Culler SD, Kutner NG (2008) Costs and effectiveness of cardiac rehabilitation for dialysis patients following coronary bypass. Kidney Int 74:1079–1084
58. Lievre MM, Moulin P, Thivolet C, Rodier M, Rigalleau V, Penfornis A et al (2011) Detection of silent myocardial ischemia in asymptomatic patients with diabetes: results of a randomized trial and meta-analysis assessing the effectiveness of systematic screening. Trials 12:23
59. Colberg SR, Albright AL, Blissmer BJ, Braun B, Chasan-Taber L, Fernhall B et al (2010) Exercise and type 2 diabetes: American College of Sports Medicine and the American Diabetes Association: joint position statement. Exercise and type 2 diabetes. Med Sci Sports Exerc 42:2282–2303
60. Fletcher GF, Ades PA, Kligfield P, Arena R, Balady GJ, Bittner VA et al (2013) Exercise standards for testing and training: a scientific statement from the American Heart Association. Circulation 128:873–934
61. Myers J, Voodi L, Umann T, Froelicher VF (2000) A survey of exercise testing: methods, utilization, interpretation, and safety in the VAHCS. J Cardiopulm Rehabil 20:251–258
62. Lazarevic G, Antic S, Vlahovic P, Djordjevic V, Zvezdanovic L, Stefanovic V (2007) Effects of aerobic exercise on microalbuminuria and enzymuria in type 2 diabetic patients. Ren Fail 29:199–205

63. Cheema BS, Smith BC, Singh MA (2005) A rationale for intradialytic exercise training as standard clinical practice in ESRD. Am J Kidney Dis 45:912–916
64. Konstantinidou E, Koukouvou G, Kouidi E, Deligiannis A, Tourkantonis A (2002) Exercise training in patients with end-stage renal disease on hemodialysis: comparison of three rehabilitation programs. J Rehabil Med 34:40–45
65. Koh KP, Fassett RG, Sharman JE, Coombes JS, Williams AD (2010) Effect of intradialytic versus home-based aerobic exercise training on physical function and vascular parameters in hemodialysis patients: a randomized pilot study. Am J Kidney Dis 55:88–99
66. Bennett PN, Breugelmans L, Barnard R, Agius M, Chan D, Fraser D et al (2010) Sustaining a hemodialysis exercise program: a review. Semin Dial 23:62–73
67. Ohmura N, Tamura H, Kawaguchi Y, Ohta M, Miyahara T (1989) The influence of dialysis solution on the exercise capacity in patients on CAPD. Adv Perit Dial Conf Perit Dial 5:46–48
68. Johansen KL, Finkelstein FO, Revicki DA, Gitlin M, Evans C, Mayne TJ (2010) Systematic review and meta-analysis of exercise tolerance and physical functioning in dialysis patients treated with erythropoiesis-stimulating agents. Am J Kidney Dis 55:535–548
69. Thompson PD, Franklin BA, Balady GJ, Blair SN, Corrado D, Estes NA 3rd et al (2007) Exercise and acute cardiovascular events placing the risks into perspective: a scientific statement from the American Heart Association Council on Nutrition, Physical Activity, and Metabolism and the Council on Clinical Cardiology. Circulation 115:2358–2368
70. Siscovick DS, Weiss NS, Fletcher RH, Lasky T (1984) The incidence of primary cardiac arrest during vigorous exercise. N Engl J Med 311:874–877
71. Painter P, Blagg CR, Moore GE (1995) The risks. In: Exercise for the dialysis patients: a guide for the nephrologist. The life options administered by the Medical Education Institute, Inc. http://lifeoptions.org/catalog/. Accessed 16 Jan 2015

Retraction Note to: Various Kinds of Bone Disease in Diabetes: Rheumatic Conditions

Hitoshi Goto

M. Inaba (ed.), *Musculoskeletal Disease Associated with Diabetes Mellitus*,
DOI 10.1007/978-4-431-55720-3_2

The chapter published in Musculoskeletal Disease Associated with Diabetes Mellitus, pages 11–25, 10.1007/978-4-431-55720-3_2 has been retracted because it contains significant parts plagiarizing another publication: Rheumatic conditions in patients with diabetes mellitus, Clinical Rheumatology, Volume 32, Issue 5, pages 527–533, 10.1007/s10067-012-2144-8. The authors would like to express their most sincere apology to the Editor and readers as well as the authors of the original article.

The online version of the original chapter can be found at
http://dx.doi.org/10.1007/978-4-431-55720-3_2

H. Goto, M.D. (✉)
Graduate School of Medicine, Osaka City University, 1-4-3, Asahi-machi, Abeno-ku, Osaka 545-8585, Japan
e-mail: goto@msic.med.osaka-cu.ac.jp

M. Inaba (ed.), *Musculoskeletal Disease Associated with Diabetes Mellitus*,
DOI 10.1007/978-4-431-55720-3_20

MIX
Papier aus verantwortungsvollen Quellen
Paper from responsible sources
FSC® C105338

If you have any concerns about our products,
you can contact us on
ProductSafety@springernature.com

In case Publisher is established outside the EU,
the EU authorized representative is:
Springer Nature Customer Service Center GmbH
Europaplatz 3, 69115 Heidelberg, Germany

Printed by Libri Plureos GmbH
in Hamburg, Germany